CANCER PREVENTION IN MINORITY POPULATIONS

Cultural Implications for Health Care Professionals

CANCER PREVENTION IN MINORITY POPULATIONS

Cultural Implications for Health Care Professionals

Edited by

MARILYN FRANK-STROMBORG, RN, EdD, FAAN

Professor, Oncology Nursing, School of Nursing,
Northern Illinois University,
DeKalb, Illinois

SHARON J. OLSEN, RN, MS

Lecturer, Department of Acute and Long Term Care, School of Nursing,
University of Maryland at Baltimore,
Baltimore, Maryland

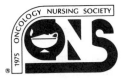

Illustrated

Mosby

St. Louis Baltimore Boston Chicago London Philadelphia Sydney Toronto

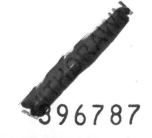

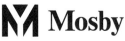

Mosby

Dedicated to Publishing Excellence

Editor: Jeff Burnham
Developmental Editor: Winifred Sullivan
Project Manager: Karen Edwards
Production Editor: Cynthia A. Miller
Designer: Gail Morey Hudson
Manufacturing Supervisor: Kathy Grone

Printed in the United States of America.

Mosby–Year Book, Inc.
11830 Westline Industrial Drive
St. Louis, MO 63146

Library of Congress Cataloging in Publication Data

Cancer prevention in minority populations : cultural implications for health care professionals / edited by Marilyn Frank-Stromborg, Sharon J. Olsen.
    p.   cm.
   Includes bibliographical references and index.
   ISBN 0-8016-6948-0
   1. Cancer—United States—Prevention. 2. Minorities—United States—Diseases. 3. Health behavior—United States. 4. Cancer—United States—Risk factors. I. Frank-Stromborg, Marilyn. II. Olsen, Sharon J.
   [DNLM: 1. Ethnic Groups. 2. Minority Groups. 3. Neoplasms—epidemiology. 4. Neoplasms—prevention & control—nurses' instruction. 5. Risk factors.   QZ 200 C215366]
RA645.C3C36394 1993
614.5'999—dc20
DNLM/DLC
for Library of Congress   92-49102
                                                          CIP

93 94 95 96 97 CL/MY 9 8 7 6 5 4 3 2 1

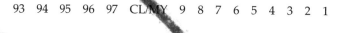

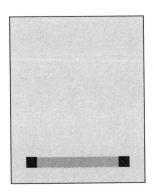

Contributors

VERONICA A. CLARKE-TASKER, RN, MS

Doctoral Student,
University of Maryland at Baltimore,
Baltimore, Maryland

REBECCA J. COHEN, RN, MSN, EDD, MPA, CPHO

Assistant Professor,
Department of Nursing, Rockford College,
Rockford, Illinois

LORETTA OBEDLYN LEINANI HUSSEY, RN, BSN

Department of Health,
Office of Hawaiian Health,
Honolulu, Hawaii

JOANNE K. ITANO, RN, PHD, OCN

School of Nursing,
University of Hawaii,
Honolulu, Hawaii

EUNICE M. LASKY, RN, MS

School of Nursing,
Northern Illinois University,
Dekalb, Illinois

CAROLE H. MARTZ, RN, MS, OCN

Elmhurst Memorial Hospital,
Elmhurst, Illinois

SHARON J. OLSEN, MS, RN

University of Maryland at Baltimore,
Baltimore, Maryland

JACQUELINE A. ROHALY, MSN, RN, OCN

Department of Nursing Service,
Edward Hines Jr VA Hospital,
Hines, Illinois

KAREN N. TAOKA, RN, MN, OCN

The Queen's Medical Center
Honolulu, Hawaii

YVONNE C. YOUNG, RN, BSN

Public Health Nurse,
Department of Health,
Honolulu, Hawaii

This book is dedicated to the late

BARNEY LEPOVETSKY, PhD, JD,

a visionary who saw the need for this project
and a steadfast advocate who enabled us to make it a reality.

This book is also dedicated to the

hundreds of nurses who attended the cancer prevention and
early detection workshops funded by the National Cancer Institute
through the Oncology Nursing Society from 1985 to 1991.

Their commitment to improving the health of ethnic and racial minorities
in this country has served as the inspiration for this work.
The reader profits from the information in this book
because so much of it is based on the unique
personal and cultural perspectives of the
participants that they willingly
shared during these
national workshops.

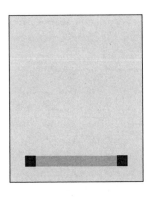

Preface

This book and the series of federally funded grants for ethnic and nonethnic nurses would never have come to fruition without the assistance of Barnie Lepovetsky, PhD, JD. In the early 1980s, Dr. Lepovetsky met with several nurses in leadership positions in the Oncology Nursing Society (ONS) and urged them to write a training grant to promote the education of minority nurses on cancer prevention and screening.

As a result, Marilyn Frank-Stromborg, RN, EdD, Judi Johnson, RN, PhD, and Ruth McCorkle, RN, EdD, wrote a relatively small grant offering a 1-day workshop on cancer prevention for 30 African American nurses held the day before the 1985 ONS Annual Congress in Houston. As few black nurses traditionally attended the annual ONS congresses, the investigators were apprehensive about whether enough nurses would apply to fill this small workshop.

The tremendous response to our call for applications—over 500 black nurses applied—quickly dispelled any doubts. The investigators were impressed with these nurses' commitment to improving the health of black people and with their involvement in community activities. In unsolicited comments, the applicants poignantly documented the need for cancer prevention/screening programs in their communities. The nurses also recognized that they needed greater knowledge and better skills in order to conduct activities on cancer prevention.

The 560 applicants were from 40 states, Canada, Puerto Rico, and Germany. They represented all nursing specialties. Many were already delivering health care to black Americans in food pantries, low income housing projects, shelters for the homeless, churches, public health departments, jails and federal correction facilities, hospitals, clinics, physicians' offices, family planning programs, inner city high schools, community organizations in remote rural areas, and the military.

Selecting just 30 participants from the hundreds of stellar applicants was a formidable task. The culmination of this process was a workshop involving 30 outstanding, socially committed black nurses who were leaders of black nursing organizations and sororities in this country.

The faculty for the workshops was comprised primarily of individuals who had attended the first workshop in 1985, had a strong interest in oncology, and were actively involved in community-based prevention programs. The faculty was located throughout the nation, enabling the Oncology Nursing Society to hold regional workshops.

In order to evaluate the success of this type of educational intervention, the developers of the workshop tested participants before and after the workshop on three topics: knowledge about cancer prevention/early detection, attitudes about cancer prevention/early detection, and participation in community-based cancer prevention/early detection activities. The evaluation showed that the participants increased their knowledge about cancer and their involvement in community-based cancer prevention/early detection activities; in addition, their attitudes toward cancer prevention were positively influenced.

In response to feedback from the workshop participants and encouragement from Dr. Lepovetsky, Dr. Frank-Stromborg designed a grant for a series of five regional two-day workshops for black nurses. The co-project director on this grant was Claudette Varricchio, RN, DNS. The National Cancer Institute funded the grant (1T14CA90554-01) from 1986 to 1988.

Each workshop was designed to accept 30 black nurses. The material from the initial workshop was expanded and content on the specifics of planning community-based programs added.

The ONS national office received 1200 requests for applications for the 2-day courses. By the entry deadline, ONS had received and processed 744 applications. The applicants were from 40 states, Puerto Rico, and the Virgin Islands.

Eighty applicants were chosen for each workshop and then assigned to one of two groups: one that actually attended the workshop; or one that served as a matched control group for purposes of evaluating the success of the workshops. Once the workshops were over, the project directors used a cross-sectional, repeated measures design to test the two groups for knowledge of and attitudes about cancer prevention, and involvement in community-based cancer prevention activities.

The investigators were able to conclude that:

1. The workshops significantly increased participants' knowledge about cancer prevention/early detection as measured by the Cancer Prevention/Early Detection Cognitive Test.

2. Participants increased their involvement in cancer prevention/early detection activities to a greater extent than did nonparticipants as measured by the Cancer Prevention/Early Detection Activities Survey.

3. Workshop participants' attitudes about cancer were more positive than the attitudes of nonparticipants.

Based on the educational model used

successfully with black nurses, Frank-Stromborg and co-investigator Sharon Olsen obtained another grant from NCI (NCI 5R25CA09554-03) to offer a series of regional workshops for 180 ethnic and nonethnic nurses working with Hispanic, Asian American, and Native American populations. The response was as strong as it had been for the previous black nurses workshops: 218 Hispanic nurses, 131 Native American nurses, and 73 Asian American nurses applied.

Typical reasons for wanting to attend the course included:

"It has been my experience, especially in the Native American populations, that though the cancer rate is apparently low, when people finally are diagnosed, the cancer is already quite advanced and often beyond cure. I need ideas for how to make this population more aware of symptoms and less afraid to come in for examinations or screenings, plus I want to hone my own skills in early cancer detection."

Family Nurse Practitioner
U.S. Public Health Service
Red Lake IHS Hospital
August, 1988

"We know that the population of adult Asian immigrants does not subscribe to the Western concept of preventive health care. Many clients also seek traditional Chinese medical care before coming to see us; therefore, we see many patients sporadically, only once or twice a year. After learning the latest screening procedures and the skills to do them, I will share what I learn with the other providers and develop protocols for systematically performing cancer screens for patients when they come in for sporadic/sick visits."

Family Nurse Practitioner
South Cove Community Health Center
381 School Street
Watertown, MA 02172
July, 1990

The need to develop an understanding of individual health beliefs and practices was underscored by the following statement from a participant at the workshop:

"I see patients who are primarily low-income, uninsured, and have various cultural and language barriers to health care. Our patients have very limited resources and often seek care for acute or chronic health problems only; health maintenance or disease prevention issues, such as cancer risk reduction, are usually not addressed. Consequently, there is a need to develop an efficient method of cancer risk appraisal that can be integrated into our existing services. By understanding the health beliefs and values of Asians and Pacific Islanders, we can develop interventions that will motivate them to acquire cancer detection skills, to seek screening by health care providers, and to obtain follow-up care when necessary."

Nurse Practitioner
Kalihi-Palama Health Clinic
766 N. King Street
Honolulu, Hawaii 96817

Before beginning the regional workshops, an extended 3-day workshop was held. Ten stellar applicants for each of the three ethnic groups were selected to attend. Culture-specific seminars were presented during the first 2 days; on the third day three culture-specific focus group interview sessions were held. Study questions and work assignments previously sent to the participants allowed them to prepare to share information about the unique health beliefs and practices of their ethnic group and how these influenced the prevention and early detection of cancer. Participants were also asked to bring patient education materials specifically designed for the ethnic groups with whom they worked.

The focus groups generated information on the health beliefs, medical practices, physical factors, and psychosocial factors to consider when assessing cancer risk and health status. The discussions were tape recorded and transcribed. The faculty for each of the five subsequent regional workshops used the information gained from this 3-day workshop and actively sought additional input from their participants. The result was a large body of practical, practice-oriented, culturally sensitive information.

In this book, the chapters on Asian Americans, Hispanics, and Native Americans contain much of the information that emerged from the focus groups and ensuing regional workshops. Thus the chapters are based not only on academic sources but also on information from health care professionals who are members of a particular ethnic group and/or have worked extensively with that group.

The focus groups and regional workshops were also the source of the wide range of educational materials described in the compendium. Nurses who participated in the focus group interview sessions have reviewed each chapter.

The editors of this book believe it is unique in terms of the information it provides on each racial/ethnic group. Federal funding enabled the editors and each author to generate a comprehensive and geographically representative book. The extensive reviews by ethnic nurses from across the United States helped to ensure that the information in each chapter was culturally relevant, timely, and would be of practical assistance to the health care professional working with members of the Native American, Hispanic, Asian/Pacific, Native Hawaiian, and African American cultures.

Marilyn Frank-Stromborg
Sharon J. Olsen

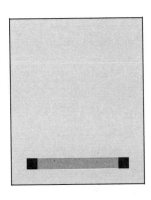

Acknowledgments

The authors would like to acknowledge the contributions of the following nurses to this text:

Iris Yuriko Ahana, RN, MN
St. Francis Hospital,
Honolulu, Hawaii

Lillian M. Chase, RN
USPHS Indian Hospital,
Rosebud, South Dakota

Priscilla Choy, RN, MPA
Chinese Hospital,
San Francisco, California

Karen Hassey Dow, RN, MS
Beth Israel Hospital,
Boston, Massachusetts

Mary Gulatte, RN, MN
Emory University Hospital,
Atlanta, Georgia

Dianne N. Ishida, RN, MS
University of Hawaii,
School of Nursing,
Honolulu, Hawaii

Ryan Iwamoto, RN, ARNP, MN, CS
Mason Clinic,
Seattle, Washington

Erna F. Burton, RN, BSN
H.H.H.I.H.S.P.H.S.,
Sells Hospital,
Sells, Arizona

Mei Chou, RN, MN
Chinese Hospital,
San Francisco, California

Fern Clark, RN, MS
Administrator,
Office of Hawaiian Health,
State of Hawaii,
Department of Health

Joyce Guillory, RN, MS
Morris Brown College,
Atlanta, Georgia

Anne Harrison, RN, BSN
Chief Andrew Isaac Health Center,
Fairbanks, Alaska

Joanne Itano, RN, MS, MEd, OCN
University of Hawaii,
Department of Nursing,
Honolulu, Hawaii

Cheryl A. Jones, RN
St. Joseph's Hospital,
Mitchell, South Dakota

Ursula Knoki-Wilson, RN, CNM, MSN
Ganado, Arizona

Mee Hoe Lee, RN, BSN
Seattle, Washington

Erma M. Marbut, RN, BSN
USPH Albuquerque Indian Hospital,
Albuquerque, New Mexico

Patricia Protho-Shepherd, RN
Veteran's Affairs Medical Center,
Philadelphia, Pennsylvania

Noma Roberson, RN, PhD
Roswell Park Cancer Institute,
Department of Cancer Control and
Epidemiology,
Buffalo, New York

Lucille Sachiko-James, RN, MSN, OCN
Straub Clinic and Hospital,
Hospital Nursing Service,
Honolulu, Hawaii

Eva Smith, RN, PhD
University of Illinois at Chicago,
Chicago, Illinois

Carolyn Beth Lee, RN, MSN, MPA, CNA
PHS, US Dept. of Health and Human
Services,
Rockville, Maryland

Frances Fen-Fang Lee-Lin, RN, MN, OCN
LAC/USC Medical Center,
Education and Consultation
Department,
Los Angeles, California

Geralyn M. Martinez, RN, BSN
Taholah Indian Health Center,
Taholah, Washington

Bonnie Rathod, RN, MN
Jamestown Klallam Tribe,
Sequim, Washington

Monica S. Rozzell, RN, BSN, OCN
Cancer Research Center of Hawaii,
Cancer Information Services,
Honolulu, Hawaii

Verna Schad, RN
USPHS Indian Hospital,
Eagle Butte, South Dakota

Yvonne Sterling, RN, PhD
Louisiana State University Medical
Center,
School of Nursing,
New Orleans, Louisianna

Karen N. Taoka, RN, MN, OCN
The Queen's Cancer Institute,
Honolulu, Hawaii

Beverly Mae Warne, RN, BSN USPHS IHS,
Phoenix Indian Medical Center,
Phoenix, Arizona

Bernadette Whitlow, RN
Creek Nation Community Hospital,
Okemah, Oklahoma

Bessie Woo, RN
Children's Hospital of San Francisco,
San Francisco, California

Luella Vann Thornton, RN, BS
Banning, California

Thomas Welty, MD, MPH
Aberdeen Area Epidemiology Program,
Rapid City, South Dakota

Gaylan Noelani Wilcox, RN, MS
State of Hawaii,
Department of Mental Health
Honolulu, Hawaii

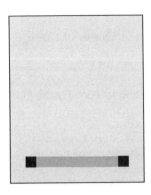

Contents

CANCER PREVENTION IN MINORITY POPULATIONS

Cultural Implications for Health Care Professionals

Cancer Prevention and Early Detection in Native American and Alaska Native Populations

I was honored by the request to write this forward for the chapter on Native Americans. I am a Native American, a member of the Mandan and Hidatsa tribes of North Dakota. I was raised on a reservation and have been involved most of my life with the health and psychosocial issues of Native Americans.

It is gratifying to see a chapter on Native Americans included in this book. In past discussions and publications on health care for Americans, the Native American has been excluded or perhaps lumped in with other minorities. Often Native Americans were considered to be too small a population for consideration or mention. Thus this chapter is remarkable not only because it considers this group but also because resource persons used were competent and knowledgeable in their fields. Many of these resource persons are Native Americans who contributed personal knowledge to this chapter.

This chapter will certainly prove helpful to the health professional who will provide care to the Native American. It offers a succinct review of the current lifestyle of Native Americans as well as an overall view of some tribal beliefs about health and health practices. It also provides an analysis of the current status of Native people on reservations. It is written in a style that would be helpful to all health care providers from physicians to CHRs.

A great deal of work and effort went into this chapter, not only the descriptions of and statistics on Native Americans, Alaska Natives, and Innuits, but also the various tribal health belief systems. Certain tribal beliefs, such as the Navajo's healing practices and use of medicine men and healers, are described in exquisite detail. The author is careful to point out that there are distinct differences between tribal groups and that cultural practices vary widely. People of other ethnic groups who have tried to deal with Native people as a single homogeneous group have found this difficult. While it seems easier to generalize and deal with Native Americans as a single entity, ignoring tribal differences can lead to the wrong conclusions or incorrect judgments. Not only are there basic differences in tribal lifestyles, but also in beliefs about life and death and about healing and religion.

The author has made extensive effort to gather together detailed and relevant data on cancer and the Native American.

She has provided a careful review of cancer statistics, tribal differences, and factors related to disease, such as diet. Of special interest are the tribal health practices that might be associated with certain cancers. Also fascinating are the various tribal beliefs associated with certain incidences of cancer.

I have always been deeply concerned about the rapid change in lifestyle experienced by many Native Americans due to acculturation, either imposed or sought. Native Americans have gone from a Stone-Age lifestyle to modern high tech in a few generations. They have been exposed to infectious disease, and toxins of many kinds, and lost almost all traditional ways of life.

Changes in basic food and diet are particularly interesting. Although the diets of different Native American groups varied widely, they now eat primarily fat, sugar, and fried foods. It is rare today to see Native Americans growing their food in gardens or hunting and gathering. Native Americans once were very active and exerted themselves physically in daily activities; now many are apathetic and exercise infrequently. Obesity is the norm for many tribes.

I am vitally interested in all of this because I see that it all fits together: the rapid acculturation, the alcoholism, the apathy, the obesity, the suicide rate, and related diseases, such as diabetes and cancer.

I am also interested in stress factors encountered by the Native American and how these factors affect the immune system. The Native American has experienced incredible stresses of oppression, rapid acculturation, poverty, and alcoholism. Could these stress factors have some effect on resistance or susceptibility to various diseases? I hope researchers will investigate this further.

The most touching part of this chapter is the instructions on how to relate to the native client. As I read it, I thought the material could apply to all patients, not only Native Americans. The suggestions to take one's time, to be kind and compassionate, to listen, and to understand are universal for nurses, especially those in oncology. So many of the suggestions made are very pertinent and timely. The authors are to be commended for including this section in the chapter.

I feel the information in this chapter contributes significantly to the literature dealing with the contemporary lifestyle of the Native American.

Phyllis Old Dog Cross, RN, MS

Sioux San IHS Hospital,
Rapid City, SD

CHAPTER 1

Cancer Prevention and Early Detection in Native American and Alaska Native Populations

SHARON J. OLSEN

Native Americans include natives of the continental United States (once called American Indians), Aleuts, Alaskan Eskimos, and native Hawaiians. Eskimos, Aleuts, and other Natives residing in Alaska are referred to as Alaska Natives; those residing in other states are referred to as Native Americans. Paula Gunn Allen, a Native American of Laguna Pueblo, Sioux, and Lebanese-American ancestry, has characterized the Native American in the following way (Wayne, 1988):

A Native American is somebody who connects with and takes responsibility for the spiritual life of this continent, who recognizes the spirit entities of the land and lives in congruence with them, who understands that every aspect of life is sacred, that is, it matters to the balance of the planet. This is what makes an Indian, not skin color (p. 68).

Native Americans are not currently, nor have they ever been, a homogeneous group. Until the 1800s, they lived in loosely formed, often nomadic bands and tribes, and spoke more than 100 languages with countless dialects. It has been only 62 years since Native Americans living on reservations became United States citizens; and it has been only 52 years—a mere two generations—since the U.S. government ceased its efforts to break up Native American reservations and adopted a policy to encourage and formally recognize tribal governments (Emery, 1986).

Many Native Americans have fought to maintain their own intricate systems of beliefs, values, and practices, often in the face of extreme adversity. Over the years, many lovingly woven threads of their own cultures have either worn out or have been forcibly ripped away. Occasionally, threads of Western-European culture are integrated into the fabric of Native American life.

3

SOCIOCULTURAL CHARACTERISTICS
Population Statistics

Descendants of the original residents of North America now number approximately 1.6 million, constituting the smallest of the defined U.S. minority groups. This group encompasses numerous tribes and over 400 federally recognized nations, each with its own traditions and cultural heritage. The federal government collects detailed data on American Indians and Alaska Natives in the 33 states that have reservations. The 17 states without reservations are Arkansas, Delaware, Georgia, Hawaii, Illinois, Indiana, Kentucky, Maryland, Missouri, New Hampshire, New Jersey, Ohio, South Carolina, Tennessee, Vermont, Virginia, and West Virginia. The largest tribes include the Navajo, Cherokee, Sioux, Chippewa, and Pueblo; the states of Oklahoma, Arizona, California, New Mexico, and Alabama have the greatest number of Native American inhabitants (Antle, 1987).

Preliminary figures from the 1990 census document a significant increase in the Native American population. The increase has been partially attributed to high birth rates and improved counting by the U.S. Bureau of the Census. However, experts surmise that a substantial portion of the increase is the result of changes in self-identification, primarily among urban Native Americans who have little connection to a tribal organization. Gay Kingman, executive director of the National Congress of American Indians, suggests "there is a renaissance . . . a return to our language our music and our dances. We're teaching Indian in our schools. Tribes are more self-governing, so more people are identifying themselves as American Indian" (Vobejda, 1991). Table 1-1 is a partial list of the 1990 Native American population statistics for selected states. It is noteworthy that the biggest population changes have occurred in states without large Native American populations, especially in Eastern cities without large concentrations of tribally based Native Americans.

TABLE 1-1   The Rising American Indian Population*

State	1980	1990	Percent Increase
Alabama	7,583	16,506	117.7%
Arkansas	9,428	12,773	35.5%
Delaware	1,328	2,019	52.0%
Hawaii	2,768	5,099	84.2%
Illinois	16,283	21,836	34.1%
Indiana	7,836	12,720	62.3%
Louisiana	12,065	18,541	53.7%
Michigan	40,050	55,638	38.9%
Mississippi	6,180	8,525	37.9%
Missouri	12,321	19,835	61.0%
Nebraska	9,195	12,410	35.0%
Nevada	13,308	19,637	47.6%
New Jersey	8,394	14,970	78.3%
New Mexico	106,119	134,355	26.6%
North Dakota	20,158	25,917	28.6%
Rhode Island	2,898	4,071	40.5%
South Dakota	44,968	50,575	12.5%
Texas	40,075	65,877	64.4%
Vermont	984	1,696	72.4%
Virginia	9,454	15,282	61.6%
Wyoming	7,094	9,479	33.6%

*American Indian population includes Eskimos and Aleuts. The states included in this table are those for which racial breakdowns from the 1990 Census have been issued.
From United States Bureau of the Census.

In order to receive government assistance that is expressly earmarked for their group, Native Americans must prove that they are enrolled members of a federally recognized tribe. Most tribes require an individual to have at least one-quarter of the blood of that tribe to belong. So a person could be a full-blooded Native American of mixed tribal heritage and yet be ineligible for membership in any tribe; such persons would be ineligible for any Native American assistance programs funded by the federal government (Emery, 1986). Regardless of whether they prove Native American heritage, Native Americans are eligible for all government assistance available to U.S. citizens.

General Demographic Characteristics

Overall, the Native American population is younger, less educated, and poorer than the U.S. population in general, according to the 1980 census (see Table 1-2, and Figures 1-1, 1-2 and 1-3). In addition, the birth rate among Native Americans is nearly twice that of other groups; and the average life expectancy is 6 years less. Nearly one in four Native American households is headed by a woman.

Twenty-four percent of Native Americans live on reservations in the West or Southwest, and an additional 8% live on historic trust areas in Oklahoma. Most reservations have fewer than 1,000 residents (Newell, 1988).

TABLE 1-2   Social and Economic Characteristics, Based on 1980 Census

Characteristics	Native American Groups	U.S. All Races
Median age	22.6	30.0
Percent female	50.7%	51.4%
Percent male	49.3%	48.6%
Average number of persons per family	4.6	3.8
Median family income	$13,700	$19,900
Average family income	$16,500	$23,100
Per capita income	$ 3,600	$ 7,300
Percent of all persons below poverty level	28.2%	12.4%
Percent high school graduates	55.4%	66.5%
Percent college graduates	7.4%	16.2%
Percent in labor force, Age 16 and over	57.8%	62.0%
Female, age 16 and over	47.7%	49.9%
Male, age 16 and over	68.6%	75.1%
Percent of civilian labor force unemployed	13.3%	6.5%
Female, age 16 and over	11.9%	6.5%
Male, age 16 and over	14.5%	6.5%

From Indian Health Service, Office of Planning, Evaluation, and Legislation, Division of Program Statistics (1990): *Trends in Indian Health*, Rockville, 1990, Public Health Service, p 18. Contains no copyright material.

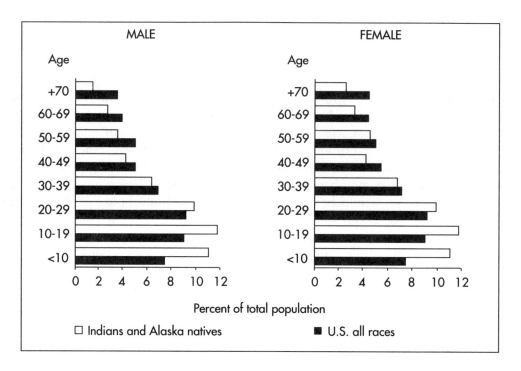

	Indian & alaska native		U.S. ALL RACES	
Age group	Male	Female	Male	Female
All ages	49,325	50,675	48,578	51,422
Under 10 years	10,762	10,502	7,460	7,127
10-19 years	11,767	11,506	8,859	8,537
20-29 years	9,451	9,645	8,990	9,036
30-39 years	6,445	6,779	6,859	7,057
40-49 years	4,248	4,565	4,898	5,148
50-59 years	3,208	3,488	4,901	5,396
60-69 years	2,024	2,343	3,784	4,545
70 years and over	1,421	1,847	2,826	4,575
NOTE: Percentages may not sum to totals due to rounding.				

Figure 1-1 Population by age and sex, 1980 Census.

(From Indian Health Service: *Trends in indian health*, Bethesda, Md, 1990, DHHS, PHS, IHS, Office of Planning, Evaluation, and Legislation, Division of Program Statistics, pp 16-17.)

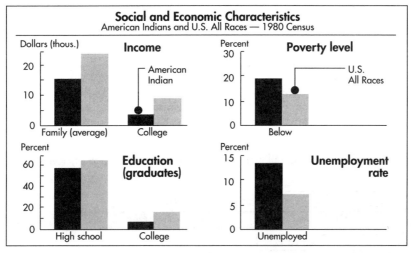

Figure 1-2 Social and economic characteristics for Native Americans and U.S. all races—1980 Census. The Indian population lags behind the U.S. All races population with respect to various income, education, and employment characteristics.

(From Indian Health Service: *Chart series book* (p. 14) by evaluation and legislation, Program Statistics Branch, Rockville, Md, 1985.)

In general, Indian people tend to value individual freedom and worth, generosity and the sharing of material goods, an orientation to the present and short-term goals, strong family ties that emphasize a respect for the elderly, patriotism, bravery and stoicism, and harmony with nature and all living things (Yuki, 1986).

Culture

The Native American today lives in a bi-cultural world that combines traditional ways and the standards of the majority culture. Since European settlement of North America, the traditional mores and cultural patterns of the Native American have been severely disrupted. This disruption and subsequent loss has left many Native Americans feeling powerless and hopeless. Some experts suggest that such feelings may account for the high incidence of alcohol abuse, suicide, depression, and obesity in this population.

Native Americans draw on strengths of the family, the tribe, and the land itself to cope with stress. Unlike the Western nuclear family, a Native American household often consists of an extended family. Many tribes are matrilineal, so women, particularly grandmothers, hold positions of power and decision making.

Among traditional Native Americans, children and elders are particularly valued and always cared for by the group. In many cases, the Native American individual lives for the group, feels free to ask for help, and does not approach

The Health of America's Native Tribes

Despite an improvement in the health status of Native Americans, disease and mortality rates are still high. Pneumonia and influenza are common causes of illness and death, and homicide mortality rates remain high.

Health care workers are also focusing efforts on early diagnosis, prevention, and treatment of high blood pressure and other risk factors for heart disease.

About half of the estimated 1.5 million Native Americans in the United States live on 162 federal reservations in 27 states. Little is known about the health status of Native Americans who live off reservations.

The following chart shows population rates, family income, and poverty levels for the 10 largest tribes.

Apache
Population: 35,861 — $12,086 Median family income — 34.1 % Living in poverty

Cherokee 232,080 — $14,809 — 20.5

Chippewa 73,602 — $12,880 — 28.2

Choctaw 50,220 — $14,542 — 21.3

Creek 28,278 — $15,287 — 19.7

Iroquois 38,218 — $15,079 — 21.1

Lumbee 28,631 — $11,933 — 27.8

Navajo 158,633 — $9,901 — 45.5

Pueblo 42,552 — $12,750 — 31.0

Sioux 78,608 — 10,608 — 38.8

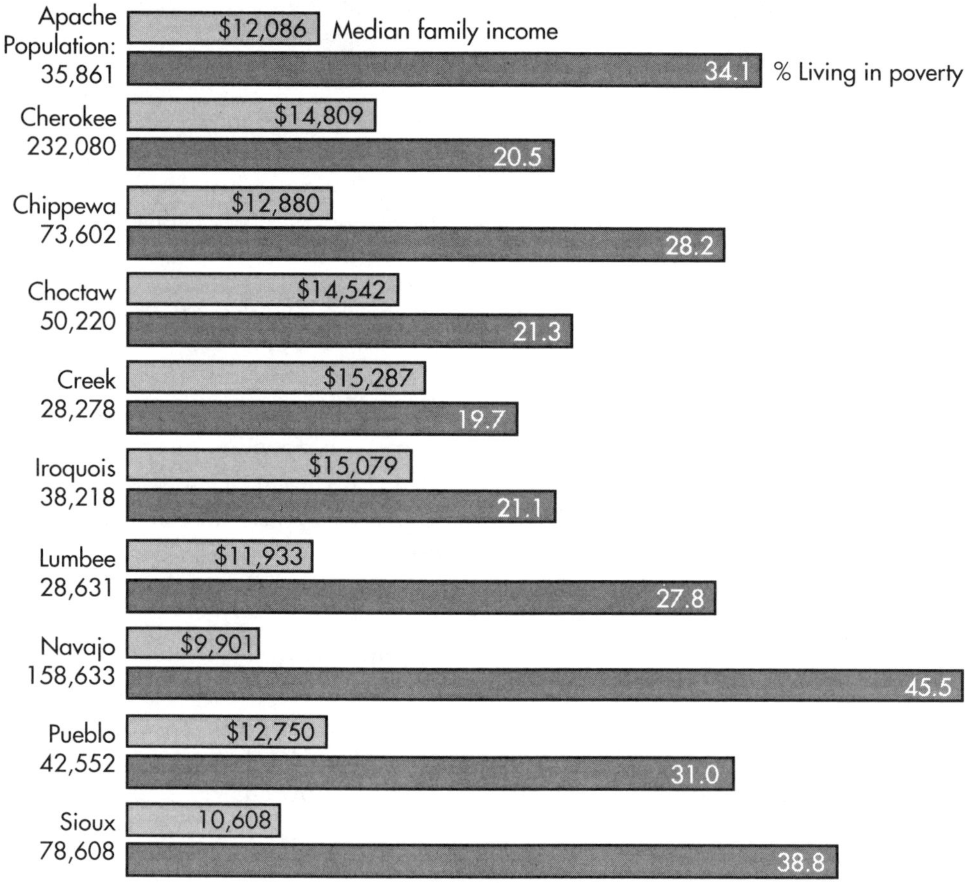

Figure 1-3 Population rates, family income, and poverty levels for the 10 largest tribes.
From Vital statistics, the Health of America's native tribes, 1990, *The Washington Post*. Copyright 1990 by *The Washington Post*. Reprinted by permission.

problems or successes alone (Antle, 1987). Despite strong family ties, however, members of this group respect individuals and their rights.

In contrast to other, more goal-oriented Americans, most Native Americans believe it unwise to plan, save, prepare, or set goals for a future that cannot be influenced. They place little emphasis on material wealth; possessions are to be used, not preserved, and shared with the group. Native Americans also strive to stay in harmony with their surroundings—picking only the crops they need, chopping just enough wood to heat the home, and killing only enough game to feed the family (Antle, 1987).

Although reservation life has been characterized by unemployment, economic dependency, and isolation from many of the twentieth century social complexities, many Native Americans find great solace in it. As Joe and Miller (1988) explained, "life seems anchored, slow-paced, and everyone has a place. Reservation life is full of relatively simple routines, and an Indian family finds some relief there from the constant pressure of the outside world" (p. 16).

Reservation populations have a high percentage of very young members as well as a growing number of residents over age 55 years. On many reservations, the land cannot support a growing and increasingly concentrated population, so poverty and welfare dependency have become common.

Urban areas offer the promise of jobs and other opportunities. In the past 25 years, the size and population of "Native American satellite communities" within the cities has increased to the point that today nearly two thirds of all Native Americans live in non-reservation communities. What began as a movement of young adults from rural to urban areas for vocational training has swelled to become a major social migration for Native Americans. This migration has produced the concomitant change from a traditional to a more modern Western lifestyle.

It is impossible to discuss all the unique qualities of each Native American tribe in this chapter. Brief discussions of the cultural characteristics of select tribes are presented in Appendices 2 to 16. Table 1-3 compares some cultural characteristics of Native Americans with those of the majority U.S. culture.

Diet

The diet of the Native American has changed significantly over time. When Native Americans were nomadic, they moved periodically, allowing stocks of wild game and wild food plants time to recover. During this period, the Native American diet was high in fiber and low in fat. Today, traditional subsistence lifestyles and confinement within reservation borders have resulted in overgrazed land and significant reductions in available game due to over-hunting. Few Native Americans have farms that produce anything beyond the subsistence needs of the family, community, or tribe.

In general, the diets of many modern Native Americans are high in refined carbohydrates, fat, and sodium and low in meat, eggs, cheese, and milk. Many Native Americans are lactose intolerant, so

TABLE 1-3   A Comparison of General Native American and European Values

Selected Traditional Native American Values	European/Industrial Values
Group life is primary	The individual is primary
Extended family is important	Nuclear family is usual focus
Respect elders, experts, and those with spiritual powers	Respect youth, success, and high social status
Orientation to the present	Orientation to the future
Personal character is the primary source of status	Educational degrees are source of status
Bilingualism; cultural pluralism	Monolingualism; assimilation
Cooperation; generosity; sharing	Competition; saving; individual ownership
Personal caution; indirect criticism	Personal openness; direct criticism
Modesty; humility; patience; calmness	Less modesty, impatience, activity
Time and place viewed as being permanent, settled. Time is always with us.	Time and place always negotiable; plans for change. Every minute should be used.
Introverted—-avoids ridicule or criticism of others if possible.	Extroverted—-seeks analysis and criticism of situations.
Pragmatic, accepts "what is."	Reformer, must change or fix problems.
Emphasizes responsibility for family and personal sphere.	Emphasizes authority and responsibility over a wide area of social life.
Emphasis on how others "behave," not on what they say. Listening and observation skills valued.	Eager to relate to others; emphasis on how they "feel" or "think." Verbal skills valued.
Work to meet needs; non-materialism	Work for work's sake (Puritan work ethic); materialistic
Incorporates supportive non-family or other helpers into family network.	Keeps network of family, friends, acquaintances separate.
Cooperation with nature; respect for tradition and subsistence skills.	Control over nature; oriented to progress and modernism.
Seeks harmony.	Seeks progress.
Religion and spirituality pervade life.	Religion is segment of life.
Holistic approach to health; illness is mental, spiritual, and physical imbalance.	Attention to physical ailment primarily; illness is physical imbalance.
Lack of or limited eye-to-eye contact is sign of respect.	Eye-to-eye contact demonstrates interest, involvement and respect.
Self-exploratory child rearing practices.	Punishment-oriented child rearing practices.

From Joe JR, Miller D: American Indian cultural perspectives on disability, *Native American Research and Training Center Monograph Series*, The University of Arizona, Tucson, Az, p 4; Ouellette J: personal communication, March 1, 1990, Munising Tribal Center, Munising Mich.

milk and milk products cause them severe intestinal distress (American Indian Health Care Association, 1992). Dried milk has been called "white man's poison." Yet this product has been regularly distributed to the Native Americans from surplus food commodities. Today many assistance programs have replaced dried milk with canned milk, which is not quite as likely to provoke the distressing symptoms of milk intolerance.

Alcoholism and obesity are significant problems in the Native American population. One group of experts estimated that 95% of Native American families are affected either directly or indirectly by a family member's alcohol abuse (Rhoades, Hammond, Welty, Handler, and Amler, 1987).

Welty (in press) reviewed the history and implications of obesity in Native American cultures. In 1967, his investigation of the nutritional status of Navajo children revealed that they were malnourished. Federal government food assistance programs subsequently started, but these provided primarily high-fat and low-fiber foods. The incidence of obesity rapidly increased among many Native American groups. Welty postulates that the rapid dietary changes resulting in obesity may have been exacerbated not only by a concurrent change from a very active to a sedentary lifestyle, but also by this group's inherent metabolic characteristics, which may differ from those of other ethnic groups.

In the past, traditional Native peoples were generally free from diseases like diabetes, cardiovascular disease, and cancer. Some experts believe the increasing,

and relatively recent, prevalence of obesity plays a major role in increasing rates of these diseases, as well as hypertension, hypercholesterolemia, and gallbladder and renal disease (Welty, in press). Welty even attributes increasing musculoskeletal problems to obesity.

Many Native Americans have said that the adoption of the white man's diet is cause for concern. Locust (1987b) notes that informants in her study of diabetes among Yaqui Indians concluded that the disease was apparently unknown to older generation Yaquis. They attributed this problem to dietary changes. One informant said:

> Eating habits have changed. The changes have made new illnesses. The human body is not as pure as it once was when all foods were natural and were prepared with love. When grains were ground by hand, vegetables were grown in the garden or harvested from the wilderness, the food was good for you. Nowadays when parents work and food comes from the grocery market, there is little love in it. And people starve; not from lack of food but lack of love that goes into nourishing the spirit as well as the body (p. 38).

Two study participants noted that they were unable to follow the diet prescribed for diabetics; one woman said she "didn't have the money to purchase the required fresh fruits and vegetables," and the other said the "diet requirements were impossible, but she did the very best she could" (p. 38).

The Apache people feel that forsaking traditional ways, in particular moving away from the traditional diet, has caused many of their health problems. Locust (1986) noted that:

Traditionally the Apache diet consisted of wild nuts made into stew, bread, and a kind of tamale. They had garden plots, but also harvested many wild plants, cacti, fruits, and roots. To this pantry they added wild game meats and eggs from wild game birds. They did not eat fish or bear meat. Today, however, their diet contains many fried foods, beef, potatoes, soft drinks, and candy bars and other sweets purchased from the tribal store. One consequence of this new diet is type II diabetes mellitus, the major health concern among tribal members. Diabetes leads to cardiovascular problems such as retinopathy, renal failure, and limb amputations. Gall stones also plague the older people, tooth decay is rampant, and heart problems—almost unknown in earlier times—have become common. 'The people are not eating right,' one elderly informant told this researcher. 'They have taken the white man's food and they have become soft like the white man. They cannot work long and hard any more. They have no endurance to stay awake the whole time of a ceremony. They get tired too easy, and get sick too much' (pp. 33-35).

Little information is available on the day-to-day dietary habits, food preparation styles, and food selection preferences of Native Americans today—traditional or otherwise. Clearly, this is an area ripe for research.

BELIEFS CONCERNING HEALTH AND UNWELLNESS

In her comprehensive study of Native Americans' beliefs concerning health and unwellness, Locust (1985) found that although no two tribes held the same beliefs about health and illness, most Native American health beliefs are closely linked to their religious beliefs. Health is both a physical and a spiritual state. For instance, for the Navajo, healing ceremonies are integral to community life; in addition, the Tohono O'Odham tribe does not distinguish between healing and worship during ceremonies.

Little information is available on Native American beliefs and attitudes about health and disease. Locust (1985) suggests this is due to the "reluctance of Indian people to discuss such personal matters with anyone, particularly non-Indians" (p. 19). She notes that because beliefs, philosophies, and religions affect "past lives, present lives, and any lives in the future . . . [there is] guilt and fear . . . [that] talking of such things may be in violation of some tribal custom and could possibly bring retaliation from other tribal members . . . [and talking about an illness] may give it the power to manifest or express itself in human form" (p. 19).

Beliefs common to most Native Americans are briefly reviewed here. The reader is referred to Dr. Locust's monograph (1985) for more in-depth study of these common beliefs (also see Appendixes 2 to 16).

1. *Native Americans believe in a supreme creator. In this belief system there are also lesser beings.* The supreme creator may be referred to as "First Being," "Father—Mother," "Giver of Life," "Grandfather," "Original Being," or by other titles. The supreme creator is spiritual, all-powerful, and generally never impersonated or personified in tribal ceremonies and rituals. Spirit beings associated with the supreme creator may be a partner, co-creator, mate, or offspring. The sons of Cherokee deities are called Thunder, the

Yaqui have a female deity called Maala Mecha (Moon Mother), and the Navajo have the Monster Slayers, twin offspring of the Navajo deities. Most tribal groups also recognize a variety of spirit helpers or lesser beings that assist humans. These are not gods and are not prayed to, but they command respect and thanks. These include Kachinas (Hopi), Ghan or Mountain Spirits (Apache), Yei (Navajo) or Pascolas (Yaqui). Locust (1985) explained that, "during religious ceremonies, humans may vest themselves in regalia symbolic of a particular spirit helper, inviting that spirit helper to incarnate in them for the duration of the ceremony, thus bringing blessings and knowledge to the group" (p. 4).

2. *A person is a threefold being made up of the body, mind, and spirit.* The physical body is a dwelling place for the spirit, and the mind—the source of one's awareness—functions as a link between the body and the spirit.

3. *The spirit existed before it came into a physical body and will exist after the body dies.* Existence is circular and continuous for most traditional Native Americans. They existed as spirit beings with the supreme creator before birth; at death their spirit being joins the creator and eventually returns to the physical world in another form (Locust, 1985). This continued existence of the spirit accounts for Native American comments such as "my (deceased) father visited me this morning." Most tribes have identified

places where spirits may rest, do penance for past deeds, or progress in spiritual understanding, and living people may encounter spirits at those places.

4. *Plants and animals, like humans, are part of the spirit world. The spirit world exists side-by-side and intermingles with the physical world.* Native Americans live side by side with the spiritual entities embodied in the physical world; the physical world intermingles with the spirit world. Medicine men can "see" into both worlds and can also see how both worlds are intermingled. Spirits may hold the power to relieve human suffering; and because all things have a spirit, a stone or plant can be powerful. For example, crystals can be used for healing or camomile can be used as a sedative. Only the medicine person knows which objects contain various powers and how to use those powers.

5. *Wellness is harmony in body, mind, and spirit.* "Harmony is not perfection, utopia, or euphoria, but an attitude toward life that creates peace" (Locust, 1985, p. 11). It is not "events" themselves, but an individual's response to them, that creates harmony, "One may not be able to change the pain of stiffening joints, but one can control his attitude about having to live with the pain" (Locust, 1985, p. 11).

6. *Unwellness is caused by disharmony between the body, mind, and spirit.* The concept of a mind-body-spirit triad influences many tribes' beliefs about the

treatment of disease. Illnesses that occur will influence the mind, body and spirit simultaneously. Locust (1985) noted that "among the Yaquis it is common for one to die because they were too sad to live, 'to die of melancholy' " (p. 11). So a Native American may consult both a medicine person and a Western doctor at the same time. Locust (1985) also noted that, "the physician treats the physical element; the medicine man helps the person heal himself by assisting him to restore harmony between his body, mind, and spirit" (p. 6).

Illness means different things to different tribes. For the Apache, alcoholism is a sickness; some Hopis, however, consider alcoholism a deliberate choice of behaviors. Other ethnic groups may label the mentally retarded, learning disabled, or emotionally ill as unwell, but many Native Americans do not see these as illnesses. Many Native American languages do not contain words equivalent to the English words "retarded," "crippled," or "handicapped."

To treat the spirit and mind, a healer must understand why the disease or disability occurred and begin to resolve the conflict occurring between the mind, body, and spirit. The medicine person helps individuals see how their spiritual needs or mental states have affected the physical body.

7. *Natural unwellness is caused by the violation of a sacred or tribal taboo.* Taboos can be moral, religious, or cultural (Locust, 1985). They may concern proper ritual observance, death, sexual relationships, incest, witchcraft, natural phenomena such as lightning or eclipse, or certain foods. Tribal taboos may also concern reptiles, insects or spiders, birds, animals, or plants. Most clans have strict procedures about touching the dead, preparing the body for cremation or burial, and disposal of their belongings. Some major taboos are associated with the menstrual cycle, which is considered unclean and associated with negative energy. Women in their "moon time" must be careful where they go, what they do, and how they discard sanitary waste for fear of contaminating something, thus bringing dire consequences upon the tribe. Whether a taboo is violated intentionally or unintentionally, the violation can affect the offender and the family.

8. *Unnatural unwellness is caused by witchcraft.* Native Americans do not have words in their vocabulary for witches or witchcraft. In the context of Native American beliefs, evil comes from "one who is on the bad side" or a person who walks at night (Locust, 1985, p. 15). Evil can be very powerful and can cause disharmony resulting in physical illness, depression, or confusion. Evil or negative energy can be premeditated, or unpremeditated. So individuals must be careful how they think or talk because "the bad thoughts we have and the bad things we say are like poisoned arrows that can pierce the heart" (Locust, 1985, p. 15), causing significant harm or injury. Many tribes believe that speaking about a deformity or illness may

give it the power to manifest or express itself in human form. They consult a medicine person to dissipate negative energy or other evil.

9. *Each of us is responsible for our own wellness.* Many Native Americans believe they are responsible for their own health or illness. From the moment of birth, each person is responsible for his or her own character. When one lives in harmony, transgressions against tribal taboos do not occur, and negative energy from witchcraft cannot penetrate the individual. One cannot blame others for one's own shortcomings (Locust, 1985, p. 17).

GROUP HEALTH
Health Care System

The U.S. Department of Health and Human Services (DHHS), primarily through the Indian Health Service (IHS) of the Public Health Service (PHS), is responsible for providing health services to Native Americans. In 1954, the PHS was charged with "all functions, responsibilities, authorities, and duties . . . relating to the maintenance and operation of hospital and health facilities for Indians, and the conservation of Indian health" (IHS, 1990a).

Figure 1-4 illustrates the structure of the IHS. In 1975, the Indian Self Determi-

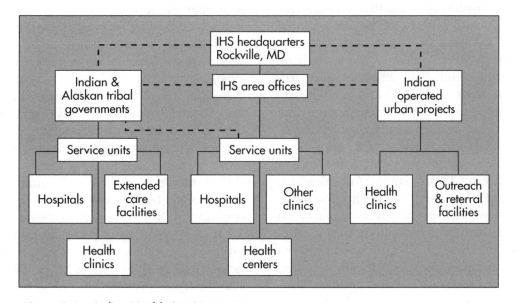

Figure 1-4   Indian Health Service structure.
(From Indian Health Service: *Trends in indian health* 1990, Bethesda, Md, 1990, PHS, p 10.)

nation Act gave tribes the option of staffing and managing IHS programs in their communities. The program now consists of 12 regional administrative units called **area offices.** The IHS Service Area offices are located in Aberdeen, SD; Anchorage, AK; Albuquerque, NM; Bemidji, MN; Billings, MO; Sacramento CA; Nashville, TN; Navajo (covers portions of AZ, NM, CO, and UT); Oklahoma City, OK; Phoenix, AZ; Portland OR; and Tucson, AZ. As of October 1, 1988, the area offices consisted of 127 basic administrative units called **service units;** of these, 52 were tribally operated. During the same time the IHS operated 43 hospitals, 66 health centers, five school health centers, and 60 health stations. Tribes operated seven hospitals, 73 health centers, two school health centers, 65 health stations, and 173 Alaskan village clinics. Both the California and Portland areas had no hospitals, while the Phoenix and Aberdeen areas had eight and nine hospitals, respectively. The Tuscon area had the fewest health centers, with three, and Oklahoma area the most, with 27.

In 1976, an amendment to the Indian Health Care Improvement Act called for efforts to improve the health status of Native Americans to levels equal with the general U.S. population. At that time, the federal government appropriated resources to expand health services, build and renovate medical facilities, construct more sanitary disposal and safe drinking water facilities, increase the number of Native American health professionals working with Native American clients, and improve health care access for urban-dwelling Native Americans.

Some have questioned the adequacy of funding for the IHS. Cooke (1990) believes that the IHS has "an absurd task that's roughly the equivalent of running a Third-World relief effort on a shoestring budget. For 35 years, the agency has been tap dancing between charges of neglect if it fails in its job, and paternalism if it succeeds" (p. 68).

IHS budgets have not been commensurate with the costs of medical care in the U.S. In 1987, the IHS had $845 per person to spend for health care; the rest of the nation spent $1,987 per person. The Office of Technology Assessment estimated that in 1988 alone 28,000 elective procedures for Native American patients were postponed. In the Billings, MT area, many deferred procedures were potentially lifesaving services, including obstetric exams, mammograms, and psychiatric care for suicidal teenagers (Cooke, 1990).

Besides the usual health care providers, the IHS makes extensive use of a unique and important category of personnel, the community health representative (CHR). CHRs are educated and skilled members of the lay community who provide health care to others in their community. In 1989, CHRs made over 3.7 million client contacts in the community, in hospitals and clinics, in the home, and in their offices (IHS, 1990b). The functions provided by these individuals include problem assessment; therapeutic and follow-up services; resolution of physical, economic, and cultural barriers to health; health education and consultation; surveillance and control of environmental factors affecting health (Table 1-4).

TABLE 1-4   Community Health Representatives Client Contacts: By Setting, Function, and Health Care Area, 1989

	Client Contacts*	
Type of Contact	Number	Percent Distribution
SETTING:		
Total client contacts	3,753,237	100.00
Community	1,175,742	31.3
Hospitals and clinics	1,035,969	27.6
Home	811,544	21.6
CHR office	729,982	19.5
HEALTH FUNCTION:		
Total client contacts	2,951,780	100.0
Problem assessment, therapeutic, & follow-up service	1,323,244	44.8
Resolve physical, economic, & cultural barriers to health care	1,061,034	36.0
Health education & consultation	314,808	10.6
Surveillance & control of environmental factors affecting health	252,694	8.6
HEALTH CARE AREA:		
Total client contacts	3,418,532	100.0
General health care	2,231,710	65.3
Maternal & child health	518,440	15.2
Environmental health care	283,192	8.3
Gerontological health care	280,930	8.2
Dental health	66,716	2.0
Mental health care	37,544	1.0

*Estimated data based on CHR reports of actual client contacts completed during July and August, 1989. Based on these reports, annual workload projections through September 1989 were prepared. The total number of client contacts reported under the headings of setting, function, and health care area vary as a result of the manner in which training and administration were reported in each category.

From Indian Health Service, Office of Planning, Evaluation, and Legislation, Division of Program Statistics (1990): *Trends in Indian Health*, Rockville, 1990, Public Health Service. Contains no copyright material.

Access to and use of the health care system. Although Native Americans living on reservations and members of tribes with access to reservation health facilities receive health care through the IHS, access to this care is still a major problem. Many live in rural areas where the number of physicians is about half that of the national average and where the IHS may not provide health care services (IHS, 1991). Little is known of the problems urban Native Americans face when trying to obtain care.

Nearly 105,000 patients were admitted to IHS and tribal direct and contract hospitals in 1988 (Figure 1-5). The number of admissions ranged from 570 in California to 23,669 in Navajo. The leading cause of

MALES

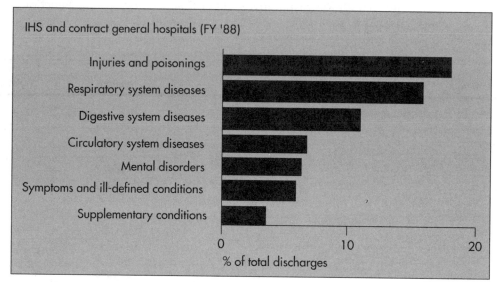

FEMALES

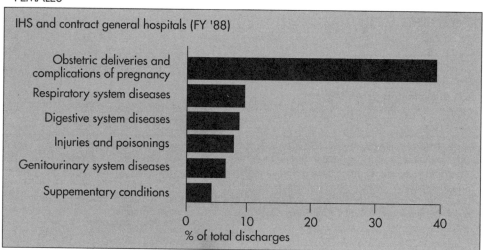

Figure 1-5 Leading causes of hospitalization.

(From Indian Health Service: *Trends in indian health*, Bethesda, Md, 1990, PHS, p 60.)

MALES

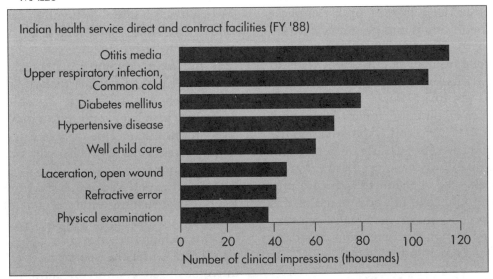

FEMALES

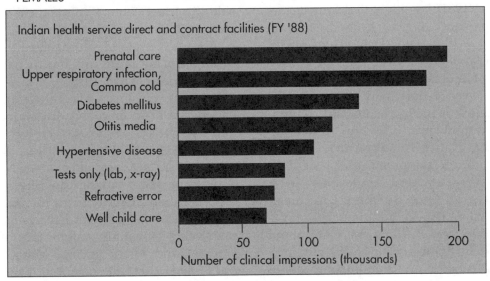

Figure 1-6 Leading diagnoses for outpatient visits.

(From Indian Health Service: *Trends in indian health*, Bethesda, Md, 1990, PHS, p 65.)

hospitalization in all but two IHS areas was "obstetric deliveries and complication of puerperium and pregnancy" (IHS, 1990a, p. 6).

The total number of outpatient visits to IHS and tribal direct and contract facilities was approximately 5 million (Figure 1-6). Tucson had the fewest outpatient visits with 87,795, and Oklahoma had the most with 898,007. Clearly, when health care facilities are available, Native Americans make use of them. Health care providers should take full advantage of this exposure and make personally relevant health education and screening programs available to each individual.

Barriers to Seeking Health Care

Antle (1987) has identified four factors that prevent Native Americans from seeking health care: lack of resources; lack of familiarity with the hospital environment and associated procedures; confusion over requirements for medical procedures or prescriptions; and communication problems. Like any other patient, the Native American may confuse certain cancer symptoms—such as diarrhea, fever, pain, and skin lesions—with symptoms of more common, less threatening ailments. In addition, these patients may fear learning the truth about their health status, or have difficulty integrating Western and traditional forms of medicine.

Lack of resources. Poverty and lack of transportation can make paying for and obtaining care difficult. Native Americans who believe in living day-to-day rather than planning for the future (Yukl, 1986) may not have insurance, savings,

or retirement funds with which to pay for health care. Often reservation inhabitants must walk, hitch-hike, or hire a neighbor to drive them. Native Americans not living on the reservation must also travel long distances to receive care at IHS hospitals or clinics. These transportation problems and traditional Native American concepts of time can cause Native Americans to be late for or miss appointments.

Hospitalization and clinic environment issues. The bustling environment of the hospital or clinic may be neither welcoming nor personable. According to DeLoria, "tribal society is holistic . . . a tribal universe is so comfortable and reasonable that it acts like a narcotic . . . Outside the tribal context you become alienated, irritable, and lonely" (in Yukl, 1986, p. 226). A warm and informal health care setting will be more inviting to the Native American (Yukl, 1986).

In some instances Native Americans experience overt or covert discrimination and prejudice (Frank-Stromborg and Olsen, 1988), which can result in delays in diagnosis and treatment. Most Native Americans will respond stoically to attacks on their integrity or to the absence of the basic respect accorded to any human being by simply walking out of the hospital and never again seeking help from that particular institution (Yukl, 1986).

Some see the hospital as a place to die and are hesitant to be admitted or put in a room where another person has died. Members of some tribes may appreciate having the room purified by burning cedar in it after the housekeeper has left.

Native Americans are generally not receptive to any invasive body procedures, including autopsy. Many will only agree to biopsy and surgery reluctantly, if the involved area cannot be cured by other means. Relatives may refuse to donate blood for surgery for fear that if the patient dies, the donor might also. Patients may also refuse to have blood drawn or may speed up intravenous infusions so they will be completed or removed (Antle, 1987).

Native Americans should always be asked if they want a body part back after amputation, surgery, or biopsy, including the breast, placenta, any limb, hair, or even nails. The Creek, Cachon, and Mohave tribes believe the body must remain intact for burial. Pueblo Indians believe the body must be returned to the village before the sun goes down. Other tribes believe body parts can be used as a means to enter the body and cause harm. Younger generations and Northwestern tribes generally do not adhere as strongly to such beliefs (Frank-Stromborg and Olsen, 1988).

Procedure and prescription compliance. When Native American healers prescribe traditional medications, they may prescribe very large quantities. In addition, traditional Native American time is relative to what needs to be done and not regulated by clocks; "Indian time" typically runs from 1 hour to a few days later than standard time (Yukl, 1986). For these reasons, health care workers should give careful instructions on how to take modern medications. Instructions to take a medication four times a day may result in four pills being taken at once or at improper intervals. A chart identifying the position of the sun in the sky to indicate the time to take a medication and color coding medication labels to correspond with the position of the sun may be helpful (Kniep-Hardy and Burkhardt, 1987).

Traditional families are generally very involved in making decisions about a member's health care, often to the point of making decisions for the patient. In matrilineal Native American societies, a patient may not give written consent for procedures or surgery until he or she obtains permission from the mother, grandmother, or aunt. On occasion, patients will give consent only after a traditional ceremony; if this cannot be done in the hospital, then the patient may leave and return after the ritual (Antle, 1987).

Phyllis Old Dog Cross, RN, MS, a member of the Mandan and Hidatsa (Sioux) tribes of North Dakota, notes that the Sioux, among other tribes, often engage in fasting and cleansing rituals before healing. These are usually required by the medicine man or woman to ensure that all aggressive, resentful, and angry behaviors are removed before healing can take place (Lammers, 1987).

Communication problems. Some Native Americans, especially older ones, speak only their traditional language; others speak some English but may be unwilling to admit any problems understanding; others are fluent in English. Younger generations, particularly those educated off the reservation, may be bilingual. Interpreters are often necessary but should be used carefully. Interpreters must understand the nature of social, cultural, and familial lines of communication and respect. Some tribes consider discussions with one individual about another inappropriate and a sign of disrespect. Worse yet, discussions about another could break a cultural taboo, leaving oneself or family member vulnerable to harm.

Cross explains that interpersonal relations are carefully spelled out among Indian tribes. "Who you speak to, when you speak to them, how you speak, and your sequence of speaking are very important . . . the mother-in-law cannot speak to the son-in-law or cannot be in the same room with him. So it is not always appropriate to have the family members together in the same room" (Lammers, 1987, p. 1211).

Diana Velasquez, a Yaqui **curandera** (medicine woman) employed by the federal health system advises health care

---

CONTRIBUTIONS OF TRADITIONAL HEALING PRACTICES TO THE KNOWLEDGE BASE OF MEDICINE

BENEFITS OF THE TRADITIONAL SWEAT

The traditional Navajo sweat benefits the body by ridding it of salt and hormones such as adrenalin. The hormones leave the body with water when a person sweats. Adrenalin in the body causes a flight or fight response making clear thought impossible. Adrenalin also makes the heart beat faster and the blood sugar go up. After the body is cleansed by a sweat, body processes slow down, including the blood pressure, pulse rate, and breathing. Following a sweat, the mind can think clearly and profoundly.

THE HEALING PROPERTIES OF THE DRUM

The rhythmic beat of a rattle or drum is also a method of healing. It not only causes a foot to tap in time, but the body's beats are affected as well. The heart rate, speed of circulation, and brain waves are actually changed by the rhythmic beat that accompanies chants. The beats actually slow the inner rhythms of the body and make clear thinking or meditation possible.

THE HEALING PROPERTY OF COLD

A Canadian tribal custom, much like the Navajo and Hopi custom of rolling in the snow, is to throw cold water on oneself in the mornings. The belief is that it will make one stronger and more resistant to cold. Modern medical research has proven that exposing the body to cold in these ways actually does cause a tremendous increase in the white blood cell count. The white blood cells, in turn, cause the body to be more resistant to infections like the common cold.

From Norrell-Kahn B; Methods come from Navajos; at long last, modern medicine is catching up with traditions, *Times Today,* 1985.

practitioners to use the "power" they have very wisely. She cautions, "if you are going to lay hands on my people, remember that you are the vessel that carries healing. Anger, hatred, bitterness, and guilt can create evil spirits in a person. If you carry evil spirits, my people will fear that" (Lammers, 1987, p. 1212).

Native Americans tend to be very private people who are comfortable with silence and do not readily volunteer information. They may consider intensive questioning to be excessive. Some may nod "yes" but actually do not understand, others may give responses they think the health practitioner may wish to hear, especially if the question is regarded as inappropriate (Antle, 1987).

Conflicts between Western and traditional medicine. Traditional Native Americans who want to integrate the practices of both Western health care practitioners and their own medicine men may find that physicians and nurses are unwilling to accept traditional healing practices of Indian culture. This lack of respect and understanding for the Native American concept of wellness and harmony may discourage many of these patients from using the Western health care system. However, the two systems are generally compatible and can lead to effective healing if health care workers have respect, patience, and tolerance. Some scientific studies have documented the value of traditional healing practices (see box).

During focus group interviews, experienced Native American nurses have described the level of suspicion that health care workers must confront: "A real medicine woman or man will know without

being told what is wrong with you. Anglo doctors ask a lot of questions and still can't figure out what is wrong;" "The IHS staff come to the reservation to 'practice' medicine on Indians;" "A person, particularly a white person should not tell you about illness if they have never had personal experience with it" (Frank-Stromborg and Olsen, 1988).

Overcoming Barriers to Health Care

Yukl (1986) has suggested several interventions that may be helpful in overcoming some of the cultural barriers American Indians may encounter when they enter the health care system. They are listed below:

1. Native American patients should feel they are accepted as whole human beings without judgment for their physical appearance, beliefs, or practices.
2. Health care workers should recognize Native Americans' orientation to the present and to short-term goals, as well as their unique cultural beliefs and behaviors.
3. Staff and services should be available to patients when the need arises rather than scheduling appointments.
4. Many Native Americans dislike standing out in a group and do value privacy, so they may prefer individual to group counseling.
5. Staff should be educated about cultural differences to facilitate understanding and appreciation.
6. Supplemental home care services rather than nursing home placement will maximize family unity and strengths while minimizing economic strain.

7. Illustrating medical problems in concrete ways will facilitate traditional learning styles, understanding, personal relevance, and retention.

NATIVE AMERICAN: HEATH STATUS AND CANCER INCIDENCE
Overview

As noted earlier, Native Americans are a youthful population, a factor that may be explained partly by the high incidence of premature deaths in this group. A large portion of this population dies before age 45. Excess deaths in a subgroup or minority are defined as deaths that would not have occurred in that group if its death rates were comparable to those of the total population. In the Native American population, excess deaths have been traced to six causes: unintentional injuries, cirrhosis, homicide, suicide, pneumonia, and complications of diabetes (Figure 1-7). Heart disease and cancer are not among the causes of excess deaths among Native Americans, probably because these are generally diseases of older age. The incidence of cancer in this group is lower overall than that of the general population. However, the incidence of lung cancer among Oklahoma Indians is double that of the total U.S. population, Southwest Indians have high rates of gallbladder cancer, and Alaska Natives suffer high rates of liver cancer (USDHHS, 1986).

In 1987, The U.S. Department of Health and Human Services identified national health promotion and disease prevention objectives for the nation. They outlined objectives for several subpopulations, including Native Americans. These objectives are enumerated in Appendix 1.

Cancer statistics for Native Americans are limited. Two sources of information are available, the Surveillance, Epidemiology, and End Results (SEER) Program and the IHS, but they contain data on different populations.

The SEER program collects data from six states (Connecticut, Hawaii, Iowa, New Mexico, New Jersey, and Utah), four large metropolitan areas (Atlanta, Detroit, San Francisco, and Seattle) and Puerto Rico. Native Americans constitute only 0.3% of the SEER population. The most recent SEER data for American Indians covers the period 1977 to 1983.

The IHS collects data from Native Americans who attend IHS and tribal fa-

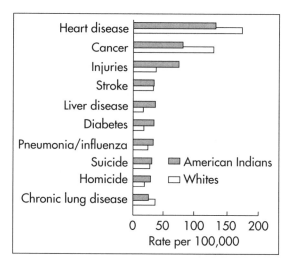

Figure 1-7 Leading causes of death for Native Americans in reservation states compared to whites (1987), age-adjusted rates.

(From DHHS: *Healthy People 2000* Washington, DC, 1991, U.S. Government Printing Office.)

cilities. Regional differences, for mortality statistics only, can be derived for each of the 12 regional health service areas (Table 1-5). The most recent cancer mortality statistics from this database cover 1986 through 1988 (Table 1-6). Only about one third of all Native Americans are accounted for in this information. Fifty percent of Indians live off the reservation, so little information on cancer incidence and mortality statistics for this population is available.

Justice (1988) suggests that regional tumor registries are needed to collect cancer data on Native Americans. Such a registry could document distinctive pat-

terns of cancer incidence among tribes, much as other databases have registered patters in different ethnic groups.

Sievers and Fisher (1983) suggest that among Native Americans, the occurrence and anatomic distribution of cancer appears to be influenced more by cultural conditions than by an inherited resistance or predisposition.

Cancer Incidence, Mortality, and Survival

Although the incidence of different types of cancers can differ among different Native American tribes (Justice, 1988), overall Native Americans have the

TABLE 1-5 Native American Deaths from Malignant Neoplasms by Sex for Each IHS Area (1986-1988)*

IHS Area	Gender			IHS Service Population	1986-1988 Crude† Cancer Rate per 100,000 Population	
	Male	Female	Combined			Rank
Tucson	18	13	31	20,702	149	(7)
Aberdeen	99	91	190	84,280	225	(3)
Bemidji	73	59	132	55,742	237	(2)
Albuquerque	52	34	86	60,667	142	(8)
Alaska	116	104	218	85,737	254	(1)
Billings	59	45	104	49,368	211	(4)
Oklahoma	252	200	452	218,262	207	(5)
Nashville	38	37	75	43,545	172	(6)
Phoenix	49	76	125	99,569	125	(11)
California	46	42	88	86,699	101	(12)
Portland	82	70	152	109,969	138	(9)
Navajo	103	141	244	190,946	128	(10)

*Absolute frequencies reported.

†Crude rates are summary rates calculated only for comparison purposes, usually based on annual data. For purposes of this report, only 2-year combined data were available; therefore, interpretation is limited to this set of data only. The purpose was only to ascertain differences between IHS population areas. Data cannot be compared to national mortality rates for any other population(s).

From Indian Health Service, Office of Program Statistics: *Indian and Alaska Native Deaths By Cause (recode 282) Sex and Age for Each IHS Area*, Rockville, Md, 1990, Public Health Service. Contains no copyrighted material.

TABLE 1-6 Native American Deaths from Malignant Neoplasms by Site (All IHS Areas Combined) (1986-1988)*

Site	Frequency
Larynx, trachea, bronchus, lung	567
(Male) 373	
(Female) 194	
Colon & rectum	209
(Male) 105	
(Female) 104	
Female breast	123
Pancreas	121
Prostate	118
Leukemia	107
Kidney	76
Cervix	75
Liver	74
Ovary	72
Gallbladder	70
Lip, oral cavity, & pharynx	46
Esophagus	32
Bladder	21
Thyroid	12
Melanoma	9
Hodgkin's disease	9
Testis	5
Eye	1
Penis & other male genital organs	1
Male breast	1

*Absolute frequencies reported.
From Indian Health Service, Office of Program Statistics: *Indian and Alaska Native Deaths by Cause (recode 282) Sex and Age for Each* IHS Area, Rockville, Md, 1990, Public Health Service. Contains no copyrighted material.

TABLE 1-7 Age-adjusted Cancer Incidence Rates per 100,000 Population by Racial/Ethnic Group by Sex—SEER Program 1978-1981

Site/Ethnic Group	Males	Females
Black, all areas	487.9	290.3
White, all areas	391.9	303.2
Hawaiian, Hawaii	390.9	336.5*
Japanese, Hawaii	300.4	214.5
Japanese, San Francisco —Oakland	225.5	210.1
Chinese, San Francisco —Oakland	293.8	230.3
Chinese, Hawaii	258.9	227.7
Hispanic, New Mexico	279.8	218.4
Hispanic, Puerto Rico	245.2	181.3
Filipino, Hawaii	235.2	191.6
Native American, New Mexico	172.3	155.5

*Indicates racial group with highest cancer rates.
From American Cancer Society: *Minority Facts and Figures*, New York, 1986, American Cancer Society. Adapted by permission.

lowest cancer incidence and mortality rates of all U.S. populations (USDHHS, 1986). SEER data indicate that the cancer incidence rates for Native Americans of both genders are about half that of the majority U.S. population (Table 1-7). In general, Native Americans have incidence rates below non-minorities for cancers of the lung, breast, and prostate (Table 1-8). Incidence rates are much higher for cancers of the oral cavity, cervix, gallbladder, colon and rectum, and kidney. Because Native Americans, as a group, are younger than the majority population and have a shorter life expectancy, they often do not live long enough to develop cancer (USDHHS, 1989). However, this group has high rates of obesity and diseases associated with alcohol and tobacco use; these risk factors could lead to higher cancer rates in the future.

Cancer is ranked as the third leading cause of death among Native Americans, preceded only by accidents and heart dis-

TABLE 1-8 Age-Adjusted (1970 U.S. Standard) Cancer Incidence Rates Per 100,000 Population by Race and Cancer Site Both Sexes 1977-1983.

Cancer Site	African American	Chinese	Japanese	Filipino	Native American	Mexican American	Native Hawaiian	Alaska Native	Caucasian
All Sites	382.8‡	247.6	242.5	212.4	137.6	245.1	346.5	314.3	358.5
Oral cavity	15.0	15.4	4.8	8.9	2.1	6.6	9.0	16.5‡	11.7
Esophagus	11.6‡	3.3	2.8	3.4	1.0	1.6	7.3	6.1	3.4
Stomach	14.5	10.5	26.6	7.8	15.1	15.3	27.0‡	15.5	8.9
Colon & rectum	50.3	40.4	48.8	30.3	9.6	26.2	31.7	62.6‡	52.8
Liver	3.6	9.6‡	3.6	5.4	2.1	3.1	5.5	6.4	2.1
Gallbladder	1.0	1.0	1.5	1.4	10.0	4.6	1.3	10.6‡	1.3
Pancreas	13.8‡	6.3	7.1	4.9	3.7	11.0	8.0	9.9	9.5
Lung	69.8‡	40.6	27.1	27.3	6.3	23.4	66.9	46.9	56.4
Melanoma (skin)	0.8	0.7	1.2	1.0	1.9	1.9‡	1.1	na	9.4‡
Breast*	75.2	57.8	55.0	41.3	21.3	52.1	106.1‡	44.2	92.9
Cervix uteri*	19.7	10.3	5.9	8.6	19.9	16.1	15.2	28.0‡	8.6
Corpus uteri*	15.0	18.0	17.7	11.3	7.2	11.3	28.2‡	na	26.6
Ovary*	10.2	9.2	8.8	9.7	7.5	11.3	14.4‡	9.5	14.1
Prostate gland†	125.5‡	29.6	43.8	44.0	31.0	76.3	56.1	34.5	73.2
Urinary bladder	9.6	9.0	8.0	4.4	1.4	7.9	8.5	6.1	18.0‡
Kidney and renal	6.8	3.5	3.6	3.1	5.7	6.4	4.2	11.2‡	7.2
Brain and CNS	3.4	2.4	2.4	1.9	1.2	3.7	3.0	2.1	6.3‡
Hodgkin's disease	1.8	0.6	0.5	1.2	0.2	2.6	1.0	na	3.2‡
Non-Hodgkin's	7.2	8.5	7.2	8.3	2.8	6.7	8.4	na	11.7‡
Leukemia	9.1	4.8	5.7	7.1	4.6	6.9	8.2	na	10.4‡

*Females only.
†Males only.
‡Indicates the racial group with the highest rate for the cancer.
Data source:African American, Caucasian—San Francisco-Oakland, Atlanta, Detroit, Connecticut.
Chinese, Japanese, Filipino—San Francisco-Oakland, Hawaii.
Native Hawaiian—Hawaii.
American Indian—New Mexico, Arizona.
Mexican American—New Mexico.
Alaska Native—State of Alaska, 1969-83.
From SEER, The National Cancer Institute Surveillance Program, Cancer Statistics Branch, Bethesda, 1991, National Cancer Institute.

ease (Figure 1-8). In general, the age-adjusted mortality rate for Native Americans is lower than the rate for all U.S. races (Figure 1-9). However, the IHS has documented excess mortality rates—that is, rates over and above those commonly expected for this population—for cancers of the cervix, gallbladder, and kidney (Table 1-9). Native Americans generally experience lower mortality rates than

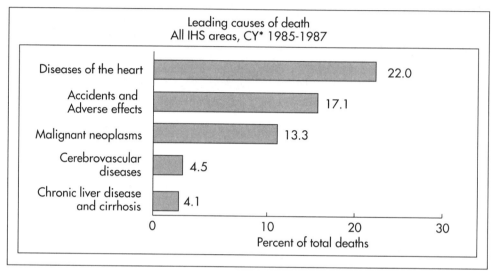

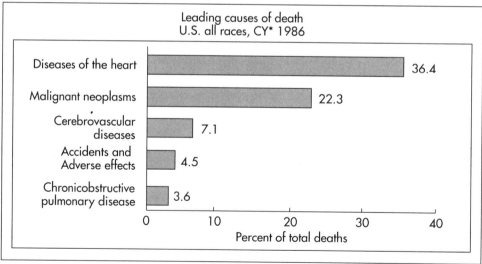

Figure 1-8   Leading causes of death; all IHS areas (1985-1987) compared to U.S. all races (1986). CY = Calendar Year.

(From Indian Health Service: *Regional Differences in Indian Health*, 1990. Bethesda, Md, 1990, PHS, p 35.)

non-minorities for cancers of the lung, breast, and prostate (Table 1-10). Native American men generally have higher cancer death rates than women (Figure 1-10).

Compared to any other ethnic or cultural group in the United States, Native Americans of both sexes have the lowest 5-year relative survival rates for cancers of the stomach, rectum, prostate, breast,

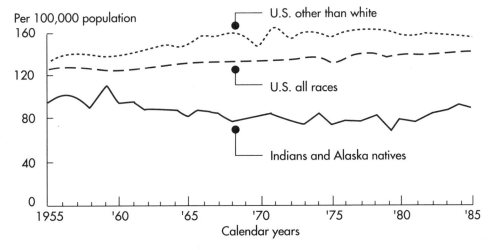

Figure 1-9 Age-adjusted malignant neoplasm death rates.

TABLE 1-9 Numbers and Standardized Mortality Ratios (SMRs) for the 10 Leading Cancer Sites among Native Americans of the 26 Reservation States, 1974-1976

Site	Male SMR	Female SMR	Total Observed (No.)	Total Expected (No.)	SMR*
Lung	39	66	153	352.1	43
Colon	51	47	89	181.8	49
Breast	—	53	78	148.0	53
Stomach	89	113	76	78.1	97
Pancreas	71	98	74	90.9	81
Cervix	—	229	66	28.8	229
Gallbladder	—	432	54	12.4	435
Prostate	57	—	53	93.5	57
Kidney and renal pelvis	145	171	52	33.8	154
Liver	101	138	29	25.3	115
All cancer deaths	55	89	1,202	1,736.9	69

Items listed in order of frequency. Data from Indian Health Service (supplied by Mozart I. Spector, Director, Office of Program Statistics.)
*SMR = (observed deaths/expected deaths) × 100.

TABLE 1-10   Age-Adjusted (1970 U.S. Standard) Cancer Mortality Rates per 100,000 Population by Race and Cancer Site, Both Sexes 1977-83.

Cancer Site	African American	Chinese	Japanese	Filipino	Native American	Mexican American	Native Hawaiian	Alaska Native	Caucasian
All Sites	209.8‡	125.0	108.0	72.0	89.3	132.0	207.2	182.1	164.2
Oral cavity	5.7	5.4	1.7	2.4	1.8	1.9	3.9	5.9‡	3.3
Esophagus	9.1‡	2.8	2.1	1.8	2.0	1.7	7.2	3.2	
Stomach	10.0	7.6	17.9	3.5	5.8	11.8	21.8‡	10.8	5.2
Colon & rectum	22.4	17.9	16.8	7.9	8.9	13.2	14.6	26.6‡	21.4
Liver	3.6	10.1‡	3.4	3.5	2.0	3.9	5.2	6.9	1.9
Gallbladder	0.7	0.7	1.1	0.6	2.6	3.2	0.5	3.6‡	0.9
Pancreas	11.2‡	6.4	7.0	3.5	4.6	10.2	10.0	8.7	8.4
Lung	51.3	31.7	19.8	14.5	18.1	9.5	56.5‡	32.1	41.6
Melanoma (skin)	0.4‡	0.2	0.2	0.3	0.3	0.4	0.3	—	2.2‡
Breast*	26.9	12.0	10.2	7.8	9.0	19.4	37.2‡	14.0	26.8
Cervix uteri*	8.7	3.3	2.2	1.9	5.5	.2	5.6	11.1‡	3.2
Corpus uteri*	6.5‡	2.7	2.4	1.7	1.8	2.3	6.3	1.1	3.9
Ovary*	6.4	3.8	4.4	2.6	3.2	5.9	8.2‡	4.0	8.1
Prostate gland†	43.9‡	7.4	8.4	8.7	11.7	19.4	15.8	10.7	21.1
Urinary bladder	3.8‡	1.7	1.8	1.4	1.0	2.3	2.9	1.7	3.8‡
Kidney and renal	2.7	1.7	1.6	0.8	2.7	2.6	2.3	5.2‡	3.2
Brain and CNS	2.4	1.3	1.3	1.1	1.3	3.2	2.0	2.4	4.2‡
Hodgkin's disease	0.6	0.3	0.1	0.3	0.3	1.0‡	0.2	0.3	0.9
Non-Hodgkin's	3.3	2.8	3.5	3.4	2.1	3.1	5.6‡	3.1	5.2
Leukemia	5.8	4.1	3.5	4.1	2.9	4.8	6.8‡	3.8	6.7

*Females only.
†Males only.
‡Indicates the racial group with the highest rate for the cancer.
Data source: African American, Caucasian, Chinese, Japanese, Filipino, Native American—United States.
Native Hawaiian—Hawaii.
Mexican American—New Mexico.
Alaska Natives—Alaska, 1969-83.
From SEER, The National Cancer Institute Surveillance Program, Cancer Statistics Branch, Bethesda, Md, 1991, National Cancer Institute.

bladder, and, for men, lung and bronchus.

Tribal Comparison of Cancer Rates

Few studies have compared the distribution of primary cancers among tribes with very different cultural, genetic, and environmental backgrounds. Justice (1989) conducted such a study to prove that cancer patterns among tribes could be unique. He compared one Southwestern tribe, the Papagos, (also known as the Tohono O'Odham) with a northern plains tribe, the Oglala Lakota Sioux. The Tohono O'Odham are generally a homogeneous population that has experienced very little intermarriage with Europeans or with other tribes; in contrast, the mi-

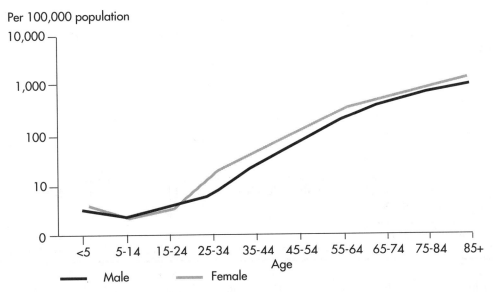

Figure 1-10   Age-adjusted malignant neoplasm mortality by age and sex. The age-specific malignant neoplasm death rate (1985-1987) for Indian males was higher for all age groups, except under 5 and 25 through 54 years, in comparison to Indian females. The rates for Indian males and females increased with age beginning with age 5.

(From Indian Health Service: *Trends in indian health*, 1990 Bethesda, Md, 1990, PHS, p 47.)

nority of Oglala are "purebloods" as a result of intermarriage with Europeans and members of other tribal groups.

Justice found distinctively different cancer profiles for each tribe. Oglala men experienced proportionately more cancers of the lung, pancreas, penis, and bladder than Tohono O'Odham men. Male Tohono O'Odham patients had proportionately more stomach, liver, and testicular cancer.

Oglala women had significantly more lung, stomach, colon, pancreas, breast, leukemia, and cervical cancer than Tohono O'Odham women. Tohono O'Odham women had excess cancers of the gallbladder, ovaries, and melanoma of the skin.

Compared with men of all U.S. races, men from both tribes had significantly lower rates of colorectal, lung, prostate, and bladder cancers. Compared to women of all U.S. races, females from both tribes had a relative lack of colorectal, breast, uterine, and bladder cancers. However, compared to females from all races, the Oglala lung cancer, cervical cancer, and stomach cancer rates appeared unusually high. In fact, the Oglala women had the highest rate of lung cancer mortality for females in the world. In addition lung cancer rates for male and female Oglalas at Pine Ridge were the highest reported for a Native American tribe.

Lung Cancer

In general, Native Americans experience lower incidence and mortality rates from lung cancer than all other U.S. populations (Tables 1-8 and 1-10). Despite the apparently favorable nature of these statistics, it must be recognized that Native Americans have the poorest survival rates when they do contract cancer (Table 1-11), and lung cancer accounts for the largest number of cancer-related deaths in this group.

TABLE 1-11 Five-Year Cancer Relative Survival Rates (%) by Race and Cancer Site, Both Sexes, 1975-84.

Cancer Site	African American	Chinese	Japanese	Filipino	Native American	Mexican American	Native Hawaiian	Caucasian
All sites	39.6	47.5	53.1	46.1	35.4‡	48.4	43.2	51.3
Oral cavity	33.0‡	55.7	44.4	46.6	38.6	60.7	42.8	49.8
Esophagus	4.2	11.5	5.8	3.4	—	0.0‡	0.0‡	6.1
Stomach	17.5	21.6	29.8	18.8	8.9‡	17.8	12.9	16.6
Colon & rectum	46.7	53.1	61.7	44.8	39.7‡	45.0	58.4	54.2
Liver	3.1	2.0	1.5	6.7	0.0‡	0.0‡	6.6	3.9
Gallbladder	8.9	—	16.2	—	2.8‡	8.5	26.2	8.8
Pancreas	3.2	0.0‡	2.6	5.2	0.0‡	1.2	0.0‡	2.3
Lung	11.7	15.1	14.3	13.2	0.0‡	10.8	13.0	14.2
Melanoma (skin)	57.5‡	—	81.0	—	—	82.1	—	81.3
Breast*	63.2	80.8	85.4	73.7	46.2‡	70.6	68.0	75.5
Cervix uteri*	61.6‡	74.6	70.2	73.0	63.5	70.5	67.7	66.7
Corpus uteri*	54.9‡	86.1	84.1	79.9	82.7	77.0	74.6	84.6
Ovary*	40.9	43.3	43.5	44.7	42.9	38.7	46.8	38.1‡
Prostrate gland†	63.4	72.5	80.5	71.7	54.2‡	72.4	72.0	7.03
Urinary bladder	53.4	78.5	80.8	58.4	—	64.6	51.4‡	75.8
Kidney and renal	56.3	60.7	63.1	47.0‡	49.7	51.4	59.0	55.2
Brain and CNS	28.5	35.9	40.6	29.6	37.6	32.2	38.9	22.6‡
Hodgkin's disease	71.0	—	—	43.5‡	—	69.0	74.1	73.8
Non-Hodgkin's	47.9	50.3	41.1	33.8	31.1‡	41.1	40.2	49.9
Leukemia	28.0	19.8‡	26.0	22.3	21.4	25.7	21.1	32.6

*Females only.
†Males only.
‡Indicates the racial group with the lowest survival rate for the cancer.
Data source: African American, Caucasian—San Francisco-Oakland, Atlanta, Detroit, Connecticut.
Chinese, Japanese, Filipino—San Francisco-Oakland, Hawaii.
Native Hawaiian—Hawaii.
American Indian—New Mexico, Arizona.
Mexican American—New Mexico.
From SEER, The National Cancer Institute Surveillance Program, Cancer Statistics Branch, Bethesda, Md, 1991, National Cancer Institute.

Regional statistics (DHHS, 1986) suggest that lung cancer rates vary across tribes and are related to different cigarette smoking practices. In an IHS study conducted from 1986 to 1988 (Table 1-12) on the frequencies of lung, larynx, trachea, and bronchial cancer deaths across IHS areas, the number of deaths reported in the areas of Tucson, Navajo, Phoenix, California, and Albuquerque was significantly lower than the number reported in Oklahoma. Oklahoma Native Americans smoke heavily, whereas Southwestern tribes smoke very little (USDHHS, 1986).

Boss (1986) reported that the four IHS areas with the highest rates of lung cancer were Aberdeen, Alaska, Bemidji, and Billings. Welty (1989) reviewed information on lung cancer among Native Americans in the Aberdeen area and found lung cancer death rates that were slightly less than the rate for all U.S. races, but almost 15% higher than the rate for the entire IHS populations. He also noted that the Aberdeen, Bemidji, and Billings area tribes (members of the Northern Plains tribes) and the Alaskan tribes had high rates of cigarette smoking. Citing studies of these tribes conducted from 1968 to 1985, Welty documented a high prevalence of smoking, from 13% to 70%.

One particular type of bronchogenic cancer, small cell, undifferentiated carcinoma, occurs more frequently among Navajo uranium miners than among other Native Americans. Samet et al. (1984) confirmed the influence of this occupational exposure. Navajos should

TABLE 1-12 Native American Deaths from Malignant Neoplasms by Sex for Each IHS Area (1986-1988)*

IHS Area	Pancreas		Larynx, Trachea, Bronchus, Lung		Melanoma	
	M	F	M	F	M	F
Tucson	1		5	2		
Aberdeen	10	7	40	25		
Bemidji	3	4	33	17		
Albuquerque	4	2	9	3		
Alaska	7	9	56	40		1
Billings		3	23	19	1	1
Oklahoma	15	13	108	34	1	3
Nashville	3	1	17	12		
Phoenix	4	3	16	12		
California	3	5	19	6		
Portland	3	2	33	19		1
Navajo	12	7	14	5	1	

*Absolute frequencies reported.
From Indian Health Service, Office of Program Statistics: *Indian and Alaska Native Deaths By Cause (recode 282) Sex and Age for Each IHS Area*, Rockville, Md, 1990, Public Health Service. Contains no copyrighted material.

therefore be cautioned of the dangers of corralling sheep or resting in abandoned uranium mines.

Five cases of malignant mesothelioma among Pueblo Indians have also been reported (Driscoll, Mulligan, Schultz, and Candelaria, 1988). An epidemiologic investigation confirmed that at one time this tribe used asbestos to make silver jewelry and to whiten leggings for ceremonial use. After this investigation, state and local public health authorities and Native American officials collected asbestos from the homes of Pueblos and began educational programs for the Pueblo communities. Alternative materials were identified for use by ceremonial dancers and silversmiths. However, health care providers should still conduct thorough occupational histories on Pueblos to identify those who may be at risk for mesothelioma.

Lung cancer prevention efforts among native Americans should include a comprehensive history of occupation and cigarette smoking followed by the recommendation to stop smoking, referral to appropriate cessation programs, and ongoing support for all efforts toward this goal. There is some evidence that Indian adolescents are increasing their cigarette smoking behavior (Schinke, Moncher, Holden, Batvin, and Orandi, 1989). This trend must be monitored to ensure lung cancer rates remain low among Native American groups that currently have low rates.

The Plains and Woodland tribes use tobacco primarily for religious ceremonies. Health care professionals should be careful about how they discuss tobacco use with these groups, as it can be embarrassing for members of these tribes to be against cigarette smoking while at the same time buying it for ceremonial use. In fact, if tobacco use is restricted to ceremonial use it represents almost no health hazard.

Smokeshops located on tribal land do sell cigarettes. This tax-free product is a source of tribal income and could make smoking cessation efforts controversial.

Stomach and Colon Cancer

During this century, mortality rates from stomach cancer have decreased markedly in the United States for Caucasians but not to the same extent for Native Americans. Incidence and mortality rates for all Native American groups are still more than double the Caucasian population (Table 1-8). Five-year survival rates for this cancer are particularly poor among Native Americans (Table 1-11). Deaths from stomach cancer appear to be highest among the Navajo and the tribes of the Oklahoma service areas (Table 1-13).

Colon cancer death rates appear to vary among tribes according to data from the IHS for 1974 to 1976 (USDHHS, 1986). Researchers found Oklahoma tribes had the highest death rates and Southwestern tribes the lowest compared to rates for colon cancer in all Native Americans (Table 1-14). Dietary factors are believed to influence this difference. Compared to the Oklahoma tribes, Southwestern tribes consume large quantities of beans, a high fiber staple that may protect against colon cancer. After the Oklahoma tribes, Alaska Natives ap-

TABLE 1-13 Native American Deaths from Malignant Neoplasms by Sex for Each IHS Area (1986-1988)*

IHS Area	Lip, Oral Cavity, & Pharynx		Esophagus		Stomach	
	M	F	M	F	M	F
Tucson			1		3	2
Aberdeen	2		1	2	5	6
Bemidji	5	3	3	2	1	4
Albuquerque	3		1		8	4
Alaska	6		4	1	8	4
Billings		1	1		4	2
Oklahoma	10	4	5	1	15	10
Nashville	1		1			
Phoenix			2	1	4	5
California	1	1		1	6	2
Portland	2		1	3	8	3
Navajo	2	4	1		19	14

*Absolute frequencies reported.
From Indian Health Service, Office of Program Statistics: *Indian and Alaska Native Deaths by Cause* (recode 282) *Sex and Age for Each* IHS *Area*, Rockville, Md, 1990, Public Health Service. Contains no copyrighted material.

TABLE 1-14 Native American Deaths from Malignant Neoplasms by Sex for Each IHS Area (1986-1988)*

IHS Area	Colon & Rectum		Liver		Gallbladder	
	M	F	M	F	M	F
Tucson	1	1	2			4
Aberdeen	10	9	1	2	1	5
Bemidji	6	2	4	2		1
Albuquerque	3	6	5	1		1
Alaska	14	16	3	1	2	6
Billings	4	6	5	1		1
Oklahoma	36	31	6	8	6	6
Nashville	5	1	1	2		
Phoenix	2	10	2	5	5	5
California	5	8	3		1	2
Portland	11	6	1	1		1
Navajo	8	8	5	13	7	16

*Absolute frequencies reported.
From Indian Health Service, Office of Program Statistics: *Indian and Alaska Native Deaths by Cause* (recode 282) *Sex and Age for Each* IHS *Area*, Rockville, Md, 1990, Public Health Service. Contains no copyrighted material.

parently have the second highest death rates from colon cancer. Traditionally, their diet has not included large quantities of fiber.

Breast Cancer

Breast cancer incidence and mortality rates among Native American women are low (Tables 1-8 and 1-10). The age-adjusted breast cancer mortality rate per 100,000 Native American women over age 24 residing within IHS areas was 12.1 during the 10-year period between 1974 and 1983 (Funk, 1986). This was 58% less than the rate for all U.S. races in 1982, 28.6. Within every age cohort, the age-specific breast cancer mortality rate for Native Americans is less than for U.S. women overall. Factors associated with a decreased incidence of this cancer such as early age of first pregnancy, multiparity, and lower socioeconomic status are more common among Native Americans than among non-minority women in the United States (USDHHS, 1986).

Looking at the geographical breakdown by the IHS service areas for the period 1986 to 1988, the greatest number of deaths due to breast cancer occurred in the Oklahoma, Navajo, and Aberdeen areas (Table 1-15). The fewest occurred in the Tucson, Albuquerque, California, and Billings areas.

Some data indicate that Native American women present with more advanced tumor stage at diagnosis. Among residents of New Mexico, the incidence of remote metastases at diagnosis was 10.2% for Caucasians, 12.5% for Hispanics, and 25.8% for Native Americans (Black, Bordin, Varsa, and Herman, 1979).

TABLE 1-15 Native American Deaths from Malignant Neoplasms by Sex for Each IHS Area (1986-1988)*

IHS Area	Female Breast
Tucson	2
Aberdeen	16
Bemidji	8
Albuquerque	3
Alaska	9
Billings	4
Oklahoma	35
Nashville	8
Phoenix	8
California	3
Portland	6
Navajo	21

*Absolute frequencies reported.
From Indian Health Service, Office of Program Statistics: *Indian and Alaska Native Deaths by Cause (recode 282) Sex and Age for Each IHS Area*, Rockville, Md, 1990, Public Health Service. Contains no copyrighted material.

Funk (1986) has questioned the rationale of the ACS guidelines for the use of mammography for Native Americans. She suggests that in the face of decreasing breast cancer mortality rates among Native Americans the costs associated with potential radiation exposure, the morbidity from negative biopsies, the number of procedures, and the money spent for each breast cancer death prevented may not be justified.

Pancreatic Cancer

Generally, the incidence of pancreatic cancer among Native Americans is lower than that for all other races (Table 1-8). Survival rates are uniformly low for all races and ethnic groups. Among Native

Americans mortality rates are also low (Table 1-10) but deaths from this cancer do vary among IHS areas. Service areas with the highest frequency of pancreatic cancer deaths include Oklahoma, Navajo, Aberdeen, and Alaska (Table 1-12). Potential risk factors for cancer of the pancreas include tobacco and alcohol use and diet, possibly fats, oils, sugar, and animal protein (Boss, 1986).

Cervical Cancer

Data from the New Mexico Tumor Registry indicate that between 1969 and 1972 cervical cancer accounted for 16.3% of all female malignancies, making it the most common cancer among Native American women (Black, Key, Carmany, and Herman, 1977). Data from the SEER registry (Tables 1-8 and 1-9) indicate that Native Americans have excess incidence of and mortality from cancer of the cervix compared to other racial and cultural groups. Mortality figures for 1974 to 1976 from the IHS (Table 1-9) document that the rate of cervical cancer deaths among Native American women is 2.29 times greater than that for other U.S. groups. Early studies of age-specific incidence and mortality suggest this excess occurs primarily among older Native American women (Bivens and Fleetwood, 1968; Jordan, Munsick and Stone, 1969).

Cervical cancer mortality rates among specific Native American tribes have been investigated by three groups of researchers, Skubi (1988), Hall and Branstetter (1990), and Horner (1990). All found elevated cervical cancer mortality rates among Native American women of the Rosebud Sioux Reservation, Fort McDowell community of Arizona, and in North Carolina state. Skubi and Horner found the Native American women in their studies had infrequent and, in some cases, no history of Pap smear screening. Follow-up for abnormal results was found to be lacking. Barriers to screening and early treatment were attributed to poverty, significant unemployment, underfunded and overburdened health care services, the lack of local treatment for abnormal Pap smears (women had to travel 200 miles for cryotherapy), public use of the health care system for treatment of acute illness rather than preventive care, and belief that the test was unnecessary due to "good health."

Jordan and Key (1981) reported the results of cervical cytologic screening conducted between 1966 and 1975 for patients at IHS hospitals and clinics in New Mexico and the Arizona Navajo reservation. Subjects included Navajos, Apaches, and Pueblos. They found that the majority of in situ and invasive cervical cancers occurred in women over age 60. They also found that after age 30, the proportion of women in each age group who were screened declined steadily. The lack of screening in this population therefore, may have contributed to the increase in the incidence of cervical cancer. The researchers attributed infrequent screenings to follow-up problems, including the patients' failure to return for visits despite repeated letters and visits from health personnel, difficulty locating women on a 25,000 square-mile reservation, and relocation out of the state or region.

Cigarette smoking has been implicated as a risk factor for cervical cancer. In 1986, Boss noted that of the four IHS areas with the highest rates of lung cancer

(Aberdeen, Alaska, Bemidji, and Billings), three also had the highest rates of cervical cancer (Aberdeen, Alaska, and Billings). More recent data (Table 1-16) suggest the two IHS areas with the greatest number of cervical cancer deaths are Oklahoma and Navajo. Native Americans from the Oklahoma area are known to have high cigarette smoking rates (US-DHHS, 1986). Reasons for the elevated cervical cancer deaths for Navajo women are unclear. Access to care may be an important consideration given that over 45% of Navajo people live below the poverty level.

The Department of Health and Human Services recently developed a new classification system for reporting cervical and vaginal cytological diagnoses, called the Bethesda System (NCI Workshop, 1989). The Public Health Service has mandated that all public health agencies use this new system, which was designed to ensure uniform reporting of all cervical and vaginal cytology. The system is detailed in the box on pp. 40-41.

Liver Cancer

Between 1986 and 1988, liver cancer was the tenth leading cause of cancer-related deaths among the IHS area populations (Table 1-17). The incidence of primary hepatocellular carcinoma (HCC) is high among Alaska Native males and particularly high among Alaska Eskimo men compared to both Greenland/Canadian Eskimos and U.S. males (Lanier, McMahon, Alberts, Potter, and Heyward, 1987; Heyward, Lanier, Bender, Hardison, Dobson, McMahon, and Francis, 1981).

Chronic Hepatitis B Virus (HBV) infection appears to be the most important risk factor in these populations, but such infection is generally uncommon in other Native American populations. Alcoholic cirrhosis and the consumption of aflatoxin-contaminated foods do not appear to contribute to the liver cancer problem. Lanier and her colleagues (1987) concluded that among liver cancer patients: (1) there was a high male-female ratio (15:4), (2) there was a high proportion of young patients (nearly 50% were younger than 30 years), and (3) there were a disproportionate number of Eskimos (most were Yupik) compared to other Native American groups. The researchers also found familial and village clustering of these cancer cases.

TABLE 1-16 Native American Deaths from Malignant Neoplasms by Sex for Each IHS Area (1986-1988)*

IHS Area	Cervix	Uterus	Ovary
Tucson	1		
Aberdeen	3	6	4
Bemidji	4	1	4
Albuquerque	4		2
Alaska	5		5
Billings	8	1	3
Oklahoma	15	8	17
Nashville	5		1
Phoenix	7	2	8
California	3	3	6
Portland	8	2	8
Navajo	12	1	14

*Absolute frequencies reported.
From Indian Health Service, Office of Program Statistics: *Indian and Alaska Native Deaths by Cause* (recode 282) *Sex and Age for Each IHS Area*, Rockville, Md, 1990, Public Health Service. Contains no copyrighted material.

In a group of 11 Alaska Native HCC patients presenting symptoms included abdominal pain and tenderness (91%), swelling of the abdomen or an abdominal mass (50%), weight loss (45%), nausea (42%), vomiting (33%), weakness (33%), and jaundice (17%) (Lanier, et al., 1987). These researchers suggested that a screening program using alpha fetoprotein (AFP) analysis would detect most new tumors while they are still resectable, and could significantly reduce the number of deaths due to HCC. A comprehensive HBV vaccination program now being conducted for Alaska Natives has markedly reduced hepatitis B infection rates, which should eventually reduce rates of liver cancer (McMahon, et al., 1987).

Gallbladder Cancer

Gallbladder cancer, as well as gallbladder disease, is common among Native Americans. Data from the New Mexico Tumor Registry between 1969 and 1972 indicated that this cancer was the third most common malignancy in Native American women, accounting for 8.5% of all female Native American cancers (Black, Key, Carmany, and Herman, 1977). An excess of gallbladder disease was reported for Native Americans as early as 1947 and since then, excesses have been reported for the Chippewa, Sioux, Arapaho, Shoshone, Pima, Navajo, and Apache tribes (Morris, Buechley, Key, and Morgan, 1978). Black and his colleagues (1977) noted three important findings: (1) gallstones had been identified in 73% of Pima Indian women between the ages of 25 and 34; (2) gall-

TABLE 1-17 Native American Deaths from Malignant Neoplasms by Site: Ranking Comparison Combined Data for All IHS Areas from 1986-1988 to SEER Cancer Mortality Rates from 1978-1981*

Rank	IHS	SEER
1	Larynx, trachea, bronchus & lung, male	Lung, male
2	Colon & rectum	Prostate
3	Larynx, trachea, bronchus & lung, female	Colon & rectum and lung, female
4	Female breast	Female breast
5	Pancreas	Stomach
6	Prostate	Cervix
7	Leukemia	Pancreas
8	Kidney	Ovary
9	Cervix	Esophagus
10	Liver	Multiple myeloma
11	Ovary	Uterus
12	Gallbladder	Bladder
	Lip, oral cavity, & pharynx	
	Esophagus	
	Bladder	
	Thyroid	
	Melanoma	
	Hodgkin's disease	
	Testis	
	Eye	
	Penis & other male genital organs	
	Male breast	

*Absolute frequencies reported.
From Indian Health Service, Office of Program Statistics: *Indian and Alaska Native Deaths By Cause (recode 282) Sex and Age for Each IHS Area*, Rockville, Md, 1990, Public Health Service. Contains no copyrighted material.

THE 1988 BETHESDA SYSTEM FOR REPORTING CERVICAL/VAGINAL CYTOLOGICAL DIAGNOSES

STATEMENT ON SPECIMEN ADEQUACY

Satisfactory for interpretation
Less than optimal
Unsatisfactory
Explanation for less than optimal/ unsatisfactory specimen:
—Scant cellularity
—Poor fixation or preservation
—Presence of foreign material (eg., lubricant)
—Partially or completely obscuring inflammation
—Partially or completely obscuring blood
—Excessive cytolysis or autolysis
—No endocervical component in a premenopausal woman who has a cervix
—Non-representative of the anatomic site
—Other

GENERAL CATEGORIZATION

Within normal limits
Other:
　　See descriptive diagnosis
　　Further action recommended

DESCRIPTIVE DIAGNOSES
Infection
Fungal
　　Fungal organisms morphologically consistent with *Candida* species
　　Other
Bacterial
　　Microorganisms morphologically consistent with *Gardnerella* species

　　Microorganisms morphologically consistent with *Actinomyces* species
　　Cellular changes suggestive of *Chlamydia* species infection, subject to confirmatory studies
　　Other
Protozoan
　　Trichomonas vaginalis
　　Other
Viral
　　Cellular changes associated with cytomegalovirus
　　Cellular changes associated with herpesvirus simplex
　　Other
　　(Note: for human papillomavirus [HPV], refer to "Epithelial Cell Abnormalities, Squamous Cell")
　　Other
Reactive and reparative changes
Inflammation
　　Associated cellular changes
　　Follicular cervicitis
Miscellaneous (as related to patient history)
　　Effects of therapy
　　Ionizing radiation
　　Chemotherapy
　　Effects of mechanical devices (e.g., intrauterine contraceptive device)
　　Effects of nonsteroidal estrogen exposure (e.g., diethylstibestrol)
　　Other

THE 1988 BETHESDA SYSTEM FOR REPORTING CERVICAL/VAGINAL CYTOLOGICAL DIAGNOSES—cont'd

Epithelial cell abnormalities

Squamous Cell

- Atypical squamous cells of undetermined significance (recommended follow-up and/or type of further investigation: specify)
- Squamous intraepithelial lesion (SIL) (comment on presence of cellular changes associated with HPV if applicable)

    Low-grade squamous intraepithelial lesion, encompassing:

    Cellular changes associated with HPV

    Mild (slight) dysplasia/cervical intraepithelial neoplasia grade 1 (CIN 1)

    High-grade squamous intraepithelial lesion, encompassing:

    Moderate dysplasia/CIN 2

    Severe dysplasia/CIN 3

    Carcinoma in situ/CIN 3

- Squamous cell carcinoma

Glandular cell

- Presence of endometrial cells in one of the following circumstances:

    Out of phase in a menstruating woman

    In a postmenopausal woman

    No menstrual history available

- Atypical glandular cells of undetermined significance (recommended follow-up and/or type of further investigation: specify)

    Endometrial

    Endocervical

    Not otherwise specified

- Adenocarcinoma

    Specify probable site of origin: endocervical, endometrial, extrauterine

    Not otherwise specified

- Other epithelial malignant neoplasm: specify

Nonepithelial malignant neoplasm: specify hormonal evaluation (applies to vaginal smears only)

- Hormonal pattern compatible with age and history
- Hormonal pattern incompatible with age and history: specify
- Hormonal evaluation not possible

    Cervical specimen

    Inflammation

    Insufficient patient history

Other

From The 1988 Bethesda System—NCI Workshop, JAMA 262(7).

stones were prevalent throughout the tribes of the Southwest; and (3) gallstones were common in the Chippewa, Sioux, Arapaho, and Shoshone tribes from Minnesota, the Dakotas, and Wyoming. Alaska Natives, in particular women, have been reported to have an increased incidence of gallbladder cancer (Boss, Lanier, Dohan, and Bender, 1970).

Between 1974 and 1976 mortality rates from gallbladder cancer among Native Americans were 4.35 times that expected for non-minorities (Table 1-10). Indians of the Southwest were found to experience 6.36 times and Oklahoma Indians 2.27 times the mortality rate of non-minorities (USDHHS, 1989).

The reason for high rates of gallbladder disease and gallbladder cancer in Native Americans is unknown, but diet and genetic factors have been implicated. Indian diets differ substantially from the typical American diet; however, they also differ substantially among tribes. Gallbladder cancer is also strongly associated with obesity, adult-onset diabetes mellitus, and gallbladder disease; the presence of cholesterol gallstones, in particular, has been implicated as a causative factor (Weiss, Ferrell, Hanis, and Styne, 1984).

The USDHHS suggests that gallbladder cancer and disease are probably linked to genetics (1989). Rates of gallbladder cancer for Hispanic Americans with some Native American heritage are midway between those for Native Americans and those for whites (Schottenfeld and Fraumeni, 1982) suggesting support for a genetic predisposition. Weiss and his colleagues (1984) discuss how the "thrifty gene" theory might explain the high incidence of gallbladder cancer in Native Americans.

Gallbladder disease is probably a result of acculturation to nonaboriginal environments, because the genetic basis of the diseases as they now manifest would have had to rise in frequency in the face of some negative selection. It is possible, considering the nature of the relationship among obesity, parity, puberty, and the initial development of gallstones, that today's susceptibility reflects genes positively selected for the efficient utilization and storage of nutrients by females. In aboriginal times, especially in the climate of the Bering land bridge, food supplies may have been unpredictable and a fertility and lactation advantage would accrue to females with such genes. Males also could have benefited from such genes (p. 1271).

In a study of patients with gallbladder cancers, Black, et al. (1977) noted that pain was the most common symptom (82%), followed by jaundice (58%), and weight loss (29%); and 15% had a palpable mass. The duration of symptoms was less than 1 month in 20 patients, 1 to 3 months in 18 and had existed for more than 3 months in seven.

Patients with this tumor have a poor prognosis. Less than 10% of patients are alive 5 years after diagnosis (Weiss, et al., 1984). Practical preventive measures for cancer of the gallbladder do not currently exist, although early detection of gallstones by ultrasonography may at least indicate those who would be at risk (Weiss, et al., 1984). Lowenfels, Lindstrom, Conway and Hastings (1985) estimate that 4% to 5% of young Indian women with silent gallstones, might eventually develop gallbladder cancer.

Nasopharyngeal Cancer

All three Alaska Native ethnic groups face an increased risk of nasopharyngeal carcinoma. Relative risks for male Eskimos, Aleuts, and Alaskan Natives are 20, 31, and 6, respectively, and for female Eskimos and Alaska Natives are 30 and 11 (Lanier, Bender, Talbot, Wilmeth, Tschopp, Henle, Henle, Ritter, and Terasaki, 1980). The Southwestern Native Americans, to whom some groups of Alaska Natives are related, have increased risks for nasal and sinus cancers but not nasopharyngeal cancer (Creagan and Fraumeni, 1972). Potential risk factors for nasopharyngeal cancer include the Epstein-Barr virus, inhaled substances such as tobacco, and consumption of salt fish as part of the childhood diet.

Other Cancers

Recent studies of Native American men from eight tribes living in North Carolina and of Alaska Natives other than Aleuts or Eskimos have documented elevated mortality from prostate cancer and cancers of the male genitalia (Creagan Fraumeni, 1972; Blot, Lanier, Fraumeni, Bender, 1974; Lanier, 1977, Bender, Blot, Fraumeni, 1982, Horner, 1990). In addition, from 1986 to 1988, 124 deaths due to prostate, testicular, and male genital cancers occurred among Native American men utilizing the IHS (Table 1-18). Dietary fat intake has been linked to cancers of the prostate; however, few studies have been conducted on the diets of these tribes.

In a study of the occurrence of retinoblastoma in Navajo children from July, 1966 to May, 1981, Berkow and Fleshman (1983) found 2.5 to three times the expected incidence of the disease. Most cases were unilateral with no family history of the disease. Since only 8,000 Navajos existed in the mid-1800s, the increased incidence of retinoblastoma in this study could be most easily explained by the limited gene pool from which these children came. According to one hypothesis, if a limited gene pool is present and the gene for the mutation that causes retinoblastoma is present in that pool, then descendants of the original population will have increased expression of the mutation (Knudson, Heth-

TABLE 1-18 Native American Deaths from Malignant Neoplasms by Sex for Each IHS Area (1986-1988)*

IHS Area	Prostate	Testis	Penis & Other Male Genital Organs
Tucson	2		1
Aberdeen	13		
Bemidji	8		
Albuquerque	12	1	
Alaska	7		
Billings	11	1	
Oklahoma	22		
Nashville	4		
Phoenix	9		
California	6		
Portland	9		
Navajo	15	3	

*Absolute frequencies reported.
From Indian Health Service, Office of Program Statistics: *Indian and Alaska Native Deaths By Cause* (recode 282) *Sex and Age for Each IHS Area*, Rockville, Md, 1990, Public Health Service. Contains no copyrighted material.

cote, and Brown [1975] cited in Berkow and Fleshman, 1983).

Melanoma is rare among Native Americans; however, it does occur and its anatomic distribution differs from that commonly associated with Caucasians. Black and Wiggins (1985) reviewed 18 cases of melanoma in Native Americans. Nine cases involved subungual areas (the sole or palm); three involved the mucous membranes (anal and nasal mucosa); two were ocular melanomas; three were skin melanomas (calf, cheek, thigh); and one was of unknown primary. Researchers could not link any lifestyle factors, including sun exposure, to these cases and there were no unusual occupational patterns, exposures to carcinogens, or evidence of a familial melanoma history. No information was available on the prevalence of atypical or dysplastic nevi within the Native American population. However, the researchers did note that 15 of the 18 patients were Navajo. Careful skin examinations clearly are indicated for the Navajo population, including education on changes in moles.

Cancer of the esophagus among Native Americans is generally rare; however, reports do suggest an elevated risk and incidence among Alaskan Natives who speak Inupiag, Yupik and Sugpiag (Lanier, Kilkenny, Wilson, 1985). Regular oral examinations for Inupiag, Yupik, and Sugpiag speaking Alaska Natives would therefore be prudent.

Oral Cancers and Smokeless Tobacco Products

The prolonged use of smokeless tobacco (ST) has been associated with oral cancer among African Americans (Winn, Blot, Shy, Pickle, Toledo, and Fraumeni, 1981) but such an association has not yet been confirmed among Native Americans. However more and more young Native Americans have begun using ST and snuff in the past two decades: the prevalence of ST use by Native American adolescents has varied from 18.4% to 42.6% in boys and from 2.7% to 34% in girls (Wolfe and Carlos, 1987; Centers for Disease Control, 1987; Centers for Disease Control, 1989).

Wolfe and Carlos (1987) also reported on the oral health effects of ST use in Navajo children. In their study of 226 adolescents aged 14 to 19, 64.2% used ST (75.4% boys and 49% girls); 62.1% of ST users consumed alcohol (generally on less than one occasion per week but taking three or more drinks on each occasion); and over half (54%) smoked, usually 1 to 5 cigarettes per week. Twenty five percent of all the ST users demonstrated evidence of leukoplakia on oral examination; the prevalence of leukoplakia was highest among subjects who used both ST and alcohol, at 36%. In a study of ST use in the Northern Plains region, Centers for Disease Control (CDC) officials found there was a higher overall prevalence of ST use among Native American adolescents than among teens of other ethnic origins; Native Americans began to use ST at a younger age than other ethnic groups; and the prevalence of ST use among adolescent Native American boys and girls was about equal (Centers for Disease Control, 1989).

To address the problem of ST and snuff use by Native Americans, the CDC suggested the IHS and tribal outreach programs should: (1) educate youth, school administrators, and parents about the adverse health effects of ST use; (2) advocate to restrict the sale and distribution of ST to children; (3) implement tobacco use cessation programs; (4) screen and monitor for adverse health effects; and (5) conduct further research to explain the high prevalence of ST.

CULTURALLY SENSITIVE RISK ASSESSMENT AND CANCER CARE FOR NATIVE AMERICANS

Adequate cancer risk assessment should include a comprehensive history of personal, family, lifestyle and occupational factors and, age- and gender-specific screening examinations. To conduct a successful and comprehensive risk assessment of the Native American client, the health care worker must also remain attentive to the cultural beliefs and values of the individual.

Variations in the incidence of specific cancers between different Native Americans is at least partially due to the diversity of their customs and the degree to which they have adopted Western culture. Health care providers working with Native Americans must have a sound understanding of the cancer rates for each tribe or IHS area (Table 1-19) with which they are working because rates may vary significantly throughout the United States. For this reason, care providers should not rely too heavily on aggregate data (e.g., national SEER data) for accurate cancer incidence and mortality rates for Native Americans, particularly when planning cancer prevention and early detection efforts (Hampton, 1989).

With this in mind, health care professionals can tailor intervention programs to the needs and the customs of different Native American groups. As a beginning, Hammond (1989) has revised the American Cancer Society's seven warning signals for the detection of cancer to reflect certain tribal and regional risks (see box).

Native American cancer incidence and mortality rates should be interpreted within a socioeconomic perspective. Many Native Americans are economically disadvantaged and therefore subject to poor living conditions, nutritional problems, and limited access to care. In addition, Western health care interventions for the disadvantaged are frequently cri-

---

CANCER'S SEVEN WARNING SIGNALS

1. Unusual vaginal bleeding or discharge (all Native Americans).
2. Indigestion or difficulty swallowing (Southwestern tribes and Eskimos).
3. Nagging cough or hoarseness (All Native Americans).
4. Change in bowel or bladder habits (Southwestern tribes and Eskimos).
5. A sore that does not heal (all Native Americans).
6. Thickening or lump in the breast or elsewhere (all Native Americans).
7. Obvious change in wart or mole (more in Caucasians but may occur in Native Americans)

TABLE 1-19   Cancers for Which Specific Tribes Have Higher Cancer Incidence

Tribe	Cancer(s)	Known or Suspected Risk Factors	Recommended Intervention
Alaskan natives			
Men	Lung	Cigarette smoking	Smoking cessation
	Nasopharyngeal		Regular head & neck exams
Men & women	Gallbladder	Diet and genetics	Screen for gallbladder disease; identify high-risk persons
Eskimo men & women	Liver	Chronic HBV infection	HBV vaccination
			AFP screening
	Renal cell		
	Thyroid		
	Colorectal	High fat diet	Annual digital rectal exam; annual hemocult; sigmoidoscopy.
Navajo			
Children	Retinoblastomas	Genetics	
Men & women	Melanoma	Unknown—perhaps sun	Skin exams, note palms and soles especially; educate about mole changes.
	Gallbladder	Diet and genetics	Screen for gallbladder disease; Identify high-risk persons
Men	Lung	Uranium mining	Occupational history
Pueblo			
Men & women	Mesothelioma	Silver jewelry making; ceremonial whitening of leggings with asbestos	Occupational history
Chippewa, Sioux, Arapaho Shoshone, Pima, Apache	Gallbladder	Diet; genetics	Screen for gallbladder disease; identify high-risk persons

sis oriented, focusing primarily on the presenting complaint.

Epidemiology experts from the IHS's Aberdeen area office have developed, tested, and implemented a health risk appraisal instrument for use with all Native American populations (Welty, 1988). This instrument (Figure 1-11) is now available on an IBM-PC compatible software program that uses an optical scanner to automatically read and enter the data. The program can be used in tribal and IHS outpatient, inpatient, and employee health settings; for community surveys; and to track health promotion and disease prevention objectives. For more information contact:

Thomas Welty, MD, MPH
Aberdeen Area Epidemiology Program
3200 Canyon Lake Drive
Rapid City, SD 57702
(605) 348-1900 Ext. 401

Interacting with Native Americans

Nurses of Native American heritage who have had extensive experience with patients from a number of tribes outlined the following guidelines for culturally sensitive history taking and physical examination (Frank-Stromborg and Olsen, 1988). When first entering the Native American patient's hospital room or the clinic examination room, the health care practitioner (HCP) can honor and show respect for the patient by knocking on the door before entering. If possible, care providers should introduce themselves in the native language of the patient and offer a handshake. However, it is important to remember that some Native Americans consider a firm handshake to be a sign of aggression. A good rule of thumb is to return what you are given. Introduce yourself in a manner that establishes your connectedness to the tribe. If Native American, this would include identifying who your mother, grandmother or father was. Care providers from other ethnic groups should take the time to explain how the agency they work for relates to the tribe.

The HCP should maintain a facial expression that is attentive, concerned and caring. Smiling and eye contact may be appropriate, but remember that some Native Americans feel that exposing the teeth or prolonged, direct eye contact are signs of aggression (Antle, 1987). At all times, the practitioner should be respectful, gentle, and unhurried; excessive familiarity may be suspect.

Care providers should also be attentive to the way they approach and speak to Native American patients: good body language is open without closing or crossing the arms, loud speech may be considered rude or angry, and speaking slowly may be interpreted as a sign of a condescending attitude. To enhance rapport and understanding, the care provider could ask what the native word for "_____" (e.g., pain, trouble breathing, blood, etc.) is and then use it during the examination.

One can initiate the visit with casual conversation about family, social functions, or about the tribe they are from. Because many Native Americans are very private people, it is important that the HCP gradually ease into discussions about personal and family health. One should never use first person language when discussing risk factors with a Native American patient, such as "If you don't stop smoking you will get cancer." This may be viewed as putting a hex on the individual. Some traditional patients believe use of first person language involves one's spirit and may cause them to get cancer. In addition, some native patients believe it is improper to talk with someone other than a family member about their breasts, testicles, examining their own body, or uterine bleeding.

1. Your Age. **2.** Your Height. **3.** Your Weight.

(If you don't know your height and weight, please ask someone to weigh and measure you.)

1. AGE	2. HEIGHT	3. WEIGHT
YEARS	FEET / INCHES	POUNDS

4. Sex. — 4. ☐ Male ☐ Female

5. Have you ever been told that you have diabetes (or sugar diabetes)? — 5. ☐ Yes ☐ No

6. Did your mother, father, brothers or sisters ever have diabetes or sugar diabetes? — 6. ☐ Yes ☐ No

7. Are you now taking medicine for high blood pressure? — 7. ☐ Yes ☐ No

8. CIGARETTE SMOKING
How would you describe your cigarette smoking habits? — 8. ☐ Never Smoked (Skip to Question 11.) ☐ I smoke now ☐ I have quit

9. IF YOU SMOKE CIGARETTES NOW:
How many cigarettes a day do you smoke?

10. IF YOU'VE QUIT:
a. How many years has it been since you smoked cigarettes fairly regularly?
b. What was the average number of cigarettes you smoked per day?

If your answer is less than 10, place the number in the second column.

9. NUMBER	10a. YEARS	10b. AVERAGE

11. How many cigars do you usually smoke per day? — 11.

12. How many pipes of tobacco do you usually smoke per day? — 12.

13. How many times per day do you usually use smokeless tobacco? (Chewing tobacco, snuff pouches, etc.) — 13.

14a. In the next year how many thousands of miles will you travel by car, truck (TRK) or van?

14b. In the past year did you ride on a motorcycle, all terrain vehicle (ATV) or snowmobile (SNB)?

14c. In the next 12 months how many thousands of miles will you travel by motorcycle, ATV or SNB?

NOTE: U.S. average for cars is 10,000 miles.
Questions 14a. and 14c. - If your answer is less than "10" place the number in the second column. If you travel between 1 and 1000 miles, enter "1".

14a CAR/TRK/VAN MILES	14b MOTORCYCLE ATV, SNB IN PAST YEAR	14c CYCLE, ATV SNB MILES
000	☐ Yes ☐ No	.000

15. On a typical day how do you usually travel? (Mark only one) — 15.
☐ Walk ☐ Small car ☐ Bus
☐ Bicycle ☐ Large car ☐ Boat
☐ Motorcycle/Snowmobile ☐ Truck/Van ☐ I Don't

16. How often do you usually buckle your safety belt when traveling by car or truck? — 16.
☐ 0-19% Rarely ☐ 40-59% Half ☐ 80-100% Almost always
☐ 20-39% Now and then ☐ 60-79% Usually

17. On the average, how close to the speed limit do you usually drive? (MPH = miles per hour) — 17.
☐ 0-5 MPH Over ☐ 11-15 MPH Over
☐ 6-10 MPH Over ☐ More than 15 MPH Over

18. How many times in the last month did you drive or ride in a vehicle or boat when the driver had perhaps too much alcohol to drink?
NOTE: If you have not drunk alcohol in the last year, fill in "0" for questions 18-21.

19. How many drinks of alcoholic beverages do you have in a typical week? (1 drink = a can or bottle of beer, a small glass of wine or a shot of hard liquor)

20. On how many days in a typical month do you have at least one drink?

21. On the days when you drank any liquor, beer or wine, about how many drinks did you have on the average?

If your answer is less than 10, place the number in the second column.

18. Drink & Drive - per month	19. Drinks per Week	20. Days per month Drink	21. Drinks per Day

22. How many times during the past month did you have 5 or more drinks on an occasion? — 22.
☐ 0 times ☐ 2-4 times
☐ 1 time ☐ 5 or more times

Figure 1-11 Health risk appraisal for Native Americans.

(From Indian Health Service: *The Groundswell Project, health promotion training for leaders of Indian communities,* Bethesda, Md, 1989, PHS, USDHHS.)

23	[ ] Never □ Yes, but not recently □ Yes, within last 2 months	23. Have you seriously considered suicide?
24	□ Less than 1 Year □ 2 Years □ Never □ 1 Year □ 3 or More Years	24. About how long has it been since you had a rectal exam?
25	□ 0 Times per Week □ 1-2 Times per Week □ 3 or More Times per Week	25. How often do you get physical exercise like running, dancing, bicycling, vigorous walking or active sports?
26	□ Brush & Floss daily □ Less than once a day □ Brush daily □ Never/No teeth	26. How often do you brush or floss your teeth?
27	□ None □ 5-10 Cups □ 1-4 Cups □ 10 or more Cups	27. How many cups of caffeinated beverages (ie., coffee, tea) do you drink per day?
28	American Indian / Alaska Native □ Full Blood □ Less Than 1/4 Blood □ 1/4-7/8 Blood □ Non-Indian	28. ETHNIC BACKGROUND. Mark the most appropriate category.
29	□ Grade School or Less □ Some College □ Some High School □ College Graduate □ High School Graduate □ Post-Grad or Professional Degree	29. EDUCATION. What is the highest grade you completed in school?
30	□ Employed-Full time □ Retired □ Employed-Part time □ Student □ Homemaker □ Unemployed ⟨ 6 mos. □ Unemployed ⟩ 6 mos.	30. EMPLOYMENT. What is your employment status? (Mark only one) ⟨ 6 mos. = Less than 6 months ⟩ 6 mos. = 6 months or more

WOMEN ONLY	Questions 31-40: WOMEN ONLY
31. □□ □□ □□ □□ □□ □□ □□ □□ □□ □□ □□ □□ □□ □□ □□	31. At what age did you have your first menstrual period?
32 □ No Children □ 20-24 Yrs. □ 30 Yrs. or Over □ Less than 20 Yrs. □ 25-29 Yrs.	32. How old were you when your first child was born?
33 □ Less Than 1 Year □ 2 Years □ Never □ 1 Year □ 3 or More Years	33. How long has it been since your last breast X-ray (Mammogram)?
34 □ None □ 2 or More □ 1 □ Don't Know	34. How many women in your natural family (mother and sisters only) have had breast cancer?
35 □ Yes □ No	35. Have you had a hysterectomy operation? (Removal of your uterus.)
36 □ Less Than 1 Year □ 2 Years □ Never □ 1 Year □ 3 or More Years	36. How long has it been since you had a pap smear for cancer?
37 □ Monthly □ Rarely or Never □ Every Few Months	37. How often do you examine your breasts for lumps?
38 □ Less Than 1 Year □ 2 Years □ Never □ 1 Year □ 3 or More Years	38. About how long has it been since you had your breasts examined by a physician or nurse?
39 □□ □□ □□ □□ □□ □□ □□ □□ □□ □□	39. How many times have you been pregnant? (Include live births, miscarriages, abortions, and stillborns.)
40. □ Yes □ No	40. Are you now or do you think you might be pregnant?

Question 41-44 should be completed with the help of a Health Professional.

41. B.P.-SYSTOLIC	42. B.P.-DIASTOLIC	43. TOTAL CHOL.	41. Blood Pressure (Systolic)	42. Blood Pressure (Diastolic)	43. Total Cholesterol (mg/dl)

44. GLUCOSE	45. Participant ID or SSN Number	44. Random Glucose (mg/dl)	45. Participant ID or Social Security Number (SSN)

Figure 1-11, cont'd   For legend see opposite page.

Some Native Americans will not speak of the dead. To obtain information about family history, phrase the question in a way that does not refer directly to a deceased relative such as "has anyone in your family ever had . . .?"

If appropriate, HCPs may wish to consider offering food during appointments. Some Native Americans refer to this as "the give away," a celebratory experience, that meets basic needs and shows welcome, concern, caring, friendship, and neighborliness. Offering food is a tangible expression of the link in a relationship; it also serves as a memory— you will always remember the person.

To determine the extent to which a patient uses traditional medicines, simply ask: "How much of your traditional tribal ways do you still practice?" Even patients who reside in urban areas may believe that "for every natural disease, the earth provides a cure." Many Native Americans keep roots in their house that they chew on to alleviate pain, clear their mind, or treat a toothache.

The health care provider may observe a variety of things that indicate the Native American patient has visited or been visited by a traditional healer: medicine bundles or small jars of medicinal solutions; reddish, grey or blackish marks on patients' skin; the smell of smoke, perhaps from burnt cedar, sage, or grasses, whatever is appropriate to the tribe; or shells, seeds, beads, or arrowhead bracelets. These items should never be removed from the patient without his or her express consent.

Because a traditional healer automatically knows what to do without having

to ask a lot of questions, some traditional Native Americans will think that the Western care provider's method of assessing a patient by intensive questioning means the provider does not know what he or she is doing.

Health care workers should try to make maximal use of the time they spend with Native American patients by weaving cancer prevention and screening efforts into each medical visit. In addition, a sound understanding of the Native American patient's health beliefs and practices, and customs, attitudes, and values can enable the health care practitioner to creatively integrate cancer prevention and screening practices within the context of day-to-day health care. For example, IHS clinics throughout the United States have instituted a comprehensive care paradigm called the Industrial Strength Triage (IST) Program in which specifically trained nurses have been successful in expediting patient care, improving recognition of health care needs beyond the presenting complaint, and improving patient follow-up (Shorr and Daniels, 1987).

Until programs similar to this become the standard, health care workers can identify alternative ways to integrate comprehensive care. For example, checkups for healthy babies can include discussions with mothers on the importance of teaching their young sons testicular self-examination. Age-appropriate adult cancer screening examinations can be discussed during medical visits for colds, broken bones, and other minor health problems. Appointments should be made on the spot and include arrangements for form of payment and transportation to the clinic.

Discussions of the relationship between diet and cancer prevention can be easily integrated into counseling sessions on diabetes or cardiovascular health, as many of the recommendations are similar. By discussing weight loss within the context of eating high-fiber traditional foods and following the Native American tradition of physical fitness and exercise, health care workers can revitalize cultural values and limit risk factors for disease while operating within the Native American concept of maintaining harmony between body, mind, and spirit.

PHYSICAL EXAMINATIONS AND PATIENT EDUCATION

Native American patients may be very modest, so during physical examination the health care worker should avoid exposing any more of the patient's body than is necessary. The examiner should ask the patient's permission to perform the examination. It also may be helpful to show exactly what the procedure will entail, explain how the procedure relates to the patient's health complaint, and explain what the patient can do to make the examination go easier.

Lung Assessment

During auscultation of the lungs, it may be helpful for the health care worker to explain how to take deep breaths. Female patients should always be provided with adequate draping for privacy. When listening to the front of a woman's chest, special attention should be given to adequate draping. Following the examina-

tion, the care provider should tell the patient what was heard, relating the findings to the patient's history and what will be done in the future.

Colorectal Examination

If possible, an examiner of the same gender as the patient should conduct digital rectal examinations, colonoscopys, and sigmoidoscopys. When questioning the patient about the nature of his or her stools, the care provider should remember that the patient may not look at his or her stool at home and so cannot relay information about its color or character. Also, when stool samples must be collected the nature of the patient's plumbing facilities should be considered: some reservations still primarily have outhouses, so procedures may need to be modified.

The Breast Examination

When conducting a breast examination never expose both of the patient's breasts. The examiner should explain normal, unusual, and abnormal features of the breast to the Native American patient. A female health care worker should always be present during breast examinations by a male practitioner.

Traditional Apache women wear a lot of layers of clothing. Often several pairs of underwear and multiple slips (half and whole slips). Advise Apache women that they do not need to remove all their clothing for a breast examination—just the top garments. Some Indian women are strict Mormons and will not remove the T–shirt-like undergarment, known as "the Garment." Breast examinations can be done over the garment or with only one arm taken out of the garment at a time. Some Native American women will cover their eyes, their mouth, or part of their face during a breast examination.

Gynecological Examination

Before a gynecological exam it is important for care providers to explain why the exam is necessary and what it will entail. Proper draping is especially important. Some Native American women will prefer that the exam be conducted by a female practitioner. During the gynecological examination the Native American patient may even want to hold the hand of the examiner or an assistant. Talking during the examination can help relieve tension.

Health care workers may want to use the gynecological exam as an opportunity to educate women about their bodies, even situating the drapes so the patient can watch the exam. The examiner should make positive comments about findings that are normal. Some tribes have taboos about the use of mirrors, so the health care worker may not want to use them to teach vulvar self-examination or identify parts of the anatomy. Alaskan women are very interested in looking at "where the baby comes from."

Pueblo women wear a wide band around their waist that acts somewhat as a girdle. If it doesn't interfere with the examination, it should be left alone. Apache women should be told exactly what clothing they need to remove during this examination; the gynecological examination can be done with multiple slips in place.

Examinations on Men and Young Boys

Native American men usually visit health care facilities only when they are very sick, so health care workers may want to talk to spouses about testicular, prostate, and colorectal examinations and provide them with culturally sensitive brochures to give to their husbands or male children. However, this should not be done without careful investigation of local customs, because such discussions may be taboo among certain tribes. The establishment of a men's clinic 1 day or night a week may be useful for some native men. Care providers may want to provide instructions on testicular self-examination when they teach new mothers about the care of their newborn boys and the importance of pulling back the foreskin for cleanliness.

Female practitioners should not perform a prostate assessment on an elderly or traditional Native American man. If there is no other option, she should not look directly into the patient's eyes. Native American men, like most men, fear an erection during the examination.

Skin Examination

During skin examinations, care providers should avoid exposing more of the body than is necessary, especially with older patients. The examiner should never ask about numbers tattooed on the body (a common practice in some tribes).

Patient Education

Some Native Americans may find it embarrassing to have anatomically correct models or pictures openly displayed in public areas and will cover their eyes or face as they walk past these displays. Such materials are best kept for private, one-on-one discussions. In addition, these patients may not accept group educational sessions. It is important to note that most IHS agencies cannot afford and therefore do not have access to breast, testicular, and other practice models.

One participant at the Native American Workshop (Frank-Stromborg and Olsen, 1988) suggested that Native American women be encouraged to keep pamphlets on breast self-examination with their menstrual pads as a reminder of when to do BSE.

The following general guidelines have been suggested when developing educational materials for Native Americans (Frank-Stromborg and Olsen, 1988):

1. Materials should be geared toward clients with elementary school education.
2. Materials should be primarily pictorial (color would be preferred), should feature Native Americans and should be simple.
3. When using educational materials, explain anatomy and physiology in culturally specific lay terms; present the patient with choices and leave control with them.
4. Always involve Native Americans in the planning and development of educational materials. Ask what they want, what they need, what they understand about the issue, and how they would like the materials presented.

When teaching self-examination techniques and performing physical examinations, Native American care providers must assess their own value systems. Many Native American practitioners have expressed concern that they feel as if they are invading the privacy of their patients when doing intimate physical examinations. According to one Indian nurse: "It's hard to ask about sexuality, to do breast examinations, or other intimate examinations. I need to put aside my own Indian values."

To be effective care givers and educators, health professionals must consider health in terms that are familiar to the Native American: as a state in which the body, mind, and spirit are in balance.

REFERENCES

1. American Cancer Society: *Minority facts and figures*, New York, 1986, American Cancer Society.
2. American Indian Health Care Association: Native Americans suffer from lactose intolerance, *Native Newsbriefs*, Winter 1992.
3. Antle A: Ethnic perspectives of cancer nursing: The American Indian, *Oncology Nursing Forum* 14(3):70-73, 1987.
4. Baquet CR, Ringen K: *Cancer among blacks and other minorities: Statistical profiles.* Bethesda, Md, 1986, National Cancer Institute, p 27.
5. Berkow RL, Fleshman JK: Retinoblastoma in Navajo Indian children, *American Journal of Diseases in Children* 137:137-138, 1983.
6. Bivens MD, Fleetwood HO: A ten-year survey of cervical carcinoma in Indians of the Southwest, *Obstetrics and Gynecology* 32(1):11-16, 1968.
7. Black WC, Bordin GM, Varsa EW, Herman D: Histologic comparison of mammary carcinomas among a population of Southwestern American Indian, Spanish American, and Anglo women, *American Journal of Clinical Pathology* 71(2):142-145, 1979.
8. Black WC, Key CR, Carmany TB, Herman D: Carcinoma of the gallbladder in a population of Southwest American Indians, *Cancer* 39:1267-1379, 1977.
9. Black WC, Wiggins C: Melanoma among Southwestern American Indians. *Cancer* 55(12):2899-2905, 1985.

10. Blot WJ, Lanier A, Fraumeni JF, Bender TR: Cancer mortality among Alaskan natives, 1960-1969, *Journal of the National Cancer Institute* 55(3):547-554, 1975.

11. Boss LP: *Closing the gap: Malignant neoplasms,* Unpublished document/draft, 1986.

12. Boss LP, Lanier AP, Dohan PH, Bender TR: Cancer of the gallbladder and biliary tract in Alaskan Natives: 1970-1979, *Journal of the National Cancer Institute* 69(5):1005-1007, 1982.

13. Butler C, Samet JM, Black WC, Key CR, Kutvirt, DM: Histopathologic findings of lung cancer in Navajo men: Relationship to uranium mining, *Health Physics* 51(3):365-368, 1986.

14. Cannelos JH: *Alaska native elders project on suicide prevention,* 1986, Alaska Native Health Board.

15. Centers for Disease Control: Smokeless tobacco use in rural Alaska, *Journal of the American Medical Association* 257(14):1861-1862, 1987.

16. Center for Disease Control: Prevalence of oral lesions and smokeless tobacco use in Northern Plains Indians, *Journal of the American Medical Association* 261(1):25-26, 1989.

17. Cooke P: Destroyer and healer, can the white man's medicine save Indian lives without killing Indian culture? In *Health* (vol 2), 65-76, 1990.

18. Creagan ET, Fraumeni JF: Cancer mortality among American Indians, *Journal of the National Cancer Institute* 49:959-967, 1972.

19. Department of Health and Human Services: *Report of the secretary's task force on black and minority health: Cancer,* vol 3, Washington DC, 1986, U.S. Government Printing Office.

20. Department of Health and Human Services: *Report of the secretary's task force on black and minority health: Cancer,* vol 3, Washington DC, 1989, U.S. Government Printing Office.

21. Department of Health and Human Services: *Healthy People 2000, National Health Promotion and Disease Prevention Objectives,* Washington DC, 1991, U.S. Government Printing Office.

22. Department of Health and Human Services: *Healthy People 2000, National Health Promotion and Disease Prevention objective,* Washington DC, 1991, U.S. Government Printing Office.

23. Driscoll RJ, Mulligan WJ, Schultz D, Candelaria A: Malignant mesothelioma, a cluster in Native American Pueblo, *New England Journal of Medicine* 318(22):1437-1438, 1988.

24. Emery G. Trail still tearful for Indian tribes, *Insight* 2(35):8-21, 1986.

25. Frank-Stromborg M, Olsen SJ: Focus group interview data, National cancer prevention and screening workshops for minority nurses. Native American workshop, 1988. Unpublished report.

26. Funk K: Breast cancer mortality and the use of mammography within the IHS, *The Provider* 11(6):136-139, 1986.

27. Hall P, Branstetter E: Pap smear examinations among Fort McDowell Indian women. *Communicating Nursing Research* 23:256, 1990.

28. Hampton JW: *The heterogeneity of cancer in Native American populations.* In Jones, A, editor: *Minorities and cancer,* New York, 1989, Springer-Verlag, 45-53.

29. Haraldson SSR: Health and health services among the Navajo Indians. *Journal of Community Health* 13(3):129-142, 1988.

30. Hardesty G: *Physician combines Indian and western medicine, Indian healers focus on spirit.* 1985. University of California at Irvine, College of Medicine.

31. Heyward WL, Lanier AP, Bender TR, Hardeson HH, Dobson PH, McMahon BJ, Francis DP: Primary hepatocellular carcinoma in Alaskan Natives, 1969-1979. *International Journal of Cancer* 28:47-50 1981.

32. Horner RD: Cancer mortality in Native Americans in North Carolina, *American Journal of Public Health* 80(8):940-944, 1990.

33. Indian Health Service: *Indian Health Service chart series book,* Washington, DC, 1988, US Department of Health and Human Services.

34. Indian Health Service: *The Groundswell Project, health promotion training for leaders of Indian communities,* Rockville, Md, Washington, DC, 1989, U.S. Department of Health and Human Services

35. Indian Health Service: *Trends in Indian health,* Rockville, Md, 1989, U.S. Department of Health and Human Services.

36. Indian Health Service Office of Planning, Evaluation and Legislation, Division of Program Statistics: *Regional differences in Indian health,* 1990a, U.S. Department of Health and Human Services.

37. Indian Health Service, Office of Planning, Evaluation and Legislation, Division of Program Statistics: *Trends in Indian health care, 1990,* Rockville, Md, 1990b, U.S. Department of Health and Human Services.

38. Indian Health Service, Office of Program Statistics: *Indian and Alaska Native deaths by cause (recode 282) sex and age for each IHS area.* Rockville, Md, 1990. U.S. Department of Health and Human Services.

39. Indian Health Service: *Years of productive life lost for preventable causes of death. American Indians and Alaska Natives residing in the IHS service area, 1982-1984 to 1985-1987, compared to the U.S. all races, 1986,* Rockville, MD, 1991, U.S. Department of Health and Human Services.

40. Joe JR, Miller D: *American Indian cultural perspectives on disability* (Native American Research and Training Center, Monograph Series), Tucson (No date given). University of Arizona.

41. Joe JR, Miller D, Narum T: *Traditional Indian alliance: Delivery of health care services to American Indians in Tucson* (Native American Research and Training Center, Monograph Series), Tucson, 1988. University of Arizona.

42. Jordan SW, Key, CR: Carcinoma of the cervix in Southwestern American Indians: Result of a cytologic detection program, *Cancer* 47(10):2523-2532, 1981.

43. Jordan SW, Munsick RA, Stone RS: Carcinoma of the cervix in American Indian women. *Cancer* 23(5):1227-1232, 1969.

44. Justice JW: *Contrasting cancer patterns in two American Indian tribes* (Native American Research and Training Center, Monograph Series), Tucson, University of Arizona.

45. Kniep-Hardy M, Burkhardt MA: Nursing the Navajo, *American Journal of Nursing* 95-96, 1977.

46. Lammers PK: How they view you, themselves, and disease, *AORN* 45(5):1211-1216, 1987.

47. Lanier A: Survey of cancer incidence in Alaskan natives. *NCI Monographs* 47:87-88, 1977.

48. Lanier AP, Bender TR, Blot WJ, Fraumeni JF: Cancer in Alaskan natives, 1974-1978, *NCI Monographs* 62:79-81 1982.

49. Lanier AP, Bender TR, Talbot M, Wilmeth S, Tschopp C, Henle W, Henle G, Ritter D, Tarasaki P: Nasopharyngeal carcinoma in Alaskan Eskimos, Indians and Aleutes: A review of cases and study of Epstein-Barr virus, HLA, and environmental risk factors, *Cancer* 46:2100-2106, 1980.

50. Lanier AP, Kilkenny SJ, Wilson JF: Oesophageal cancer among Alaskan Natives, 1955-1981, *International Journal of Epidemiology* 14(1):75-78, 1985.

51. Lanier AP, McMahon BJ, Alberts SR, Popper H, Heyward WL: Primary liver cancer in Alaskan natives, 1980-1985, *Cancer* 60(8):1915-1920, 1987.

52. Locust CS: *American Indian beliefs concerning health and unwellness* (Native American Research and Training Center, Monograph Series), Tucson, 1985. University of Arizona.

53. Locust CS: *Apache beliefs about unwellness and handicaps* (Native American Research and Training Center, Monograph Series), Tucson, 1986. University of Arizona.

54. Locust CS: *Hopi beliefs about unwellness and handicaps,* (Native American Research and Training Center, Monograph Series), Tucson, 1987, University of Arizona.

55. Locust CS: *Yaqui Indian beliefs about health and handicaps* (Native American Research and Training Center, Monograph Series), Tucson, 1987b, University of Arizona.

56. Lowenfels AB, Lindstrom CG, Conway MJ, Hastings PR: Gallstones and risk of gallbladder cancer. *Journal of the National Cancer Institute* 75(1):77-80, 1985.

57. McMahon BJ, Rhoades ER, Hegward WL, Tower E, Ritter D, Lanier AP, Wainwright RB, Helminiak C: A comprehensive programme to reduce the incidence of hepatitis B virus infection and its sequelae in Alaskan Natives, *Lancet* 1134-1136, 1987.

58. Morris DL, Buechley RW, Key CR, Morgan MV: Gallbladder disease and gallbladder cancer among American Indians in tricultural New Mexico, *Cancer* 42(5):2472-2477, 1978.

59. National Cancer Institute Workshop: The 1988 Bethesda System for reporting cervical/vaginal cytological diagnoses, *Journal of the American Medical Association* 262(7):931-934, 1989.

60. Oncology Nursing Society/National Cancer Institute: Cancer Prevention and Screening Workshops for Minority Nurses. Native American Workshop, 1988. Unpublished report.

61. Newell GR Screening: potential for cancer prevention, *Biomedicine and Pharmacotherapy* 42(7):435-437, 1988.

62. Norrell-Kahn BC: Methods come from Navajos: At long last, modern medicine is catching up with traditions. *Times Today,* 17, January 1985.

63. Pathak DR, Samet JM, Howard CA, Key CR: Malignant melanoma of the skin in New Mexico, 1969-1977, *Cancer* 50(7):1440-1446, 1982.

64. Rhoades ER, Hammond J, Welty TK, Handler AO, Amler RW: The Indian burden of illness and future health interventions. *Public Health Reports* 102:361-368, 1987.

65. Samet JM, Key CR, Kutvirt DM, Wiggins CL: Respiratory disease mortality in New Mexico's American Indians and Hispanics, *American Journal of Public Health* 70:492-497, 1984.

66. Schinke SP, Moncher MS, Holden GW, Batvin GJ, Orandi MA: American Indian youth and substance abuse: Tobacco use problems, risk factors, and preventive interventions, *Health Education Research* 4(1):137-144, 1989.

67. Schottenfeld D, Fraumeni JF: *Cancer epidemiology and prevention,* Philadelphia, 1982. WB Saunders Co.

68. Shorr G, Daniels S: *Improving outpatient care with concurrent visit planning: The case for industrial strength triage,* Unpublished manuscript, 1987.

69. Sievers ML, Fisher JR: Cancer in North American Indians: Environment versus heredity [Editorial], *American Journal of Public Health* 73:485-487, 1983.

70. Skubi D: Pap smear screening and cervical pathology in an American Indian population, *Journal of Nurse Midwifery* 33(5):203-207, 1988.

71. Sobralske MC: Perceptions of health: Navajo Indians, *Topics in Clinical Nursing* 7(3):32-39, 1985.

72. The Council. (1981). Do's and don'ts of village travel. *Tanana Chiefs Conference, Inc.,* (pp. 1-2).

73. Vital Statistics. (1990) The health of America's native tribes. *The Washington Post,* p. 4.

74. Vobejda (1991). *The Washington Post.* A4.

75. Wayne P: Recovering spiritual reality in Native American traditions, *Women of Power* 8:68-70, 1988.

76. Weiss KM, Ferrell RE, Hanis CL, Styne PN: Genetics and epidemiology of gallbladder disease in new world native peoples, *American Journal of Human Genetics* 36:1259-1278, 1984.

77. Welty TK: Indian-specific health risk appraisal being developed, *The IHS Primary Care Provider* 13(7):136-138, 1988.

78. Welty TK: Cancer and cancer prevention and control programs in the Aberdeen Area Indian Health Service. Paper presented at the First National Cancer Conference on Native Americans, Tucson, October, 1989.

79. Welty TK: Health implications of obesity in Native Americans (Prepublication draft), *American Journal of Clinical Nutrition,* (in press).

80. Welty TK, Tanaka ES, Leonard B, Rhoades ER, Hurlburt WB, Fairbanks ML: Indian Health Service facilities become smoke-free, *Morbidity Mortality Weekly Report* 36(22):348-350, 1987.

81. Winn DM, Blot WJ, Shy CM, Pickle LW, Toledo A, Fraumeni JF Jr: Snuff dipping and oral cancer among women in the Southwestern United States. *New England Journal of Medicine* 305:745-749, 1981.

82. Wolfe MD, Carlos JP: Oral health effects of smokeless tobacco use in Navajo Indian adolescents, *Community Dentistry and Oral Epidemiology* 15:230-235, 1987.

83. Yuki T: Cultural responsiveness and social work practice: An Indian clinic's success, *Health and Social Work* 11(3):223-229, 1986.

Healthy People 2000 Objectives Targeting Native Americans

OBJECTIVES TARGETING AMERICAN INDIANS AND ALASKA NATIVES

2.3d* Reduce overweight to a prevalence of no more than 30 percent among American Indians and Alaska Natives. (Baseline: An estimated 29-75 percent for different tribes in 1984-88)

Note: For people aged 20 and older, overweight is defined as body mass index (BMI) equal to or greater than 27.8 for men and 27.3 for women. For adolescents, overweight is defined as BMI equal to or greater than 23.0 for males aged 12 through 14, 24.3 for males aged 15 through 17, 25.8 for males aged 18 through 19, 23.4 for females aged 12 through 14, 24.8 for females aged 15 through 17, and 25.7 for females aged 18 through 19. The values for adolescents are the age- and gender-specific 85th percentile values of the 1976-80 National Health and Nutrition Examination Survey (NHANES II), corrected for sample variation. BMI is calculated by dividing weight in kilograms by the square of height in meters. The cut points used to define overweight approximate the 120 percent of desirable body weight definition used in the 1990 objectives.

2.10d Reduce the prevalence of anemia to less than 10 percent among Alaska native children aged 1 through 5. (Baseline: 22-28 percent in 1983-85)

Note: Iron deficiency is defined as having abnormal results for 2 or more of the following tests: mean corpuscular volume, erythrocyte protoporphyrin, and transferring saturation. Anemia is used as an index of iron deficiency. Anemia among Alaska Native children was defined as hemoglobin <11 gm/dL or hematocrit <34 percent. For pregnant women in the third trimester, anemia was defined according to CDC criteria. The above prevalences of iron deficiency and anemia may be due to inadequate dietary iron intakes or to inflammatory conditions and infections. For anemia, genetics may also be a factor.

3.4f* Reduce cigarette smoking to a prevalence of no more than 20 percent among American Indians and Alaska Natives. (Baseline: An estimated 42-70 percent for different tribes in 1979-87)

Note: A cigarette smoker is a person who has smoked at least 100 cigarettes and currently smokes cigarettes.

3.9a Reduce smokeless tobacco use by American Indian and Alaska Native youth to a prevalence of no more than 10 percent. (Baseline: 18-64 percent in 1987)

Note: For males aged 12 through 17, a smokeless tobacco user is someone who has used snuff or chewing tobacco in the preceding month. For males aged 18 through 24, a smokeless tobacco user is someone who has used either snuff or chewing tobacco at least 20 times and who currently uses snuff or chewing tobacco.

4.1a Reduce deaths among American Indian and Alaska Native men caused by alcohol-related motor vehicle crashes to no more than 44.8 per 100,000 American Indian and Alaska Native men. (Age-adjusted baseline: 52.2 per 100,000 in 1987)

4.2b Reduce cirrhosis deaths among American Indians and Alaska Natives to no more than 13 per 100,000 American Indians and Alaska Natives. (Age-adjusted baseline: 25.9 per 100,000 in 1987)

6.1d* Reduce suicides among American Indian and Alaska Native men in Reservation States to no more than 12.8 per 100,000 American Indian and Alaska Native men. (Age-adjusted baseline: 15 per 100,000 in 1987)

7.1f Reduce homicides among American Indians and Alaska Natives in Reservation States to no more than 11.3 per 100,000 American Indians and Alaska Natives. (Age-adjusted baseline: 14.1 per 100,000 in 1987.)

8.11 Increase to at least 50 percent the proportion of counties that have established culturally and linguistically appropriate community health promotion programs for ra-

cial and ethnic minority populations. (Baseline data available in 1992)

Note: This objective will be tracked in counties in which a racial or ethnic group constitutes more than 10 percent of the population.

9.1a Reduce deaths among American Indians and Alaska Natives caused by unintentional injuries to no more than 66.1 per 100,000 American Indians and Alaska Natives. (Age-adjusted baseline: 82.6 per 100,000 in 1987)

9.3d Reduce deaths among American Indians and Alaska Natives caused by motor vehicle crashes to no more than 39.2 per 100,000 American Indians and Alaska Natives. (Age-adjusted baseline: 46.8 per 100,000 in 1987)

13.1b Reduce dental caries (cavities) so that the proportion of American Indians and Alaska Native children aged 6 through 8 with one or more caries (in permanent or primary teeth) is no more than 45 percent. (Baseline: 92 percent in primary teeth and 52 percent in permanent teeth in 1983-84)

13.1d Reduce dental caries (cavities) so that the proportion of American Indian and Alaska Native adolescents aged 15 with one or more caries (in permanent or primary teeth) is no more than 70 percent. (Baseline: 93 percent in permanent teeth in 1983-84)

13.2b Reduce untreated dental caries so that the proportion of American Indian and Alaska Native children with untreated caries (in permanent or primary teeth) is no more than 35 percent among children aged 6 through 8 and no more than 40 percent among adolescents aged 15. (Baseline: 64 percent of American Indian and Alaska Native children aged 6 through 8 in 1983-84; 84 percent of American Indian and Alaska Native adolescents aged 15 in 1983-84)

13.5b Reduce the prevalence of gingivitis among American Indians and Alaska Natives aged 35 through 44 to no more than 50 percent. (Baseline: 95 percent in 1983-84)

13.11b Increase to at least 65 percent the proportion of American Indian and Alaska Native parents and caregivers who use feeding practices that prevent baby bottle tooth decay. (Baseline data available in 1991.)

14.1b Reduce the infant mortality rate among American Indians and Alaska Natives to no more than 8.5 per 1,000 live births. (Baseline: 12.5 per 1,000 live births in 1984)

14.1i Reduce the postneonatal mortality rate among American Indians and Alaska Natives to no more than 4 per 1,000 live births. (Baseline: 6.5 per 1,000 live births in 1984)
Note: Infant mortality is deaths of infants under 1 year; neonatal mortality is deaths of infants under 28 days; and postneonatal mortality is deaths of infants aged 28 days up to 1 year.

14.4a Reduce the incidence of fetal alcohol syndrome among American Indians and Alaska Natives to no more than 2 per 1,000 live births.

(Baseline: 4 per 1,000 live births in 1987)

14.9d* Increase to at least 75 percent the proportion of American Indian and Alaska Native mothers who breastfeed their babies in the early postpartum period, and to at least 50 percent the proportion who continue breastfeeding until their babies are 5 to 6 months old. (Baseline: 47 percent at discharge from birth site and 28 percent at 5 to 6 months in 1988)

14.11b Increase to at least 90 percent the proportion of pregnant American Indian and Alaskan Native women who receive prenatal care in the first trimester of pregnancy. (Baseline: 60.2 percent of live births in 1987)

17.2b Reduce to no more than 11 percent the proportion of American Indians and Alaska Natives who experience a limitation in major activity due to chronic conditions. (Baseline: 13.4 percent in 1983-85)
Note: Major activity refers to the usual activity for one's age-gender group whether it is working, keeping house, going to school, or living independently. Chronic conditions are defined as conditions that either (1) were first noticed 3 or more months ago, or (2) belong to a group of conditions such as heart disease and diabetes, which are considered chronic regardless of when they began.

17.9b Reduce diabetes-related deaths among American Indians and Alaska Natives to no more than 48 per 100,000 American Indians and Alaska Natives. (Age-adjusted baseline: 54 per 100,000 in 1986)

Note: Diabetes-related deaths refer to deaths from diabetes as an underlying or contributing cause.

17.10b Reduce end-stage renal disease due to diabetes among American Indians and Alaska Natives with diabetes to no more than 1.9 per 1,000 American Indians and Alaska Natives with diabetes. (Baseline: 2.1 per 1,000 in 1983-86)

Note: End-stage renal disease (ESRD) is defined as requiring maintenance dialysis or transplantation and is limited to ESRD due to diabetes. Blindness refers to blindness due to diabetic eye disease.

17.11a Reduce diabetes among American Indians and Alaska Natives to a prevalence of no more than 62 per 1,000 American Indians and Alaska Natives. (Baseline: 69 per 1,000 aged 15 and older in 1987)

20.3g* Reduce hepatitis B (HBV) among Alaska Natives to no more than 1 case. (Baseline: An estimated 15 cases in 1987)

20.4d Reduce tuberculosis among American Indians and Alaska Natives to an incidence of no more than 5 cases per 100,000 American Indians and Alaska Natives. (Baseline: 18.1 per 100,000 in 1988)

20.7a Reduce bacterial meningitis among Alaska Natives to no more than 8 cases per 100,000 Alaska Natives. (Baseline: 33 per 100,000 in 1987)

21.2k Increase to at least 70 percent the proportion of American Indians and Alaska Natives who have received, as a minimum within the appropriate interval, all of the screening and immunization services and at least one of the counseling services appropriate for their age and gender as recommended by the U.S. Preventive Services Task Force. (Baseline data available in 1991)

21.8 Increase the proportion of all degrees in the health professions and allied and associated health profession fields awarded to members of underrepresented racial and ethnic minority groups as follows:

1985-1986 Baseline   2000 Target
American Indians and Alaska Natives   0.3%   0.6%

Note: Underrepresented minorities are those groups consistently below parity in most health profession schools—blacks, Hispanics, and American Indians and Alaska Natives.

22.4 Develop and implement a national process to identify significant gaps in the nation's disease prevention and health promotion data, including data for racial and ethnic minorities, people with low incomes, and people with disabilities, and establish mechanisms to meet these needs. (Baseline: No such process exists in 1990)

Note: Disease prevention and health promotion data includes disease status, risk factors, and services receipt data. Public health problems include such issue areas as HIV infection, domestic violence, mental health, environmental health, occupational health, and disabling conditions.

From DHHS: *Healthy People 2000, National Health Promotion and Disease Prevention Objectives,* Washington, D.C., 1991, US Government Printing Office, pp 602-604.

Hopi Health Beliefs

THE HOPI PEOPLE AND THEIR WAY

There are over 30 groups of people collectively called "Hopi" who live on the reservation of the same name in Northern Arizona. The Hopi have existed as a distinct tribe for over 2000 years. Although their beliefs and values are similar, they may vary from village to village on the reservation. In the past, the Hopi were famous for their runners, who had a great deal of stamina and endurance in long-distance races.

In recent years, some of the Hopi people have been greatly affected by Western influences. However, Hopi ceremonies, taboos, and tribal teachings have not been lost. Deep spiritual ideals and values have endured as strong, reliable guides for living and dying.

The word Hopi refers to living positively; the "Hopi Way" is living in harmony. Kachinas, benevolent spirit helpers, teach peace and goodness of heart and guide daily life. The proper living of one's life, the doing of good, enables one to remain strong so as to resist any negative forces (death, disease, disability, disharmony, unwellness).

Members of the tribe who are unwell or unhappy are taught to examine their thoughts and actions to determine where they may have failed in the Hopi Way. Transgressions against the Hopi Way cause natural unwellness and witchcraft can cause unnatural unwellness. Transgressions that lead to natural unwellness include breaking such taboos as marrying one's kin, breaking a Kachina taboo, mistreating an animal, marital unfaithfulness, or quarreling. Witchcraft, the evil use of power, can cause sudden illness, misfortune, unusual happenings, or chaotic emotions.

HOPI MEDICINE PEOPLE

The Hopi tend to use both Western physicians and traditional healers. The Hopi medicine system has specialists who may concentrate on broken bones, internal medicine, obstetrics, or other areas of medicine. "Seers" are tribal visionaries; some may just do divining, while others may be able to both "see" the problem and cure it. According to one Hopi man,

There are those who only work with herbs, [and] there are others who are like chiropractors. There are many more in different sodalities [religious groups, i.e., the Antelope sodality] who, by reason of their particular powers—spiritual powers—claim within that sodality that they can do certain kinds of curing by laying on of hands and such things, or by doing a ritual around a patient [like members of the Ghost clan who can cure ghost sickness]. And there is the practitioner who, like a shaman, does magic things, taking out objects from the body. There are those practitioners who are counselors, who just talk, so you have all these different kinds of practitioners. (Locust, 1987a, p. 33)

From Locust C: *Hopi Beliefs About Wellness and Handicaps*, Native American Research and Training Center. Tucson, Az. 1987a, The University of Arizona.

Yaqui Health Beliefs

THE YAQUI PEOPLE

The Yaqui have their roots in Mexico, having only crossed the border into the U.S. in 1887 to escape persecution. As a result, their modern culture has been greatly influenced by Mexican culture. The Yaqui were originally Sun worshippers, but were influenced in the 1600s by the Jesuit priests and have incorporated many Christian concepts and symbols into their belief system.

There are three major Yaqui villages in the Tucson, AZ area: Old Pascua, Barrio Libre, and New Pascua. Other villages can be found throughout Arizona, California, and New Mexico. The Yaqui were recognized as a sovereign Indian Nation of the United States in 1978. Today, most Yaquis speak Spanish as their first language and English as their second language. Locust (1987b) describes the Yaqui people as "fiercely independent, hard working, dedicated to their Old Way, and wary of all interference from 'outsiders'. . . they tend to work at unskilled or semiskilled jobs or depend on government assistance . . . the Pascua Yaqui Tribe had an unemployment rate of 73% in 1981, and a median family income of $7,000" (p. 5).

YAQUI BELIEFS ABOUT HEALTH

Yaquis, according to Locust (1987b), believe in the power of personal and family energy to affect a cure or illness. To the Yaqui, a person who has a need, whether financial, personal, spiritual, or medical, is assisted by family members to meet that need. When a Yaqui experiences illness or spiritual weakness he or she can be sustained by the energy of his or her relatives. Relatives can transfer their energy by touching, verbal and nonverbal communication, staying in close proximity to the ill person, or placing sacred objects near or on the patient. In this culture, traditional Western medical approaches may endanger a Yaqui patient by limiting visitor numbers and visiting time (extended kin can be as important as immediate family in recovery) and by requiring the removal of all articles of clothing and personal belongings. For these reasons, Yaquis may be suspicious of Western medical approaches.

Yaqui women have important taboos regarding modesty. Females are not permitted to expose intimate body parts for extended periods of time. According to Locust (1987b), "hospital personnel who do not understand this moral taboo often insist that female patients remove their undergarments for the duration of their hospital stay. Asking a Yaqui female to break a moral taboo in favor of hospital regulations is placing her in jeopardy, and frequently a confrontation will result. Most Yaqui women will refuse to violate this taboo" (p. 9).

Locust (1987b) also notes that most traditional Yaquis are unaware of the association between primary disease and secondary complications that could develop from that disease. In the case of diabetes, she found that:

Although the people were aware of the secondary complications stemming from diabetes (retinopathy, renal problems, cardiovascular problems, etc.), they were unsure about the relationship and did not seem convinced that there really was a correlation between diabetes and secondary complications. Decubital ulcers, amputations, and visual failures were attributed to taboo breaking . . . or witchcraft (pp. 38-39).

YAQUI BELIEFS ABOUT UNWELLNESS AND HANDICAPS

The Yaqui people view the handicapped simply as physically incomplete; spiritually, however, the handicapped are perceived as perfect. Illnesses and handicaps are caused by natural processes—such as lunar and solar eclipses, intra-clan marriages, and the violation of religious, cultural, or social taboos—and unnatural processes, such as witchcraft.

The Yaqui believe that lunar eclipses contribute to birth deformities, especially missing limbs because the force that "eats" the moon also eats an unborn child's limb. Women protect themselves from this destructive force by wearing dark garments and metal objects such as crosses, keys, and safety pins. Marrying within the clan has been associated with having handicapped children. To avoid intermarriage, each Yaqui household maintains a *Book of the Dead* that contains several hundred names of adult dead and deceased children. Families consult this book when boys and girls show interest in each other to see if any relationship between the two families exists.

Deliberately violating cultural, social, and religious vows can lead to long term illnesses such as diabetes and stroke. The Yaqui consider such vows so important that they may quit their job if it interferes with their ability to adequately perform duties associated with these vows. Locust (1987b) described the belief that breaking a religious or ceremonial vow could contribute to cancer development.

One young Yaqui explained a rather complicated event in which he felt a woman's death was directly related to her breaking her vows. The woman, a grandmother, had always been active in the church and in religious ceremonies, but she began attending another church and left the Old Way. "She did not believe anymore," he said. "That same year she started to get sick. She got more sick, and they found she had cancer. She died recently. . . . She died because she broke her vow to the church" (p. 24).

Dishonoring a handicapped person by staring, laughing, quarreling, or acting any way that would dishonor the handicapped individual would risk bringing the same handicap on oneself or a family member. Finally, the Yaquis have a very strong taboo against handling sacred objects. For instance, touching or seeing sacred masks can risk unwellness.

Witchcraft is the primary unnatural cause of unwellness; it can contribute to headaches, ulcers, leg pains, sudden attacks of dizziness, going "crazy," and bad luck. It can also cause death. Yaquis believe that to protect themselves from witchcraft, they must keep their "energy" strong. They may also keep the "ojo de venado," a large seed resembling a deer's eye, wrapped and carried on their body to ward off evil. Abalone shell, a medicine bag, a rosary, or an object made from horse hair may also serve this function.

From Locust C: *Yaqui Indian Beliefs About Health and Handicaps*, Native American Research and Training Center. Tucson, Az, 1987b, The University of Arizona.

APPENDIX 4

Apache Health Beliefs

The Apache tribe is a coalition of several bands of Apache: the Coyotero, Pinal, Tonto, and Warm Springs Chiricahua. Traditional Apache families were extended and matrilineal, moving, foraging, raiding, and warring. When confined to reservations in the 1900s, their traditional way of life broke down and many adopted Western ways. Many held witchcraft responsible for the social disruption.

The Apache language, Southern Athabaskan, is related linguistically to Navajo, Chippewa, and Alaskan native languages. Today most of the young speak English, although many adults do not. Cattle raising is one of the more lucrative industries on the reservation; Apache women are noted for their fine bead work and basketry. Many reservation homes still have outhouses; most have running water but not all is drinkable. Apaches still do much of their cooking outside on a wood fire or inside on a wood stove. Locust (1986) notes that today, more young people receive an extensive education and more are returning to the reservation and to traditional ways. She believes that "the future of the tribe is strong with the promise of progress, prosperity, and achievement of its goals without the loss of cultural heritage" (p 3). However, she notes that conflict between the "Old Way" and "New Way" still causes concern:

A lot of the young people today are facing conflict in the culture. It seems as if the parents and older ones still believe the Old Way and some of the younger ones have fragments of the old . . . in the modern educational process, students will be asked to do something that is considered taboo in the Old Way (like dissecting a frog), which they cannot do because their early training teaches them that if you do it, bad things will happen. They have that bit of information, what to do and not do, and the consequences of their choice, and it is in conflict with educational policies of today. Yet, they do not have a firm basis in the Old Way to explain it to the teachers what they feel and why. This conflict, that of the Old Way and New Way, causes problems at school, at home, and in the social life of the students (pp. 4-5).

The usefulness of Western medicine is well recognized by the Apache and they generally "show little reluctance to bring the sick to the attention of medical doctors. But they also recognize that the Western physician is deficient in such critical areas as the discovery of disease causes and the bestowal of 'protection' against the recurrences of these causes. Such critical matters require Apache ceremonials and medicine people," (p. 11).

THE APACHE MEDICINE MEN AND THE CONCEPT OF POWER

The Apache concepts of health and unwellness are closely linked with their beliefs about the powers held by all natural objects. Flora, fauna, celestial objects, water, clouds, lightning, and to some extent, all things have power. Power is bestowed by the creator or "Giver-of-Life" and is attracted and manipulated, with respect, through ritual. Power can cause good or evil to occur, can lead to wellness and strength, and can cause death.

The medicine man or woman or shaman serves as a mediator between supernatural power and the individual. The shaman uses an important and strong power, called "word power," telepathically to influence the environment or persons around him. Witches both male or female control the dark side of power. They can make people ill or crazy, or they can kill them. Cibeque Apaches have characterized the differences between medicine men and witches in this way:

(1) Medicine men conduct ceremonials and use their power in public. Witches do not conduct ceremonies, and they use their power in private. (2) The medicine men employ chants to control their power. Witches do not; they resort to other techniques. (3) Medicine men make sand paintings; witches do not. (4) Medicine men use their power to diagnose and cure illnesses. Witches do neither; they use their power to perpetrate sickness, death, and certain forms of insanity (Locust, 1986, p. 11).

CAUSES OF UNWELLNESS

The Apache believe witchcraft and the violation of taboos are the two major causes of illnesses. Taboos concern power (for example, lightning), some animals (for example, birds of prey, foxes, coyotes, wolves, snakes; bears are viewed as the embodiment of evil but they might also be a reincarnated relative); plants, foods (especially during pregnancy), tribal customs (marriage within the clan, mutilation, quarreling), and religion. Violations against these can lead to stomach ailments, arthritis, weakness, lethargy, headache, pain, blindness, deafness, Down's syndrome.

There are many types of witchcraft including love witching, hate, revenge, jealousy, ghost sickness, and lightning-power. Illnesses that can be caused by witchcraft include physical and mental disorders, accidents, sudden illness and/or pain, psychosis, emotional problems, depression or suicide, sleeplessness, and fear. Locust (1986) noted that to avoid being witched, the Apache must:

live in harmony with his family, relatives, neighbors, and tribal members. He must be willing to share what he has, to help when asked, to provide transportation when needed, and to fulfill his obligations as required by his position in his clan and his wife's clan. In doing so he becomes well thought of by those around him, and therefore no one would have reason to harm him. By observing all the taboos of his culture, he avoids the consequences of violating some 'power' and can keep his family and himself free from disharmony (p. 30).

From Locust C: *Apache beliefs about unwellness and handicaps,* Native American Research and Training Center, Tucson, Az, 1986, The University of Arizona.

Pima-Maricopa Health Beliefs

THE PEOPLE

The Salt River Pima-Maricopa Indian Community is located on 52,000 acres in Maricopa County, Arizona, immediately adjacent to Scottsdale, Mesa, and the Phoenix metropolitan area. The majority of its citizens are employed in the adjacent metropolitan area (50.8%), or in the government (34.1%), reservation commercial and industrial enterprises (9.0%), and agriculture (6.1%) (Arizona Department of Commerce, 1978).

The Papagos of southern Arizona and the Opatas, now of northern Sonora, Mexico, are related to the Pimas. The Pimas and the Papagos were deadly enemies of the Apache, who often raided their villages.

Traditionally, the Pima people have survived in one of the more inhospitable desert regions of the United States. They developed irrigated farming techniques, with each community digging and maintaining irrigation canals. The Maricopas joined with the Pimas early in the nineteenth century. Although they had different languages, they intermarried and today have the same general habits and customs. The original Pima/Maricopa reservation was created in 1859 and covered 100 square miles. As farmers, their main crops were corn, beans, squash, and melons. They also raised cotton, which the men wove for clothing. In dry seasons when irrigated crops failed, they turned to natural resources and hunted deer, rats, antelope, and jackrabbit.

Wheat has traditionally been the main staple in the Pima diet. It was ground to make tortillas, or a very heavy bread baked in ashes. Pancakes were also made from this flour. The pancakes were eaten dipped in saguaro fruit syrup. The whole grain is mixed with tapari beans and boiled into a delicious dish. Wheat was roasted in live coals and ground into pinole which was mixed with water and was drunk. The pinole could be mixed to any consistency. It was kept in a can and used for a snack at any time. When used for the main meal, it was thickly mixed and eaten with jerky or cholla (cactus) buds. Some parched wheat in a clay pot, ground it and used it in the same manner. It was a thirst quencher when mixed very thin.

The women of the tribe are basket makers. Art experts consider Pima baskets among the finest in quality and design.

In the past, members of a village interacted like an extended family. When a member of the village was ill, neighbors, friends, and relatives supported the sick person and family by donating food, taking care of the patient, and running errands for the family. The dead are buried with their belongings, water and food, and their best walking sandals. This is done to prepare the deceased for the journey to the "land of the rising Sun," where friends and relatives await his or her arrival.

Claire Seota explains that today's Pima/Maricopa Indians are different:

We are surrounded by cities today and no matter which way you go there are houses crowded together, cars going in every direction, the air loaded with smelly pollution. Food stores that are a necessity today are stocked with instant foods which we use, and more numerous are the descendants of the people who invaded our country years ago [the white man]. Today we could care less what is happening to our neighbors, relatives and friends because we are so busy rushing around selfishly doing for ourselves. The Pimas no longer take pride in helping each other as the early Pimas did before the white eyes told us what was good for us, taking away what was sacred. Telling us our way of life is inferior. The religion of nature is all but forgotten. That the Earth is our Mother, that we are made from her, that to her bosom we will return when our life is over, that she will embrace us as she did over our life time by providing us a place to live, bring forth food to feed us. That the Sun is our father, giving us warmth and guiding us from overhead. That all living creatures are our brothers and sisters and these creatures sacrifice their lives that we might have food.

One nurse who works regularly with the Pima Maricopa Indian of Salt River noted that:

My people are very urban, they do not seem to have ceremonies. They are quite assimilated into the dominant society. Many work outside the reservation. We do not have healing or medicine men as a cushion to fall back on. We rely on allopathic or western medicine. However, I do recall a 30 year old Pima Maricopa woman who first went to a western doctor for healing. When she did not get better, she ultimately sought help from a medicine man (Frank-Stromborg and Olsen, 1988).

From White TB: History of Creating the Salt River Reservation 1879, *Salt River Pima-Maricopa Indian Community Paper*, Special Centennial Edition, June 14, 1979.

Alaskan Native Health Beliefs

THE PEOPLE

The native population of Alaska composes 16% of the total Alaskan population and is divided into three distinct groups: Eskimos, Aleuts, and other American natives (Lanier, McMahon, Alberts, Popper, and Heyward, 1987; Boss, Lanier, Dohan, Bender, 1982). Eskimos are 53% of the native population. On the basis of linguistic studies, two types of Eskimos are recognized: Yup'ik-speaking Eskimos (52% of all Eskimos), who live in Southwestern Alaska, and Inupiat-speaking Eskimos (36%), who live in Northwestern Alaska and across the Canadian Arctic as far east as Greenland. Linguistic studies indicate that Aleuts and Eskimos are related and that Aleuts are most like Yup'ik-speaking Eskimos. Aleuts constitute 13% of the Alaska native population; most live on the Alaskan peninsula and the Aleutian Island chain.

The other Native American groups in Alaska account for 34% of the native population. Just over half are from the Tlingit, Haida, and Tsimshian tribes of southeastern Alaska. These tribes are also found in Canada and the northwestern United States. Athabaskans, who live mainly in the interior of Alaska, make up slightly less than half of this group and appear to be linguistically related to the Navajo and Apache tribes of the southwestern United States. Approximately half of the Alaskan native population lives in urban areas and the other half lives in more remote villages.

CUSTOMS, HEALTH BELIEFS, AND PRACTICES

Wilma Manual, RN, MN, a certified family nurse practitioner and Public Health Nurse III with the Alaska Native Health Board has worked among the Aleuts (Athabaskan Indians in the Iliamna area, south of Anchorage) and the Yup'ik Eskimos in the Yukon-Kuskokwin area. She shared a few of her observations regarding the health beliefs and practices of Alaska Natives garnered over 15 years of work with them (personal communication, February 4, 1990):

About the People

One cannot assume that generalities fit all areas of Alaskan culture. It is a big place and cultural groups vary. What may be true in one village may not be true in a neighboring village.

Elders are highly regarded by most villagers and children are highly valued.

Villagers are pleased to have you visit their home and share their food (or coffee or tea). Most are very courteous and generous with whatever they have and expect the health care practitioner to be the same.

Most of my clientele welcome a comforting touch, including hugs, hand holding, and kissing, especially during periods of stress or after a long absence.

Health Beliefs and Practices

Traditional medicines are still used but 'clinic' medicines are also respected.

Many Native women are uncomfortable with male examiners and prefer female examiners.

They are not uncomfortable undressing before a female practitioner as it is their custom to share saunas with other nude females.

Avoidance of eye contact has never been noted among my clientele although some authors have suggested that prolonged eye contact is considered extremely rude among some indigenous cultures of Alaska. Some health professionals have even noted that some of the Yup'ik Eskimo tend to hold eye contact longer than is comfortable for the professional.

'Our time' (that of the Western world) is not 'theirs'. This is changing somewhat, but weather conditions, home, and family may interfere and time schedules are usually not adhered to. The appointment system is gradually becoming accepted.

The health care provider has a special place in the culture, even if he or she is 'gussak' (white). Care providers have the respect of the Alaska Native patient until they do something to destroy that respect.

Many people say the health care provider talks too fast and does not give the Alaska Native enough time to answer. Chief complaints sometimes are not expressed as the professional is in too much of a hurry and the client has not had time to tell them what the real problem is. Language frequently must be processed from English to Yup'ik and back to English; this takes time and the care provider must be patient.

Most villagers 'understand' if the health care practitioner cannot help with their health problems, but expect the professional to be able to tell them where to go for help and to continue to support them and care about the outcome.

Cannelos (1986) also noted certain Alaska Native health beliefs in a study on preventing suicide:

The indigenous cultures of Alaska consider the arbitrary act of categorically isolating physical health from mental health [a common Western practice] deviant behavior . . . In fact, elders view departmentalizing as rather amusing (p. 18).

Each village has a Health Aide who is trained in routine and emergency medical care (p. 9).

Elders are highly respected, they have a reputation for having a wealth of knowledge of traditional norms and values . . . [but] they must fully understand what the information will be used for before they permit interviews. They are known to lead exemplary lives and although they have a limited knowledge of the English language, they are considered to be scholars by their colleagues and other villagers. All Elders possess an ambiance that is difficult to explain. They exert a calming effect on anyone who spends time with them. This may be due to their total self-acceptance, self-assurance, and self-knowledge (pp. 11-13).

Manual (personal communication, February, 1990) suggests the following constitute major barriers to seeking and obtaining modern health care: language differences, a focus on today rather than on the future and preventive care, a concept of time that differs from that of the Western culture, geographic factors, travel and climate, poverty and subsistence living.

In *The Council*, a community tribal newspaper (1981), a local resident suggested several procedures that health care workers should follow when working with Alaskan Native clients:

DOs

Introduce yourself to village residents.

Listen non-defensively to what village residents say.

Be aware of the culture and life style of the village.

Follow up visits with a card or letter.

Pay for meals and lodging; partial payment in fresh fruits/vegetables taken with you is often welcome.

Establish a specific contact person in the village.

DON'Ts

Expect others to take care of you or drop everything for your visit.

Promise what you cannot deliver.

Expect others to admire or thank you for doing what you get paid for.

Count on buying food or other items in the village.

Navajo Health Beliefs

THE PEOPLE

The Navajo, or the "Dineh" in their own language, are a subgroup of the Athabascan linguistic group that migrated to the Southwest United States from Eastern Alaska and Canada about 1000 to 1200 A.D. Between 1864 and 1868, when the tribe was interned at Fort Sumner, NM, by the U.S. government, the Navajo population decreased to approximately 8,000. Scientists have suggested that this reduction of the Navajo gene pool might account for the unusually high incidence of certain cancers among Navajos. By 1980, the population had grown to approximately 146,000. The Navajo now reside primarily on the largest reservation in the United States, covering portions of Arizona, New Mexico, Colorado, and Utah.

The Navajo are not a homogeneous tribe. They range from those who are uneducated in Western ways, poor, and speak their own language almost exclusively, to those highly educated in both their own and the Western culture. The extended family is important: families care for their elders and for orphaned children. The woman is the center of the Navajo family, and descent is traced through her. Despite close family ties, the Navajo highly respect individual rights. They operate on the premise that no person has the right to speak for or to direct the actions of another.

Uranium mining is an important source of income for the Navajo. Other sources include oil, coal, and federal grants and contracts. Many raise sheep and supplement their family income by weaving. Despite these sources of income, the Navajo are plagued by high levels of unemployment (Haraldson, 1988).

Perhaps because of their work with uranium and their limited gene pool, malignant neoplasms are the third leading cause of death among the Navajo, preceded only by accidents or injuries and heart disease (Haraldson, 1988). Navajos describe cancer as "the sore that doesn't heal." Some believe that the disease is the result of the burning of ancient medicine bundles by early Christian missionaries. Members of the tribe are making new medicine bundles but this is a very laborious procedure (Frank-Stromborg and Olsen, 1988).

RELIGION

Many Navajo are members of the Native American Church. Haraldson (1988) describes this church as "a blend of the ancient Mexican Indian rites utilizing the hallucinogenic cactus, peyote, all-night ceremonies with some fundamentalist Christian elements, and pan-Indian moral principles" (p. 134).

Traditional Navajos believe that some of their "life spirit" is lost if their particular story is written and published (Kniep-Hardy and Burkhardt, 1977).

HEALTH CARE PROVIDERS

Traditional health care providers include shamans and medicine men and women (singers, curers, prayer makers, and diagnosticians). A cure may require hiring several specialists, which may be very expensive.

The Navajo area IHS is divided into eight service units. Six of these have hospitals and two offer only ambulatory clinics. The hospital that opened in 1983 in Chinele, AZ, the center of the reservation, has a specially constructed room for traditional healing ceremonies (Haraldson, 1988).

Today, a system of paved main roads, telephone communication, and air travel links the health care centers. Community and home health services are provided by public health nurses. Travel to homes may be difficult on unmarked dirt roads; some homes lack telephones, thereby hampering communication. In 1988, 40% of Navajo residences did not have piped running water (Haraldson, 1988). Even today, outbreaks of bubonic plague still occur among the Navajo in rural areas.

Community health representatives, lay workers who collaborate with the public health nurses, sanitarians, and clinics, serve an important function in Navajo health care. They form vital links with the families and communities and relay their health needs and demands to the Navajo IHS.

The Western physician is regarded as a type of herbalist who can cure symptoms but, unlike Navajo herbalists, cannot restore an individual's harmonious relationship with nature because they lack knowledge of important rituals.

HEALTH BELIEFS AND PRACTICES

Sobralske (1985) found that as with most Native Americans, the Navajo concept of health is intimately linked to religious beliefs, goodness in day-to-day living, and harmony with the surrounding environment. Illness, therefore, is a sign of one's lack of harmony.

The Navajo conduct "sings" with elaborate ritual, chants, and sand paintings to restore a sick person's harmonious relationship with nature. They commonly perform sings before a member of the tribe is hospitalized.

The Navajo believe some illnesses are caused by the violation of a cultural taboo or by witchcraft, and can only be cured by a particular ceremony. The following example was offered by a Navajo nurse (Frank-Stromborg and Olsen, 1988):

> A Navajo woman came in with uterine cancer. She believed it had come about because she had been promiscuous and had had relations with another man. She had not told her husband or anyone else in her family. She did, however, tell an Indian health care practitioner who went to the medicine man and asked him to perform the appropriate ceremony (the Moth Way Ceremony, also known as, the Prostitution Way Ceremony) to help heal her.

Navajos use many types of traditional medicines such as cedar incense for purification and corn pollen for blessings. The Navajos consider a "sweat" in a sweat lodge as a form of purging that is useful for both preventing and treating illness. Traditional Navajos perform a monthly sweat because they believe the body periodically builds up bad or negative spirits that block energy. If there is an illness, a ceremony may often accompany a trip to the sweat lodge. Navajo women do not do sweats.

Generally, Navajos will not touch a person whom they know is dying because they must let the person go. Touching the individual could "ground" them, delaying the soul's journey to the next world. They may also fear that if they do touch a dying loved one, the patient's ghost will come back and bother them (Frank-Stromborg and Olsen, 1988).

IMPLICATIONS FOR THE HEALTH CARE PROVIDER

Health care workers may have difficulty obtaining a Navajo patient's history from the patient's relatives because even close family members may believe they have no right to give personal information concerning another. Translation may also be difficult because there are no comparable terms in the Navajo language for many terms used in a medical history.

It is rare for a Navajo to agree to a procedure, operation, or transfer without first consulting the family and asking English-speaking family members for further explanation. The family, in turn, provides much support and assurance to the patient.

Some Navajos are shy in unfamiliar groups, so health care workers may need to provide them with educational materials on an individual basis. When providing care instructions to some traditional Navajos, relating human body parts to those of sheep may be appropriate as many have acquired this familiarity through butchering.

The health care worker should be cautious when color coding medications or directions, because colors have special meanings (Kniep-Hardy and Burkhardt, 1977).

Navajo patients may not acquiesce to immediate or emergency treatments. For example, if a Navajo patient comes in with advanced or metastatic disease, the health care worker may want to begin a course of intensive chemotherapy and radiation therapy right away; but the Navajo patient may want to ensure that things at home are in order and to participate in a traditional healing ceremony with the medicine man before starting therapy. Health care professionals may have to explain the reason for the urgency and negotiate a schedule with the patient (Frank-Stromborg and Olsen, 1988).

APPENDIX 8

Jamestown Klallam Health Beliefs

During focus group interviews in the Native American Workshop (Frank-Stromborg and Olsen, 1988), the following limited information on the Jamestown Klallam was provided:

The Jamestown Klallams have a fatalistic attitude toward health. They see no reason for taking preventive measures because they believe that what will happen will happen. They consider illness a natural and expected part of life. The tribe does espouse the germ theory of illness causation, and believes that respiratory problems are associated with bad air. This tribe has a strong Christian faith but many retain some of their traditional beliefs.

APPENDIX 9

Health Beliefs of the Sioux of Rosebud, SD

During focus group interviews in the Native American Workshop (Frank-Stromborg and Olsen, 1988), the following information on the Rosebud Sioux was provided:

The Rosebud reservation of North Dakota is located in the second poorest county in the United States Members of this tribe may not receive regular health care, consequently they often present with advanced stages of disease, including cancer. Most Rosebud Sioux speak English and they frequently seek medical attention off the reservation.

One nurse spoke of a female Sioux patient with lung cancer whom she saw three days before the woman died:

The medicine man believed that if he tried to heal her the cancer would lodge in his body rather than passing through him. He instructed the family not to touch the sick woman for fear the same fate would happen to them.

Health Beliefs of the Creek

During focus group interviews in the Native American Workshop (Frank-Stromborg and Olsen, 1988), the following information on the Creek was provided:

The Creek speak of good medicine and bad medicine. Good medicine is preventive. For example, in the spring they use certain herbs and take baths outside. Bad medicine entails getting a medicine man to put a hex on someone to make something bad happen to them. The Creek believe that if you practice bad medicine you may be punished for it when you get older.

The number of medicine men in the Creek tribe is dwindling. These healers are always male. Today, the tribe is attempting to attract young boys into training as medicine men but because of the attraction of the armed services and the rigor of the traditional training process few Creek boys have shown interest.

Health Beliefs of the Tohono O'Odham

During focus group interviews in the Native American Workshop (Frank-Stromborg and Olsen, 1988), the following information on the Tohono O'Odham was provided:

The Tohono O'Odham were formerly known as the Papago. Today members of this tribe usually use the Western health care system. However, they may seek out medicine men or women when they do not understand something regarding life or illness.

Many Tohono O'Odham have incorporated traditional Hispanic customs and beliefs of the "Sonoran Way," into their lives. The Tohono O'Odham also celebrate Catholic ways more than their traditional tribal ways. Usually, only the traditional members of the tribe, such as those who are old or middle aged, will seek out the medicine man.

Health Beliefs of the Quinault

During focus group interviews in the Native American Workshop (Frank-Stromborg and Olsen, 1988), the following information on the Quinault was provided:

The Native American groups known as the Quinault actually consist of several little tribes. For instance, of these tribes, one consists of only 73 individuals (the Schoalwater Tribe). Many of those in the smaller tribes are in very poor health.

Most Quinault have adopted the culture of the dominant society. However, some do practice more traditional ways. Health care workers with Quinault patients should ask them about their cultural practices.

One Quinault nurse spoke of how she employs the phrase 'genetic memory:' 'we have always known how to birth babies.' She believes that Native Americans have always practiced prevention and that they need to be encouraged to go back into themselves because some of the old practices are still viable. She believes it is empowering to encourage her people to go back or think back to the old days and bring the good that was useful then back into today's world.

Health Beliefs of the Lakota Sioux

G. M. Ellis, RN, a nurse who works with the Lakota Sioux in Black Hawk, SD, provided the following information on the health beliefs of the Lakota Sioux (February, 1990, personal correspondence):

In the Lakota philosophy, all things are related. They believe each person has three elements: mind, body, and spirit and the mind links the body and spirit. Illness is believed to affect all three elements. Consequently, the Lakota believe healing is not complete unless the individual is treated holistically.

The Lakota Sioux have two kinds of medicine men, both of which treat holistically. The most revered are those who commune with the spirits. These men know medicines, understand psychological principles, and bring the whole family and members of the community into the healing process. The other type, the "Pejuta Wicasa," work only with herbs and plants and are considered the lesser of the two healers. All medicine men help natives to regain harmony in their life, they do not necessarily work to prolong life. Their goal is to try to assure that harmony is obtained before death.

The Lakota feel that medicines used by the medicine men are sacred and must be shown proper respect or they will become ineffective. In traditional medicine, specific plants are used to treat specific problems, diseases, or affected areas. Once the appropriate plants, herbs, and sacred items are chosen, the medicine man gives thanks with a ceremony to ensure their strength and purity. Spiritual presences augment the effects of these medicines. Strict rules must be observed; among these are abstinence from negative influences, including certain persons or things.

The Lakota have lost a great deal of their culture. In part, the loss of this knowledge accounts for some of the fear the Lakota feel about cancer and other major diseases. This tribe also believes that cancers can be caused by breaking sacred tribal taboos or committing a violation against nature because these actions disrupt the harmony between body, mind, and spirit. For example, the use of pesticides or other chemicals in the soil or in the environment is a violation against nature. The Lakota believe those who eat the crops from this contaminated soil may get cancer. The traditional belief is that cancer can be healed, but only if one's faith, trust in the kind of care given, and the presence of family support are strong.

Within the Lakota concept of health, the occurrence of cancers, diabetes, heart disease, and mental illnesses can be related directly to the patient's experiences. For instance, a woman attributed cervical cancer to the suppressed negative experiences of her past including rape, sexual abuse, and the pain and anguish associated with these events. In addition, diabetes is seen as a result of excessive and negative dietary habits.

APPENDIX 14

Health Beliefs of the Yankton Sioux

Focus group interviews during the Native American Workshop (Frank-Stromborg and Olsen, 1988) provided the following information concerning the Yankton Sioux:

Many Yankton Sioux over the age of 60 are very private and do not seek health promotion on their own. Members of this age group may restrain some of their traditional tribal beliefs such as wearing protective bundles, but usually are practicing Christians.

Yankton Sioux below age 60 years are used to attending clinics or hospitals not associated with the IHS and are comfortable with Western health promotion techniques.

It is common among the Yankton Sioux for members of the extended family to live together; so if a health care worker visits the home and wants to discuss something with only one person, that person may be encouraged to come out to the car. Generally, that person is then more comfortable discussing personal health concerns.

Health Beliefs of the Cherokee

The Cherokee Nation is situated in Oklahoma. Personal communication with D. C. Adler, RN, a nurse working with the Cherokee people, provided the following cancer-related information concerning this tribe (October, 1988):

The Cherokee had a category of disease labeled 'cancer' as far back as 1891. The following were used in the treatment of cancer (in *Sacred Formulas of the Cherokees*, quoted by D. C. Adler):

Beggar lice (*Cynoglossum morrisoni*)—the tribe used the bruised root mixed with bear oil as an ointment for cancer (p. 324);

Milkweed (*Euphorbia hypericifolia*)—the juice of milkweed was mixed with other herbs and rubbed on the affected area (p. 325);

Tassel flower (*Cacalia atriplicifolia*)—the Cherokee bruise the leaves and bind them over the spot, changing them frequently (p. 326).

Health Beliefs of the Chippewa Indians

June Ouillatte, RN, a community health nurse who works with the Sault Saint Marie Tribe of the Chippewa at the Munising Tribal Center in Munising, MI, explained several of the tribe's characteristics and general beliefs about health (personal communication, 1990):

The Chippewa reside both on and off the reservation. Art, music, dance, and recreational therapy are an important part of their culture. The use of color is important, with each color having significant meaning. Extended families are the norm, with the eldest held in highest esteem.

The Chippewa are reserved in their behavior as well as their speech. As a group they express more through nonverbal communication than through verbal forms. They have little or no eye contact. Each feels he or she is responsible for their own life and if faced with a difficult situation, will remove themselves from a source of conflict rather than risk escalation of the problem by staying.

The Chippewa use both traditional and Western forms of health care. Generally, the elders follow the more traditional health practices of the medicine man, whereas the younger members of the tribe may opt for more modern [Western] health care methods. Some will use modern [Western] facilities and the medicine man simultaneously. It is important that the Western health care provider is careful not to impose his or her beliefs on the individual Chippewa.

Some Chippewa have difficulty thinking in terms of health promotion. They tend to think if they seek out the health professional when well, they are asking for trouble. Many seek help only when very ill. Many dislike admission to hospitals because they experience feelings of confinement, isolation, loss of control, and a high level of powerlessness.

The Asian/Pacific Islander Population in the United States: Cultural Perspectives and Their Relationship to Cancer Prevention and Early Detection

This chapter brings to mind some issues discussed at the East West Center Association's conference on "The Asian Pacific Experience in California: Trends and Prospectives for the Year 2000" (January 24-26, 1991, Long Beach, Calif). Dr. Snehendu Kar discussed psychosocial factors in the health care of Asian-Americans. He described two major global and national movements: (1) the focus on the primary health care provider and (2) the movement to control diseases like cancer, heart disease, and AIDS through lifestyle changes in the areas of diet, sexual practices, smoking, and the like. The American paradigms of health promotion and disease prevention do not fit the cultures of the Asian and Pacific Island immigrants. New strategies need to be devised that are congruent with Asian and Pacific Islander values.

To help us understand value differences and their implications for the health care of Asian-Americans and of Pacific Islanders, Dr. Harry Kitano explained that the Western health care system presents its services based on its own models of human behavior. For that reason, Asians and Pacific Islanders are less likely to use the services of Western health care providers. Models of human behavior are of different types. The fate orientation models of human behavior are characteristic of many Asian/Pacific Islander cultures. This model of behavior does not incorporate change, therefore, it is not popular with the Western health care system. The Western deterministic model of behavior incorporates change by assuming that if you can find the causes of behavior you can change behavior. This is the basis of science and so is valued by the Western system. The free will model is characteristic of the Western values espoused in the 1960s and 1970s when youth felt that traditions were no longer valid. Free yourself, become someone that will go beyond what your parents were. This free will model is also incompatible with many Asian/Pacific Islander cultures. These different models of behavior explain some of the difficulties experienced by health care providers in the Western system when providing services to Asian/Pacific Islanders.

Dr. Kakit-Hul gave specific examples of the difference in Western and Chinese traditional medicine. He emphasized the advantage of combining traditional Chinese with current Western medicine. However, the principal barrier to this interdisciplinary approach to health care delivery lies in the difference between the Chinese model of medicine, which focuses on maintaining health, and the Western model of medicine, which focuses on curing ills. This chapter by Eunice Lasky and Carole Martz, helps to bridge the gap between differing cultures so that cancer prevention and early detection might be more successful in Asian/Pacific Islander groups.

Geraldine V. Padella, Ph.D.

Professor and Associate Dean for Research
UCLA School of Nursing

The Asian/Pacific Islander Population in the United States: Cultural Perspectives and Their Relationship to Cancer Prevention and Early Detection

EUNICE M. LASKY
CAROLE H. MARTZ

Asian/Pacific Islanders (A/PI) make up one of the smallest but fastest growing minority groups in the United States. Between 1970 and 1980 the A/PI population increased 141%. In addition, this group has the largest proportion of foreign-born persons (58%) migrating to this country of any minority group (Newell, 1988). Recent changes in United States immigration policies have allowed millions of Asian/Pacific Islanders to relocate to the United States. In the past, many people from this region came to the United States seeking better education and economic advancement. More recently, immigrants and refugees from these areas have relocated due to social and political oppression. Today, one of every seven Asian/Pacific Islanders is a recent refugee from southeastern Asia (the term "Indochinese" is sometimes used to refer to the refugee populations). These individuals often arrive destitute, illiterate, and in poor physical and mental health (Flaskerud and Soldevilla, 1986; Lin Fu, 1988). Despite the rapid growth of the Asian/Pacific Islander population, it remains one of the most diverse and poorly understood minority groups.

GENERAL DEMOGRAPHICS AND HEALTH STATISTICS

The A/PI population is distinguished by extreme heterogeneity. Experts estimate that over 30 different A/PI groups reside in the United States, the largest of which are the Pilipinos, Chinese, and Japanese. Most of the A/PI population is concentrated in urban areas of the West Coast and in large cities across the United States. Chinese, Japanese, and Pilipinos who immigrated earlier in this century tended to be well educated, but this may not be the case for many recent immigrants who were forced to leave their countries under dire circumstances.

Fitzpatrick (1987) noted that many U.S. health care workers assume that the health status of A/PIs as a group is good. Operating on this assumption, health professionals may overlook the serious health problems and needs that have been identified in certain A/PI subgroups. For example, Southeast Asian refugees, who have migrated to the United States in great numbers recently, tend to experience high rates of tuberculosis, malaria, and parasitic infections. Many test positive for hepatitis B surface antigen, and are in generally poor mental and physical health (Fitzpatrick, 1987).

Another challenge to assessing the health problems of this population is that until very recently, A/PIs were not identified as a separate minority population due to their low numbers in the United States. As a result, scant information is available on the incidences of various illnesses, including cancer, in A/PI subgroups (Lin Fu, 1988). The incidence data that are available (Table 2-1) illustrate that A/PIs, with the exception of native Hawaiians, have a lower incidence of most major cancers than the U.S. population in general (Baquet, 1990). Data on the Pilipino population are limited to those residing in Hawaii, due to the paucity of studies performed in the United States on this group to date. The Korean population's statistics are based on data from the World Health Organization (1989). Information on cancer incidence

---

TABLE 2-1 Age-adjusted Cancer Incidence Data for Asian Pacific Americans Compared to the American Population.[†]

Asian Pacific Group	All Sites	American Whites	All Sites
Hawaiians	346.5[†]	Whites*	349.6
Japanese	242.5	Whites	349.6
Chinese	247.6	Whites	349.6
Pilipino	212.4	Whites	349.6
Korean	150.6	Whites	349.6

*Whites in Hawaii
[†]Rates are per 100,000
From Baquet CR: *Cancer data,* Paper presented at the meeting of the American Society of Clinical Oncologists 1990. Adapted by permission.

rates in Vietnam, Laos, and Cambodia is not available. Many developing nations do not yet have tumor registries, so cancer risks can only be inferred from information on the prevalence of other illnesses in these and other Asian countries. Tables 2-2 to 2-4 illustrate the cancer incidence rates for various A/PI groups in the United States from two periods of time, 1977 to 1983 and 1980 to 1990.

Ethnic groups with a high incidence of cancer and their associated risk factors are listed in Table 2-5. It must be remem-

TABLE 2-2 Age-Adjusted (1970 U.S. Standard) Cancer Mortality Rates per 100,000 Population by Race and Cancer Site, Both Sexes, 1977-1983

Cancer Site	Chinese	Japanese	Pilipino
All sites	125.0‡	108.0	72.0
Oral cavity	5.4	1.7	2.4
Esophagus	2.8	2.1	1.8
Stomach	7.6	17.9	3.5
Colon and rectum	17.9	16.8	7.9
Liver	10.1	3.4	3.5
Gallbladder	0.7	1.1	0.6
Pancreas	6.4	7.0	3.5
Lung	31.7	19.8	14.5
Melanoma	0.2	0.2	0.3
Breast*	12.0	10.2	7.8
Cervix uteri*	3.3	2.2	1.9
Corpus uteri*	2.7	2.4	1.7
Ovary*	3.8	4.4	2.6
Prostate†	7.4	8.4	8.7
Urinary bladder	1.7	1.8	1.4
Kidney and renal	1.7	1.6	0.8
Brain and CNS	1.3	1.3	1.1
Hodgkin's disease	0.3	0.1	0.3
Non-Hodgkin's	2.8	3.5	3.4
Leukemia	4.1	3.5	4.1

*Females.
†Males.
‡Racial group with the highest rate for cancer [Black, Chinese, Japanese, Pilipino, American Indian, Mexican American, Native Hawaiian, Alaska Native].
From Harras A: Personal correspondence (1991). The National Cancer Institute, Surveillance Program, Cancer Statistics Branch, Executive Plaza North, Room 343J, Bethesda, Md 20892.

TABLE 2-3 Age-adjusted (1970 U.S. Standard) Cancer Incidence Rates per 100,000 Population by Race and Cancer Site, Both Sexes, 1977-1983

Cancer Site	Chinese	Japanese	Pilipino
All sites	247.6‡	242.5	212.4
Oral cavity	15.4	4.8	8.9
Esophagus	3.3	2.8	3.4
Stomach	10.5	26.6	7.8
Colon and Rectum	40.4	48.8	30.3
Liver	9.6	3.6	5.4
Gallbladder	1.0	1.5	1.4
Pancreas	6.3	7.1	4.9
Lung	40.6	27.1	27.3
Melanoma	0.7	1.2	1.0
Breast*	57.8	55.0	41.3
Cervix uteri*	10.3	5.9	8.6
Corpus uteri*	18.0	17.7	11.3
Ovary*	9.2	8.8	9.7
Prostate†	29.6	43.8	44.0
Urinary bladder	9.0	8.0	4.4
Kidney and renal	3.5	3.6	3.1
Brain and CNS	2.4	2.4	1.9
Hodgkin's disease	0.6	0.5	1.2
Non-Hodgkin's	8.5‡	7.2	8.3
Leukemia	4.8	5.7	7.1

*Females.
†Males.
‡Racial group with the highest rate for cancer (Black, Chinese, Japanese, Pilipino, American Indian, Mexican American, Native Hawaiian, Alaska Native).
From Harras A: Personal correspondence (1991). The National Cancer Institute, Surveillance Program, Cancer Statistics Branch, Executive Plaza North, Room 343J, Bethesda, Md 20892.

bered, however, that the longer the individual has lived in this country the more likely he or she will experience the types of cancers found in the American white population due to their adoption of American dietary patterns.

CULTURE AND HEALTH CARE

Within the A/PI group, each nationality may contain multiple subgroups whose beliefs and behaviors about health and illness differ widely. As Leininger (1977) pointed out, cultural beliefs, values, and experiences all influence "a person's reaction to illness, health maintenance, daily activities, body discomforts, changes in life, food preferences, and various caring and curing treatment practices." Some researchers (Lin Fu, 1988; Newell, 1988) propose that health practices may differ more between various

educational and class levels within an ethnic category than between ethnic groups.

While cultural variations are the norm rather than the exception, A/PI groups share a few basic cultural similarities. These similarities result from common religious practices and the prominent Chinese influence throughout the Asian region. For instance, more traditional A/PIs tend not to be prevention oriented in the sense embraced by Western medicine. Their traditional diets do tend to be healthier, however, and some A/PIs perform certain health practices in the belief they can prevent illness or "bad luck." The most common beliefs that affect the health practices of A/PIs are listed in the box on p. 84.

To meet the cancer prevention and early detection needs of A/PIs health care

TABLE 2-4   Asian or Pacific Islanders in the United States: 1980 and 1990

Race	1980		1990		Number Change	Percent Change
	Number	Percent	Number	Percent		
Asian or Pacific Islander*	3,500,439	1.5	7,273,662	2.9	3,773,223	107.8
Chinese	806,040	0.4	1,645,472	0.7	839,432	104.1
Pilipino	774,652	0.3	1,406,770	0.6	632,118	81.6
Japanese	700,974	0.3	847,562	0.3	146,588	20.9
Asian Indian	361,531	0.2	815,447	0.3	453,916	125.6
Korean	354,593	0.2	798,849	0.3	444,256	125.3
Vietnamese	261,729	0.1	614,547	0.2	352,818	134.8
Hawaiian	166,814	0.1	211,014	0.1	44,200	26.5
Samoan	41,948	0.0	62,964	0.0	21,016	50.1
Guamanian	32,158	0.0	49,345	0.0	17,187	53.4

*The 1980 number for Asians or Pacific Islanders shown in this table are not entirely comparable with 1990 counts. The 1980 count of 3,500,439 Asians or Pacific Islanders based on 100% tabulations includes only the nine specific Asian or Pacific Islander groups listed separately in the 1980 race item. The 1980 total Asian or Pacific Islander population of 3,726,440 from sample tabulations is comparable to the 1990 count these figures include groups not listed separately in the race item on the 1980 census form.
From Census Bureau Press Release CB91-215.

TABLE 2-5   Cancers With High Cancer Incidence Rate in the Asian Pacific/Islander Population and Associated Risk Factors

Ethnic Group	Cancer	Risk Factors
Chinese	Nasopharyngeal	Epstein-Barr virus exposure
		Consumption of salt fish
		Genetic predisposition(?) (descendants of immigrants from southern China)
	Liver	Polluted drinking water
		Chronic hepatitis B infection
		Low intake of vitamin C
	Esophageal	Descendants of immigrants from eastern and central China
		Consumption of foods high in salt
		Drinking hot teas
		Consumption of grains contaminated with silica fibers
	Lung	Previous lung disease
		Indoor pollutants
		Smoking
		Passive smoke
		Vitamin A deficiency
	Stomach	Chronic gastritis and ulcers
		Family history of gastric cancer
		Consumption of salt-cured and moldy foods
		Loss of gastric acidity
Japanese	Stomach	Age over 65
		Diet high in salt-cured foods
		Low vitamin C intake
		Type A blood
		Conditions causing decreased gastric acidity
		Family history of gastric cancer
		History of gastric ulcer

COMMON ASIAN BELIEFS AND PRACTICES

Respect for authority
Respect for elders
Self-control
Stoicism
Humility
Fear of hospitalization
Family orientation
Fear of bodily intrusive procedures
Use of traditional medicines

From Frank-Stromborg, Olsen, 1988; Fong, 1985.

workers must become aware of and sensitive to their own cultural backgrounds, health beliefs, and practices and how these affect their practice. To increase the likelihood that an A/PI client will accept Western concepts of cancer prevention and early detection, health care providers must incorporate the target population into the planning and development of strategies. This culturally specific information should be disseminated to community and church groups, and carried

TABLE 2-5   Cancers With High Cancer Incidence Rate in the Asian Pacific/Islander Population and Associated Risk Factors—cont'd

Ethnic Group	Cancer	Risk Factors
	Esophagus	Rice gruel cooked in hot tea
		Chronic esophagitis
		Consumption of foods contaminated with molds
	Liver	Chronic hepatitis B infection
		Consumption of foods high in mold content
		Low vitamin C intake
	Gallbladder	Gallstones
		Consumption of foods high in fat
Korean	Liver	Chronic hepatitis B infection
		Consumption of foods high in mold and aflatoxin B1 content
	Stomach	Diet high in salt-cured foods
		Low vitamin C intake
		History of chronic gastritis
Pilipino	Liver	Chronic hepatitis B infection
		Consumption of foods high in mold and aflatoxin B1 content(?)
	Biliary	History of gallstones
		Consumption of fatty foods
	Lymphoma	Not known
	Thyroid	Not known

Sources:

Chinese: Chang, 1986; Gayal, 1983; King and Locke, 1980; Namura, 1982; Shimizu, et al., 1985; Yu, 1986; Wanebo, Falkson and Order, 1989.

Japanese: Gayal, 1983; Locke and King, 1980; London and McGlynn, 1990; Nomura, 1982; Frank-Stromborg, 1989; Tominaga, 1985; Wanebo, Falkson and Order, 1989.

Korean: Frank-Stromborg, 1989. London and McGlynn, 1990; World Health Organization, 1989.

Pilipino: Anderson, 1983; Kolonel, 1984; London and McGlynn, 1990.

(or published) in ethnic newspapers (Frank-Stromborg and Olsen, 1988).

A/PI patients may be more likely to accept and comply with recommended Western medical treatments if the treatments incorporate the patients' ethnic practices (as long as they are not life threatening). Health practitioners should avoid using Western strategies that may be contrary to the medical beliefs of the patient's country of origin (Benoliel, 1987; Hoang, 1985; Lin Fu, 1988; Muecke, 1983).

Language barriers can deter A/PIs from obtaining health care. This situation is complicated by the fact that individuals of the same nationality may speak different dialects. High unemployment rates among recent immigrants also serve as a barrier to health care access as they are not entitled to employer-provided insurance. They also may be unaware of social service agencies that could provide guidance regarding application for local, state, or federally funded health care programs (Lin Fu, 1988; Newell, 1988).

ASSESSMENT OF CANCER RISK

Assessment of cancer risk is discussed here in the context of the experiences shared by many members of the A/PI population. The generalized statements used to describe shared cultural experiences are meant, however, to serve only as guidelines for the evaluation of cancer risk. Health professionals should expect individual variations and should elucidate these through history taking and physical assessment. The box on pp. 87-89 offers one tool for assessing A/PI cancer risk. Use of this tool may be tailored (e.g., by asking questions from only one section) to accommodate individual clients, families, or health care settings.

PILIPINOS

Pilipinos currently make up the largest population of Asians in the United States, having recently surpassed the Chinese. (Notice that there is no "F" in the word Pilipino; this is because there is no "F" in the Philippine language. The word Filipino is an anglicized version.)

The Pilipino population consists of three major cultural subgroups and languages: Ilocano, Tagalog, and Visayan. The differences among these groups tend to be more linguistic than cultural, yet many have strong local loyalties (Baysa, Cabera, Camilon, and Torres, 1980; Flaskerud and Soldevilla, 1986). The national language of the Philippines is a mixture of Tagalog with Malayo-Indonesian, Chinese, Spanish, and English words intermixed. English is the Pilipino's second language, so a significant number of immigrants may be fluent.

In order to understand the health beliefs and health practices of Pilipino patients, health care professionals must consider how long the patient has been in the U.S. and the subgroup to which he or she belongs. It is important to remember that the patient may not ascribe to their ethnic groups' traditional beliefs (Baysa et al., 1980).

Epidemiology

Pilipino cancer incidence rates (Anderson, 1983) are relatively low compared to those of the general Caucasian American population. Pilipinos have low incidence rates for cancers of the larynx, stomach, colon, kidney, lung, and brain. They have moderate incidence rates for cancers of the tongue, mouth, pharynx, esophagus, rectum, pancreas, bladder, and leukemia. Relatively high incidence rates for liver and biliary cancers, as well as lymphomas, have been noted in the Pilipino population. Pilipino women in Hawaii also have a high incidence of thyroid cancer (Kolonel, 1984).

Several factors may place Pilipino Americans at risk for liver cancers. Chronic hepatitis B infection, which is endemic in many parts of Asia, has been implicated as a cause of hepatocellular carcinoma. Many Pilipinos also eat foods with high levels of aflatoxin B1 due to poor storage techniques, and this has also been implicated as a possible cause of liver cancer. Recent evidence indicates that aflatoxin exposure and chronic hepatitis B infection may have a synergistic effect on the development of liver cancer (London and McGlynn, 1990; Stoloff, 1989). Biliary tract tumors are generally associated with a history of gallstones and a lifestyle of fatty food consumption. Risk factors for lymphoma have not been

ASIAN CANCER RISK ASSESSMENT TOOL

DEMOGRAPHIC DATA

Name_____Age_____Marital Status_____

Religious Preference_____Weight_____

Asian Ethnic Group: Pilipino___Hmong___Chinese___

(Please check one): Japanese___Korean___Vietnamese___

       Other (please specify)_____

When did you or your family immigrate to this country?_____

From what part of Asia did you or your family immigrate? (province, island, etc. where ap-

   plicable)_____

How long have you lived in the United States?_____

Which generation?_____

Who lives in your household?_____

What languages are spoken in your home?_____

How do you explain illness? (cause and meaning of illness)_____

_____

Are you currently being treated by a traditional healer?_____

What type of traditional medicine or tools have you used?

   herbs ___ teas ___ foods ___ acupuncture ___ massage ___ moxibustion ___ medicines ___

   cupping ___ scraping ___

Other (please specify)_____

What types of foods are eaten at home?_____

_____

Are there any foods that you eat or avoid eating during periods of illness?_____

_____

At this point, a general health physical assessment should be performed.* If suspicious

   signs are noted, the nurse should refer to the specific site questions.

CANCER ASSESSMENT

Nasopharyngeal cancer (NPC)

Have you experienced any of the following problems:

   ___ facial pain ___ headaches ___ tinnitus ___ recent ear infection ___ foul taste ___ epistaxis

   ___ diplopia ___ hoarseness ___ sore throat ___ swelling lymph glands ___ toothaches

   ___ change in smell

Do you consume a diet high in salt-cured foods?_____

Is there a history of NPC in your family?_____

Did your family migrate from southern China?_____

Do you drink alcohol?_____How much per day?_____

Have you ever been tested for the Epstein-Barr virus?_____

Do you or have you ever smoked or used tobacco products?_____

How much?_____

*If any findings are suspicious do a complete evaluation of the head and neck area if not

   already done.

ASIAN CANCER RISK ASSESSMENT TOOL—cont'd

CANCER ASSESSMENT—cont'd
Gastric cancer
Have you experienced problems with any of the following:
___ indigestion ___ recent weight loss ___ abdominal pain ___ easy satiety ___ nausea
___ vomiting ___ blood in stools ___ chronic ulcers
Have you ever had stomach surgery?_____
Do you have a history of stomach ulcers?_____
Do you have to receive vitamin B_{12} injections?_____
Do you have Type A blood?_____
Is there a family history of gastric cancer?_____
Do you consume a diet high in salt-cured foods?_____
Do you eat fruits and vegetables regularly?_____
If any findings are suspicious, perform a thorough abdominal assessment.
Liver cancer
Have you had problems with any of the following?
___ abdominal pain   ___ yellowing of your skin
___ abdominal bloating   ___ yellowing of the whites of your eyes
___ recent weight loss   ___ fever of unknown origin
___ hemochromatosis
___ easy bruising
Has anyone in your family had liver cancer?_____
Have you ever had a blood test for hepatitis?_____
   When (date)?_____
   What were the results of this test?_____
   Have you ever been tested for alpha-fetoprotein? yes ___ no ___
   What were the results of this test?_____
Do you drink alcohol?   yes ___ no ___
   How many drinks per day?_____
Have you noticed any change in the color of your stools?_____
Have you noticed any change in the color of your urine?_____
Do you feel you are more weak and tired?_____
Did your family immigrate from eastern or southern China?_____
How old were you when you came to this country?_____

---

clearly identified; specific risk factors for thyroid cancer in Pilipino women residing in Hawaii have yet to be identified either (Kolonel, 1984).

Culture

Pilipinos migrated to the United States in two waves: one occurred in the early 1900s, and another began in the mid-60s and is still continuing (Anderson, 1983; Flaskerud and Soldevilla, 1986). Earlier immigrants tended to be primarily male and continue to reside in rural areas with limited financial means. Immigrants who settled in the eastern states (Anderson, 1983) may be better educated and speak

ASIAN CANCER RISK ASSESSMENT TOOL—cont'd

What kind of food did you eat in your country?_____

    Do/did you eat a lot of salt-cured foods?_____

    Do you eat fruits and vegetables routinely?_____

    Did you have any refrigeration for foods in your old country?_____

Have you been exposed to polyvinyl chloride?_____

Did you have an injection for a cerebral angiography or liver/spleen scan between the years 1930-1955 in Japan or Europe (Thorotrast)?_____

If any suspicious findings, do a complete abdominal assessment.

Biliary cancer

Have you ever had problems with the following:

    __ gallstones __ yellowing of your skin or whites of your eyes

    __ RUQ abdominal pain that radiates to your back __ recent weight __ loss of appetite

Did you ever have an injection (of Thorotrast) for a cerebral angiogram or liver-spleen scan between 1930-1955?_____

Do you eat a lot of fatty foods?_____

Esophageal cancer

Have you had problems with any of the following:

    __ chronic esophagitis __ indigestion __ heartburn __ difficulty swallowing __ regurgitation

Do you drink a lot of hot tea or eat hot cereals?_____

Do you eat a lot of "hot rice?"_____

Did you immigrate from eastern or central China?_____

Do you eat fruits and vegetables regularly?_____

Do you eat a lot of salt-cured foods?_____

Do you drink alcohol? _____How many drinks per day?_____

If suspicious findings are noted, do a thorough thoracic and abdominal assessment.

Lymphoma

Have you noticed any of the following:

    __ swollen lymph glands __ night sweats __ recent weight loss __ loss of appetite

    __ increased fatigue

If suspicious findings are noted a complete physical assessment will need to be performed.

Lung cancer

Have you noticed any of the following:

    __ cough __ change in color or odor of sputum __ dull chest pain __ persistent cold

    __ recent weight loss __ loss of appetite __ shortness of breath __ malaise

Have you been exposed to any of the following:

    __ passive smoke __ indoor pollutants __ coal stove smoke __ kerosene __ Radon

Do you now or have you ever smoked?_____How many packs per day/years?_____

Do you have a history of chronic lung disease such as:

    __ bronchitis or __ pneumonia?

Do you eat vegetables and fruits regularly?_____

If suspicious findings are noted, do a thorough chest assessment.

English. Many are professionals or persons with technical backgrounds who have at times found it difficult to find employment commensurate with their education and experience. Most of the more recent Pilipino immigrants live in urban areas of the West Coast. Pilipino Americans may appear very westernized, but are often still influenced by their cultural roots (Anderson, 1983; Flaskerud and Soldevilla, 1986).

Because the Philippine Islands have been invaded frequently by other countries throughout the ages, Pilipinos have adopted many of the cultural beliefs of other countries, especially those of the Chinese and Spanish (Baysa et al., 1980). The Spanish, in particular, introduced the concepts of barrios, close-knit inner city communities, and Roman Catholicism. Before these invasions, Pilipinos were primarily animists whose religious practices centered around the spirits of dead nonhuman creatures. Some Pilipinos may still hold these beliefs. As a result of the Islamic invasion during the 1300s, the southern Philippine islands have been strongly influenced by the Muslim religion, and some Pilipino Americans may still hold these beliefs.

Religion plays a very important role in the Pilipino Americans' lives and influences their health beliefs (Baysa et al., 1980). Because most Pilipinos are Roman Catholic, they value the authority of their priests. Guilt and divine retribution account for a somewhat fatalistic attitude in this culture: many Pilipinos consider illness and suffering unavoidable in certain circumstances. The common attitude that illness "is in God's hands" also stems from a Catholic influence.

Barrio life has also had a great impact on the culture of the Pilipino American population (Baysa et al., 1980). In these close-knit communities, families are large and place high value on neighborliness and family solidarity. The Pilipino American male often believes it is his responsibility to take care of his neighbor and his family, especially his elders. Because family ties often extend past the nuclear family, baptized children may have multiple godparents with whom they share a special relationship.

The diet of the traditional Pilipino American is similar to that of most Asians (Baysa et al., 1980). Pilipinos' daily diet usually consists primarily of rice, fish, and vegetables. Traditionally, Pilipinos tended to consume less fat and alcohol than other Asians. However, their consumption of chicken, pork, sweets, and beef has increased as Pilipinos adopt American ways. Pilipinos rarely consume milk products because many are lactose intolerant.

Health Beliefs and Practices

Beliefs about the cause of illness vary widely in the Pilipino American population (Baysa et al., 1980). Some believe in the Western, scientific view of illness. Individuals who have assimilated American culture will have little if any difficulty using the country's health care system.

The more traditional Pilipino may think that illness is caused by an imbalance in spirit or morals. These individuals believe in a range of principles concerning the balance of body elements and the diet. According to the humoral theory, sickness results from an excess or a deficiency of one or more primary humoral elements (Baysa et al., 1980). Rapid shifts from hot to cold may cause illness and mental disorders; a warm condition is healthiest. Traditional Pilipinos also believe that imbalances in the air to which they are exposed can also be unhealthy. Some illnesses are attributed to the entry of air into the body during childbirth and surgery; even a wind blowing on the body may induce colds, fever, and pneumonia. Similarly, weather changes are thought to lead to imbalances and cause fevers, pain, and disorientation.

Many Pilipino people believe in the orderliness of the universe (Baysa et al., 1980; Flaskerud and Soldevilla, 1986). They believe that most people get what they deserve: if a person behaves badly, then bad things will happen to them.

Another common Pilipino belief is that social or emotional stress, worry, anxiety, or grief can cause or contribute to a loss of equilibrium, thereby resulting in an increased susceptibility to illness (Anderson, 1983; Baysa et al., 1980). The traditional Pilipino does not feel there is a clear dichotomy between mental and physical illness. However, mental illness is seen as a shameful disease and is thought to be a punishment for misdeeds.

Use of Health Services

Underutilization of health care is a chronic problem in the Pilipino population (Baysa et al., 1980). Many newer immigrants do not have health insurance, are reluctant to accept assistance, or are simply unaware of services available. Health care professionals must consider these factors when planning cancer screenings and educational programs; they should seek out places where groups gather, such as churches, to better disseminate the information.

Pilipinos will often suppress signs of suffering and appear stoic in order to maintain their dignity in front of strangers. Within the family, however, the sick person may express himself freely and gain full support. Pilipinos may also avoid seeking medical care at the new year because their traditions hold that if they do so they'll be inclined to be ill all year (Frank-Stromborg and Olsen, 1988). For this reason they will delay seeking treatment for illnesses which might be potentially serious.

Cancer diagnoses are often kept secret from those outside the family. These patients may not seek treatment until later signs of bleeding or extreme weight loss have occurred. They often try to care for themselves and turn to hospitalization only as a last step.

In order to save face, Pilipino families tend to deal with a member's mental illness, which is thought to be a payment for bad deeds, by themselves. Pilipinos with mental illnesses who do come to health facilities for treatment will generally present with physical symptoms such as insomnia, headache, dizziness, or fatigue. It is up to the health care provider to gently uncover the root of the patient's problems. Since it is against these patients' customs to discuss their emotions, questions of a hypothetical nature often work best (Flaskerud and Soldevilla, 1986).

When traditional Pilipinos do seek treatment, they may turn to either a healer or a physician. Hilots are traditional healers who use herbal medicines, massage, manipulation of body parts, and prayer to heal the patient and restore balance to the patient's system (Frank-Stromborg and Olsen, 1988). Pilipinos may rely on such healers for a variety of reasons: tradition, familiarity, nationality, accessibility, and cost. These patients may also combine treatments suggested by healers with Western medical care.

It is not uncommon for Pilipino Americans to rely heavily on their religious beliefs to help them through an illness (Frank-Stromborg and Olsen, 1988). Patients may bring religious statues to the hospital and make pilgrimages to holy sites in order to be cured. They may continue such practices while under the care of a physician. Once health care is sought, the traditional Pilipino generally complies very well with the prescribed regimen.

Pilipinos typically have great respect for authority, so they may avoid confrontation if they do not agree with suggestions made by the health care team (Baysa et al., 1980). A smile and a response of "Yes, doctor," may not mean that the patient understands, but may instead indicate embarrassment about not understanding the instructions or a desire to avoid confrontation (Baysa et al., 1980).

Family involvement in decisions about health care is essential, and Pilipino patients may not comply with the instructions of health care workers who disregard the family's opinions. This is particularly important when planning cancer prevention and early detection programs. Families often depend on their children

educated in the United States to interpret information.

Physical Assessment and Cultural Implications

To increase the likelihood that Pilipinos will participate in routine screenings for cancer and learn about cancer prevention, it is important to be culturally sensitive during interviews and the examination process. Including family and individuals of similar backgrounds in the education process will not only increase the likelihood of compliance but also assist the patient in feeling at ease. Compared to Caucasians, Pilipinos tend to be smaller in stature, with almond shaped eyes, brown skin color, and less body hair. Health care professionals should consider generational differences when planning cancer screening examinations.

Both Pilipino men and women tend to be very modest. Even in general discussions, health care workers should start with less sensitive issues first and then explain what will be done before exposing a body part or performing a test.

It is important that care providers conducting a physical exam of a Pilipino patient expose only one body part at a time, be particularly careful about exposing genitalia, and provide privacy at all times. The clinician should attempt not to chill the patient and keep him/her covered as much as possible. Whenever possible, clinicians of the same gender as the patient should perform pelvic and rectal examinations. A Pilipino health care provider speaking the same dialect as the patient should be involved if it is unclear whether the patient understands English;

this can be particularly important during physical examinations.

Because Pilipinos tend not to be prevention-oriented, it will be important to conduct as many screening examinations during one visit as possible. For example, combining a Pap smear with a mammogram on the same day may increase compliance and, of course, minimize the patient's time away from work and family responsibilities.

Cigarettes are available at a young age in the Philippines, so immigrants from those countries should be monitored closely for signs of lung cancer possibly appearing at a younger age. The patient's family and social group should be involved in smoking cessation programs if possible.

Health care providers should also be aware that many Pilipinos are lactose intolerant and prone to develop hyperuricemia. Other conditions seen commonly in the Pilipino population are tuberculosis, Hansen's disease, thalassemia minor, hypertension, and stomach ulcers. See the box on pp. 94-95 for cancer risk assessment questions to ask Pilipino clients.

CHINESE

Many Chinese arrived in the United States before the turn of the century as laborers. After 1981, an increase in immigration occurred when a law was passed allowing separate immigration quotas from Taiwan and mainland China (Yu, 1986). As with other A/PIs, the Chinese tend to settle on the West Coast and in the larger cities of the United States. Cantonese and Mandarin are the major Chinese dialects. Chinese Americans' social and economic status varies from financially successful to below the poverty level.

In order to best assess a Chinese American patient's ideas about health care and cancer risks a health care worker must determine how many years the patient and family have lived in this country, and from which part of Asia or China they immigrated. Persons who have been in the country more than 20 years, are first or second generation Chinese Americans or are recent immigrants, tend to accept Western medicine but are still influenced by traditional modalities. Knowledge of personal or family beliefs and health practices will help the health professional plan care that is sensitive to the patient's cultural needs and distinct cancer risks (Leininger, 1977; Louie, 1985).

Epidemiology

The overall cancer mortality rate for Chinese Americans is lower than for white Americans in general: cancer accounts for only 27% of Chinese male and female deaths. Specific cancers that are found in Chinese Americans less frequently than in Caucasian Americans include prostate cancer and leukemia in males, and lymphomas (particularly Hodgkin's), breast, and genital cancers in females. Cancers that occur more frequently in the Chinese American population include nasopharyngeal and liver cancer among both sexes, esophageal cancers in men, and lung and stomach cancers in women (King and Locke, 1980; Yu, 1986).

The incidence of nasopharyngeal cancer (NPC) in Chinese Americans has de-

RISK ASSESSMENT QUESTIONS

PILIPINOS

Where do you live? (urban/rural)

With whom do you live? (extended family)

When was the last time you saw a medical doctor?

What medicines are you currently taking?

Are you using any traditional medicines or herbs? (drug interactions)

What types of foods do you eat? (traditional/American)

Do you smoke cigarettes?

Where do you work? (occupational exposure risks)

Has anyone in your family been diagnosed with liver cancer? Biliary cancer? Lymphoma?

Do you drink alcohol? How much?

Have you ever had a blood test for hepatitis done? Results? (liver cancer)

Have you ever had gallstones? (biliary cancer)

Have you ever had surgery for gallbladder problems? (biliary cancer)

Have you had any abdominal pain?

Does your abdomen appear bloated?

Have you noticed any change in the color of your urine or stool?

Have you experienced recent weight loss?

Has your neck felt swollen?

Have you experienced difficulty swallowing?

CHINESE

What religion do you practice? (health beliefs)

How long have you lived in this country? (assimilation)

With whom do you live and where? (urban vs. rural) (extended family influences)

What language is spoken at home?

Are there any ethnic foods you prefer when you are not feeling well?

What are some of your important social customs?

Are there any subjects that you would like to avoid discussing?

When you are sick do you seek the care of a faith healer/medicine man?

Are you taking any herbal or traditional Chinese medicine?

What do you believe causes illness?

Have you ever been hospitalized?

What types of foods do you eat? (traditional/American)

Where in China is your family from?

Where were you born? (risk factors)

Do you or does someone in your family smoke cigarettes? (risk factor)

Do you use incense or burn kerosene or coal in your stove at home?

What type of work do you do? (occupational exposures)

Has anyone in your family ever had cancer? If so, which kind?

clined since the 1960s, but this disease continues to be a leading cause of cancer deaths in this group. Genetic predisposition, exposure to the Epstein-Barr Virus (EBV), and dietary practices have been implicated as causes of NPC. Data suggest nasopharyngeal cancer occurs more commonly in immigrants from the southern portion of China, where elevated EBV titers are endemic (Chang, 1986; Kunz, Lam, Siu and Yeung, 1980).

Researchers have proposed that the increased incidence of lung cancer among Chinese American women is associated with previous lung disease, indoor pollutants such as kerosene or coal burning

RISK ASSESSMENT QUESTIONS—cont'd

CHINESE—cont'd

Have you ever had stomach surgery? (risk factor)

Do you have stomach problems? (risk factor)

Have you ever been tested for hepatitis B? (risk factor)

Do you have pain in your abdomen?

Have you been experiencing sore throats, hoarseness, a change in hearing, or earaches?

Have you noticed a change in your urine or stool color?

Have you had a recent weight loss?

Do you have trouble swallowing your food? Liquids?

Have you had problems with chronic esophagitis or gastritis?

Do you have any problems with cough?

Have you been running a fever?

JAPANESE

Where do you live? (urban/rural)

How long have you or your family lived in the United States?

With whom do you live? (extended family)

Do you see a medical doctor regularly?

Do you use any traditional medicines or treatments?

What kinds of foods do you eat? (traditional/American, risk factor)

Do you smoke cigarettes?

What kind of work do you do? (occupational risks)

Has anyone in your family ever had cancer? What kind?

Have you ever been treated for ulcers or stomach problems? (risk factor)

Have you ever had stomach surgery? (risk factor)

Have you ever been tested for hepatitis B? (risk factor)

Do you have any abdominal pain?

Have you had any difficulty swallowing food or liquids? Regurgitation?

Have you noticed any change in the color of your urine? stools?

Have you had a recent weight loss?

How is your appetite?

Have you had any indigestion?

Have you ever been tested for occult blood in your stomach secretions?

Have you ever had gallstones or gallbladder surgery?

stoves, passive cigarette smoke exposure, and vitamin A deficiency (Shimizu, Wu, Koo, Gao and Kolonel, 1985).

Risk factors related to the higher incidence of liver cancers in Chinese descendants include consumption of foods contaminated with mold and aflatoxin B, polluted drinking water, chronic hepatitis B infection, ingestion of foods high in nitrosamines, and vitamin C deficiency. Immigrants from the coastal and northeastern portions of China appear to be at greater risk of developing primary liver cancer (London and McGlynn, 1990; Wanebo, Falkson, and Order, 1989).

The incidence of esophageal cancer among Chinese American males is particularly pronounced in immigrants from eastern and central China, where the disease appears to be endemic in certain rural communities. Risk factors include: vitamin and mineral deficiencies; consumption of foods high in salt, sour pancakes, and fish paste; contamination of food grains with siliceous macrohairs (silica fibers); and consumption of large quantities of very hot tea (Gayal, 1983; Van Rensburg, 1987).

Risk factors for stomach cancer in the Chinese population include increasing age, the consumption of salt-cured and moldy foods, familial history of stomach cancer, emotional stress, smoking, a history of chronic gastritis, and stomach ulcers. Loss of gastric acidity has also been implicated as a risk factor (Namura, 1982).

The traditional Chinese diet consists primarily of complex carbohydrates such as rice and potatoes, salted foods, and cured fish, and includes few fruits and vegetables. Chinese Americans who follow this diet may be at greater risk for the development of diet-related cancers. As with most immigrant populations, Chinese Americans who have been exposed to the traditional Western lifestyle for several years seem to exhibit cancer incidence rates similar to the general U.S. population. Incidence rates for colorectal cancer among Chinese Americans have reached rates similar to those for U.S. whites in recent years (Whittemore et al., 1985).

Culture

As is the case with most Asian cultures, the Chinese tend to be very family-oriented (Kunz et al., 1980; Louie, 1985). Children are taught to show respect and deference to their parents and authority figures; grandparents hold a special place of honor in the family. Chinese Americans cherish their heritage. They often send their children to Chinese language classes and encourage socialization with persons of the same ethnic background.

Traditional families often expect personal sacrifice for the good of the family group, as opposed to individual achievement. A sense of duty or the need to avoid embarrassing the family may all be strong influences in the traditional Chinese American family. Confrontation and social assertiveness are viewed negatively, so many Chinese families stress the need for politeness and emotional restraint to their children.

Religion plays a major role in the life of the Chinese, including their health beliefs and practices (Kunz et al., 1980; Louie, 1985). Chinese may adhere to one of several religious philosophies, including Confucianism, Buddhism, or Taoism. Taoism espouses the idea of non-action and detachment from the world in order to allow things to be. Buddhism calls for adherence to natural changes or following the order of nature. The tenets of Confucianism state that fate guides one's life. All these religions value the balance and harmony of existence and the avoidance of extremes (Kunz et al., 1980; Louie, 1985).

Health Beliefs and Practices

Many Chinese accept Western forms of health and medical care. They espouse the concept of health promotion but not specifically cancer prevention. Members of this population may hold a variety of health beliefs, depending on their distance from their ethnic-cultural origin and their subsequent environmental and cultural exposure to American ways (Kunz et al., 1980; Louie, 1985).

The Chinese tend to be crisis-oriented in their use of westernized medicine, generally seeking health care from a physician only when absolutely necessary and often after having attempted to treat the illness themselves or with the aid of a herbalist. Many Chinese (as well as other Asians) avoid seeking health care at the beginning of the new year because they believe that to do so will cause them to be ill the entire year. As a result, these patients may delay the diagnosis and treatment of illnesses requiring immediate attention, such as cancer. Chinese patients often "doctor shop" until they find someone with whom they can relate. This often contributes to further delay in diagnosis of illness.

Traditional Chinese believe that spirits and fate determine health. They also espouse the practice of moderation to avoid the excesses that cause illness. Self-control is considered extremely important, so Chinese individuals may suppress strong negative feelings, anger, and expressions of pain.

Traditional remedies used by the Chinese include dietary and behavioral modifications to balance the extremes that lead to health and illness. In the traditional sense these practices may be considered preventive behaviors. The Chinese concepts of health and illness may also be based upon the principle of two forces, Yin and Yang, that determine the dynamic nature of the universe. Yang influences protect the body from outside elements and are represented by light and fullness, positiveness, and warmth. Yang conditions include hypertension, infection, upset stomach, and venereal disease. Yin influences are equated with darkness, cold, and emptiness. Cancer, pregnancy, and menstruation are considered Yin conditions.

Traditional Chinese believe foods have Yin or Yang properties that have a direct effect on health (Kunz et al., 1980; Louie, 1985). Yin conditions require Yang foods, and vice versa, to restore balance (Louie, 1985). In general, the Chinese prefer hot and warm beverages to cold beverages and usually do not eat raw vegetables and meats. Soy sauce, which is very high in sodium, is also used frequently.

Traditional Chinese commonly turn to folk medicine before seeking Western medical attention, especially when they do not think the condition is life threatening. They rely heavily on herbs to maintain health or treat illness, including ginseng, Chinese yam, and honeysuckle flower.

Some Chinese herbs have been found to have antibiotic and immunomodulating properties and are used in the treatment of cancer, often with good results

(Sun, 1988). Not all of the herbal teas and drinks are innocuous, however. Some have been found to have high concentrations of mercury and arsenic, leading to toxicity in some instances (Chiu, 1986). For these reasons, it is essential for the health care provider to be aware of all health preparations the Chinese patient may be using and the drug interactions that may occur (Louie, 1985). The smart health practitioner, however, will continue to allow the patient to use those remedies that are not contraindicated.

Massage, skin scraping or coin rubbing, cupping, moxibustion, balm application, and acupuncture are important elements of traditional Chinese medicine. Massage is used to stimulate circulation of energy and blood, to increase movement of stiff joints, and to increase the body's resistance to disease. There are two types of massage—pushing and grasping and palpating and massaging (Louie, 1985).

Cupping is a technique used to treat arthritis, stomach aches, abdominal pain, and abscesses. In this technique, heat is injected into a cup, which is then placed on the particular part of the body in need of healing, where it adheres firmly to the skin. Skin scraping is used to treat heatstroke, indigestion, and colic. In this technique, a coin or blunt smooth object is dipped in water or oil and scraped over the skin surface in a back and forth motion (Louie, 1985).

Moxibustion involves placing a burning moxa plant directly on the skin. It is used to treat mumps, convulsions, and nosebleeds and is often used in conjunction with acupuncture. Topical ointments and balms are often used for pain (Louie, 1985).

Traditional Chinese respect authority and believe that the physician is the leader of the health care team. They are unlikely to disagree with recommendations made by health professionals so as not to create conflict even if they are not clear about what has been suggested. Because they are small in stature, many Chinese tend to cut medication doses in half without consulting the physician. They are also very unfamiliar with the use of a pill as a means of administering medicine.

Because the Chinese have stigmatized mental or emotional illness, those with such problems will often seek medical care for somatic illnesses such as headaches, insomnia, dizziness, and other vague complaints such as difficulty with role performance or marital problems (Kunz et al., 1980; Lowe, 1985). Only those Chinese with severe emotional problems are admitted into psychiatric facilities because the family will try to care for these individuals at home to avoid shame.

Many Chinese limit the number of showers and baths they take during periods of illness because they believe extremes in temperatures cause illness or arthritis in later years. Some patients may try to avoid invasive diagnostic procedures, venipunctures, and surgeries because they fear that these procedures will release their spirits. Radiation therapy is viewed as a hotness, and is therefore considered a treatment that will weaken the body. Because many families believe in the need for body wholeness while in heaven, autopsies are rare, and if an amputation does occur, the family may wish to retain the limb so that it may ultimately be buried with the body (Kunz et al., 1980; Yu, 1987).

Physical Assessment

Health practitioners may need to tailor their physical assessment techniques to accommodate the attitudes of Chinese Americans. Maintaining a greater physical distance than one might with a Western patient is appropriate when possible. These patients tend to value modesty and privacy, so care providers should try not to expose more than one body part at a time. Exposure of the genitals, in particular, should be kept at a minimum. Care should be taken to avoid making the person feel chilled; elderly patients may even wish to keep a hat on during the examination. Most traditional Chinese will not want to talk about rectal or vaginal bleeding because they consider this dirty. The inclusion of family members of the same gender in discussions of medical and nursing interventions and health education will help promote knowledge retention as well as decrease the patient's anxiety, and increase the likelihood of compliance.

The Chinese client should also be informed about what the clinician plans to do before each step of the assessment process. Clinicians should avoid the use of complex technical expressions and should have an interpreter present when necessary to enhance communication if there is a chance that the patient does not understand English sufficiently. Ask the interpreter to repeat what he or she said so that you can be certain points are explained correctly. If a Chinese American patient has children who understand English, they can help interpret health information when necessary and promote their parents' acceptance of cancer prevention and early detection methods.

Chinese tend not to be very expressive and are socialized to avoid talking about their emotional problems. As a result, their silence may signify a multitude of situations, including an attempt to change the subject, to translate what you have said into Chinese, or to respond in English. Clinicians should not directly question these patients about moods, but rather use hypothetical situations. Again, with this population many somatic complaints can be rooted in psychological problems.

Due to the prevalence of nasopharyngeal cancer in the Chinese, it is important to begin screening for this neoplasm as early as 20 years of age. Inspection of the head and neck, paying close attention to complaints of hoarseness, sore throat, hearing changes, and earaches, is important.

Stomach and liver cancers are also prevalent among Chinese, so complaints of abdominal pain, fullness after meals, slight nausea, blood in the stools, indigestion, weight loss, or vomiting should be followed closely. Care providers should also assess the conjunctiva and fingernails for signs of anemia.

Health professionals working with identified high-risk groups for hepatitis should be vaccinated (Keehn and Frank-Stromborg, 1991). Persons at high risk for hepatitis B virus (i.e., individuals from

China, Southeast Asia) need to be screened and included in vaccination programs for the virus.

JAPANESE

The Japanese first came to the United States as poorly paid laborers. In recent years they have successfully integrated into the American mainstream, yet many still hold traditional beliefs. Like other A/PI populations, Japanese Americans tend to live along the West coast and in larger U.S. metropolitan areas. The Japanese American is familiar with Western medicine and tends to be more prevention-oriented than some of the other A/PI populations. Japanese may differ in their health beliefs and values depending on their gender, generation, and degree of identification with different cultural influences.

Epidemiology

The Japanese in America tend to have lower cancer incidence rates than do whites, and their cancer survival rates tend to be higher. Cancers that occur least frequently among the Japanese include cancers of the lung, genitourinary and nervous systems, and lymphomas and leukemias (Locke and King, 1980; Young, Ries, and Pollack, 1984). Cancers of the stomach, esophagus, liver, and gallbladder occur more frequently among Japanese Americans than among Caucasian Americans (Tominaga, 1985). In recent years Japanese Americans have experienced an increased incidence of breast, prostate, and colorectal cancers (Locke and King, 1980); this increased incidence has been correlated to the adoption of Western dietary and lifestyle habits.

Risk factors for stomach cancer in the Japanese population are linked to socioeconomic status, physical changes in the mucosa of the stomach, and environmental factors (Frank-Stromborg, 1989). A predisposition for gastric cancer appears to develop during the first two decades of life as a result of eating dried salted fish as a young child (Nomura, 1982). In addition, diets high in salt-cured foods and nitrites, and poor vitamin C intake are commonly associated with a greater incidence of stomach cancer. In many parts of the world, screening tests such as occult blood tests and gastric analyses are often performed on individuals considered at high risk for gastric cancer (Frank-Stromborg, 1989). Advancing age, Type A blood, history of gastric ulcers, and prior medical conditions that demonstrate a predisposition for decreased gastric acidity may also be important risk factors.

The Japanese often eat rice gruel cooked in hot tea, and this may elevate their risk for gastric cancer. Researchers have suggested that long-standing thermal injury may contribute to the development of esophageal cancer. A history of chronic esophagitis and the ingestion of foods contaminated with molds have also been implicated as risk factors (Gayal, 1983; Van Rensburg, 1985).

Many Japanese immigrants have been exposed to the same risk factors for liver cancers as are common among other Asians (see pp. 84-85). The risk of gallbladder cancer appears to be associated with a history of gallstones and ingestion of foods high in fat.

Culture

Traditional Japanese retain their cultural ties and maintain strong social support systems, including family and community ties. On the other hand, second-generation Japanese Americans, called Nisei, and third generation Japanese, called Sansei, tend to adopt more Western ways. They may be less likely to retain their parents' and grandparents' values. Even those Japanese who appear acculturated, however, may still maintain many traditional customs and values.

Close family ties are important to the Japanese American. Children are raised to maintain the dignity of the family at all costs. The worst of all situations is bringing shame upon one's family (haji). If an individual dishonors the family, he or she will live under the fear that a curse (bachi) might befall them in the form of a hereditary disease, physical handicap, mental illness, or a string of misfortunes (Lee and Takamura, 1980).

In traditional Japanese families the men are the formal decision makers and are responsible for the economic well-being of the family. Women are expected to care for the young and elderly, as well as the household. Japanese are taught not to question authority either within or outside the family. Japanese families also value harmony, conformity, and the avoidance of conflict. As a group, they prize self-control and are very reserved (Lee and Takamura, 1980).

Health Beliefs and Practices

The traditional Japanese believe that illness represents an imbalance or disorder. Like many Chinese, Japanese believe that the balance between Yin forces and Yang forces has an impact on health. In the concept of Yin and Yang the universe and the human being are composed of two opposite forces: the masculine, or Yang, as represented by light, strength, and heat; and the feminine, or Yin, as represented by darkness, softness and cold. Extremes in either direction will produce disease (Hoang, 1982). Certain diseases are said to result from an excess of the cold element, such as diarrhea that results from a "cold" stomach. Other diseases are ascribed to an excess of the hot element: pimples or pustules, for example, are a manifestation of an excess of a hot element erupting through the skin. Similarly, foods are divided into two groups; hot foods include spices, coffee, beef, and wild game; cold foods include tea, fruits, chicken, duck, and fish. Likewise, drugs and medicinal herbs are also classified according to their properties along a scale of hot and cold effects (Nguyen, 1985).

Some Japanese also believe that disease results from contact with pollutants or from reneging on family obligations. They also believe that the psyche and body are one; Confucianism holds that if the body is healed so will be the soul.

More acculturated Japanese tend to accept Western medicine more readily. However, the health practitioner should still assess whether the patient is also using traditional therapy. Many traditional

Japanese medical practitioners utilize pharmacotherapy, acupuncture, moxibustion, and massage to restore balance between the Yin and Yang elements in the body. In addition, they may use massage and herbal medicines similar to those of the Chinese (see p. 94).

In traditional Japanese culture the family assumes most of the responsibility for health. Physicians are thought to be skilled and sympathetic but are expected to allow patients to keep their innermost feelings to themselves. The role of the physician is to give the treatment and disclose the "bad news" to the family— although children are seldom informed about the severity of their parent's illness. When hospitalization is necessary, the family should be involved in the patient's care as much as possible in order to relieve the patient's anxiety and promote his or her emotional and physical comfort.

Many Japanese practice Buddhism, which reinforces the principle that one should avoid verbal analysis of one's emotions. Therefore, health care providers should consider using somatopsychic therapies such as biofeedback, autogenic training, and behavior modification with Japanese patients.

Out of respect for authority, Japanese American patients may not question physicians' decisions about treatment even if they conflict with patient's wishes. Clinicians should explain to these patients that they are allowed to voice their opinions; only then can the practitioner determine whether the patient will comply with recommended treatment.

Physical Assessment and Cultural Implications

The Japanese tend to value modesty. It is important for the health care practitioner to take care not to expose too many body parts, particularly the genitalia. Whenever possible, a clinician of the same gender as the patient should perform pelvic and genital examinations.

Japanese tend to be smaller than white Americans and so may need doses of medication adjusted accordingly. Japanese have slightly yellow skin color, so clinicians should assess jaundice by looking at the sclera of the eyes and the excreta.

Care providers may need to reassure Japanese American patients that they are allowed to express pain; they should explain that other patients in similar situations would do so, or that this information will aid in diagnosis. Also, because these patients tend to be less verbal, it is important to give them the opportunity to disagree with care suggestions or planned treatments. When patients are asked what they think is wrong and how it should be treated, they may be more receptive to suggestions and more likely to take an active role in their health care management.

If care providers are unsure whether their Japanese American patients understand English sufficiently, the providers should arrange for an interpreter to be present. Inclusion of the family, especially the eldest son, in medical discussions with older Japanese American clients will help ease their anxiety, increase their comprehension of information discussed, and encourage compliance with therapy.

VIETNAMESE

Approximately 1.4 million Indochinese refugees fled their homelands between 1975 and 1982. Nearly 40% of these were Vietnamese refugees who settled in the United States. They, like other Indochinese refugees, confronted multiple problems upon their arrival: They could not turn to a previously established group of Vietnamese in the United States for initial support; their culture was significantly different from American culture; and they were often identified with the unpopular Vietnam war (Nguyen 1985). In addition, most Vietnamese were political refugees who still hoped to return to their homeland one day. These problems seriously impeded their access to social, economic, and political opportunities in American society, and to health care resources.

Epidemiology

National health care statistics contain very little about the health care status and needs of the Vietnamese people. Because the Vietnamese American population is small, no cancer incidence or mortality statistics are currently available for this group; however, this will change, because they are the fastest growing A/PI group in the United States. As the Vietnamese adopt certain Western behaviors, including cigarette smoking, increased intake of dietary fat, and consumption of alcohol, their risk for cancer increases significantly (Jenkins, McPhee, Bird, and Bonilla, 1990).

There is also a high incidence of infection with hepatitis B virus (HBV) among Vietnamese, which puts this population at significant risk for liver cancer (see p. 81 and p. 84) (Jenkins et al., 1990). Lin-Fu (1988) documented in 1987 that as many as 14% of Vietnamese refugees tested positive for HBV, and 8% were chronic carriers of the virus. Persons who test positive for HBV may not have active hepatitis; however, chronic carriers are both a source of infection and at high risk for developing cirrhosis and hepatoma. The latency period from time of HBV infection to onset of liver cancer may be as long as 35 years (Frogge, 1990). Perinatal transmission from carrier mothers to their infants poses a particularly serious problem; about 90% of infants infected perinatally will become chronic carriers.

The goal of primary prevention measures for HBV infection is to prevent transmission of the virus to newborns, thus reducing their risk for liver cancer (Jenkins et al., 1990). Neonates born of HBV-positive mothers can be immunized at birth with hepatitis B immune globulin and then placed on an immunization regimen with hepatitis B vaccine.

Secondary prevention measures target adult hepatitis carriers. Adults who test positive for the HBV surface antigen should be monitored every 6 months with the alpha-fetoprotein (AFP) assay. After birth, healthy persons synthesize only small quantities of AFP, concentrations less than 50 ng/ml. Liver tumors frequently synthesize large quantities of AFP; concentrations in excess of 400 ng/ml are diagnostic of primary hepatocellular carcinoma. Therefore, health care providers should monitor adult carriers of HBV for increases in serum AFP to detect liver tumors early (McGlynn, 1986; London and McGlynn, 1990). If detected early, surgical removal of the tumor is possible.

Culture

The Vietnamese have few family names; Nguyen is the most common. Although Vietnamese are traditionally addressed by their first names, they usually write their names in the following order: family name, middle name, and first name. This may create confusion in medical record keeping.

In Vietnamese culture, the family is the fundamental social unit (Nguyen, 1985). Vietnamese place high value on family loyalty: children are raised to honor their parents and learn early that their behavior reflects on their family as well as on themselves.

If a Vietnamese dishonors his family, that person can "lose face," which is called "mat mat." If one person wrongs another, bad luck, or "xui" is believed to occur.

The Vietnamese have been strongly influenced by several sets of religious beliefs. Buddhism was introduced to Vietnam from India and China as early as the second century A.D. Many Vietnamese believe strongly in karma, the concept that an impersonal force or a law of causality determines human life. Such a belief leads to fatalistic attitudes toward health and illness. Accepting one's destiny may mean resignation, but it may also provide hope; things may be destined to improve at anytime (Gordon, Matousek, and Lang, 1980).

According to traditional Buddhist beliefs, suffering is caused by desire. Desire can be eliminated and suffering thus avoided, through correct behavior. That behavior is dictated by the "Eight-Fold Path": right understanding, right purpose, right speech, right conduct, right vocation, right effort, right thinking, and right meditation (Hoang, 1982).

Confucianism, imported from China, is more a way of life based on a code of morals and ethics than it is a true religion. This philosophy emphasizes the hierarchy of societal members and stresses ancestor worship. In the Confucian world view the head is a sacred part of the body, so it is impolite to pat the head of a Vietnamese adult. Because the feet are the lowest part of the body, it is offensive to point one's foot toward another. To signal for someone to approach by using an upturned finger is considered a provocation because Vietnamese commonly use that gesture with dogs; waving with the whole hand is considered more proper (Nguyen, 1985).

A third religion that has influenced Vietnamese culture, Taoism, originated from the sixth century B.C. philosopher Lao-tzu. This philosophy stresses that when things are permitted to assume their natural course, they move toward perfection and harmony (Hoang, 1982).

The Vietnamese' esteem for harmony has influenced their specific communication practices. The Vietnamese cannot easily answer "no" because they feel such an answer would create disharmony. Therefore, any "yes" answer should be cautiously interpreted because it could reflect an attempt to avoid confrontation or to please the addressee, rather than a valid affirmation (Gordon, Matousek, and Lang, 1980).

Whatever their religious beliefs, most Vietnamese value self-control and modesty (Nguyen, 1985). Emotions are considered weaknesses in that they interfere with self-control. As a result, most Vietnamese rarely complain of pain or express emotion. Such stoicism can contribute to denial and even difficulty assessing health problems.

Health Beliefs and Practices

The Vietnamese will frequently use folk treatments (traditional medicines) either before seeking or while using Western medical care. These folk treatments are influenced by the concepts of Yin and Yang, from which a number of folk medicine techniques (Nguyen, 1985) have evolved:

1. Cao gio, or "coin rubbing" with hot balm oil, produces ecchymotic marks and petechiae on the chest and back, and is done in hopes of bringing "bad wind" or toxicity to the body surface so it can escape. Unfortunately, some health professionals have mistaken these markings for signs of physical abuse.
2. Be bao, "skin pinching," is a derivative of the above practice.
3. Giac, "cup suctioning," is a procedure in which a cup is heated and then placed on the skin. As it cools it contracts, bringing bad wind or toxicity into the cup; a circular ecchymotic area is left on the skin.
4. Xong, "herbal steam inhalation," is done with the whole body covered by a heavy blanket; patients may also ingest herbal concoctions.
5. Tiger balm or MacPhsu Cula oil may also be applied to the skin.

These folk medicine techniques are important self-care practices for the Vietnamese. They rarely present a health threat, and can serve to make the person feel cared for and able to respond to disturbing symptoms. Besides using folk medicine, many Vietnamese will readily use Western medicine, particularly drugs. Most are familiar with the beneficial effects of Western medicine, but few understand the risks of overdosing or inadequate doses. Vietnamese may believe "more is better" and therefore prefer drastic treatments; they also think injections are more powerful and will provide relief more rapidly than an oral drug.

Because medicine usually deals with invisible elements, Vietnamese rarely feel a need for invasive techniques or surgical procedures (Nguyen, 1985). Cutting the flesh is thought to disrupt harmony, so surgery is associated with death and therefore considered only as a last resort. Vietnamese refugees may also fear bloodletting and need clear explanations about its necessity. The health professional should take as much blood as is needed for all tests during one procedure in order to minimize the number of punctures.

Clinicians should remember that folk medicine and Western medicine can usually be used together without harm to the patient. The Vietnamese are more likely to trust their care providers and comply with suggested care if those providers demonstrate understanding and respect for Vietnamese cultural beliefs. Vietnamese families may also want to be involved in any major decisions concerning the health care of an individual member (Nguyen, 1985).

Physical Assessment and Risk Factor Assessment

Specific cultural beliefs and practices of Vietnamese Americans can affect their attitudes about modesty, nudity, and the touching or invasion of one's body. Clinicians should be aware of this when they conduct a physical assessment of a Vietnamese patient. The box to the right reviews specific cultural implications for the physical assessment of Vietnamese clients.

Because physical examination should be as complete as possible, the box at the top left of p. 107 summarizes the areas of physical assessment to which health care workers need to pay particular attention with Indochinese patients. The box at the top right of p. 107 summarizes important screening and laboratory tests.

The box at the bottom of p. 107 provides a general guide for gathering information about the cultural beliefs and practices of each client. A comprehensive risk-factor assessment guide is provided on pp. 87-89.

CAMBODIANS AND LAOTIANS

While the term Indochinese is often used to refer to refugees from Vietnam, Cambodia (now named Kampuchea), and Laos, the countries are quite different. The

---

CULTURAL IMPLICATIONS FOR PHYSICAL ASSESSMENT WITH VIETNAMESE, HMONG, CAMBODIAN, AND KOREAN INDIVIDUALS

1. Explanation of all procedures and the necessity for them should be given in a clear and simple manner.
2. The human head is regarded as the seat of life, so examination of the head and its orifices should be done in a respectful and gentle manner.
3. Avoid complete disrobing of the female patient. Adults are more comfortable with health care providers of their own gender.
4. Pelvic examinations of unmarried Southeast Asian women should not be routinely undertaken because premarital sex is condemned and virginity in a bride is of great importance. When there is a medical indication for a pelvic exam, the woman may want her husband present; if possible the practitioner and the interpreter, if needed, should be female.
5. An interpreter is of great value, but avoid the visible presence of an interpreter of the opposite sex during breast or genital examinations.

Adapted from Muecke, 1983; Gordon, Matousek, and Lang, 1980.

Hmong of Laos and the Khmer of Cambodia have many distinct cultural attributes that health care workers should know. According to the 1980 census, the Laotians and Kampucheans made up only about 2% of the Asian American population, but estimates showed that they doubled in number in the United States by 1985 (Disease Prevention/Health Promotion: The Facts, 1986).

PHYSICAL ASSESSMENT AREAS REQUIRING SPECIAL ATTENTION WITH INDOCHINESE POPULATIONS

1. Skin—superficial fungal infections or scabies have been found in 10% to 15% of refugees.
2. Dental—moderate to severe dental problems occur in 90% of refugees.
3. Eye and Ear—otitis media and conjunctivitis are common; screening for hearing and vision defects should be done.
4. Endocrine—thyroid disease, particularly euthyroid goiters, have been found.
5. Cardiovascular—mitral valve disease, hypertension, and rheumatic heart disease have been detected.
6. Abdomen—special attention to assessment of the liver for cirrhosis and/or hepatoma.

SCREENING LABORATORY TESTS OF PARTICULAR IMPORTANCE IN INDOCHINESE POPULATIONS

1. Complete blood cell count: to screen for anemia and hemoglobin disorders, such as thalassemia and hemoglobin E, which are common in Southeast Asians.
2. VDRL: checked on entry to U.S., but needs to be rechecked for accuracy.
3. Urinalysis: check for microscopic hematuria.
4. Hepatitis B surface antigen: overall hepatitis prevalence rate among Indochinese refugees is 13%. If positive, do alpha-fetoprotein assay.
5. Stool: for intestinal parasites; ascaris, hookworm, giardia, and trichuris are most common.
6. Tuberculosis: Rate among Southeast Asian refugees is 14 to 70 times higher than that among Americans.

From Lin-Fu, 1988

Epidemiology

As with the Vietnamese population, there are no national health statistics or cancer incidence rates for the Laotians or Kampucheans. However, these two groups face the same magnitude of risk for liver cancer from infection with the hepatitis B virus as the Vietnamese do (see p. 103).

Culture, Health Beliefs, and Practices

Kampucheans speak the language of Khmer; the population of Laos is a mixture of many ethnic groups that speak a number of different dialects. The Hmong, a hill tribe of Laos, speak only their own dialect and do not understand the dialects of other Laotians. Such language differ-

INTERVIEW QUESTIONS FOR CULTURAL ASSESSMENT

1. What are your health care experiences?
2. Family composition: Who lives at home? Are you a first, second, or third generation immigrant?
3. What family member should be present to assist in decision-making?
4. Religion: What is your religion? What religious practices or rituals do you follow that affect your health practices?
5. Illness beliefs and healing practices: Do you use any herbs, traditional folk medicine techniques, or healers?
6. When you are sick, who do you go to first?

From Neiderhauser, 1989.

ences can become a barrier to adequate health care.

Many Hmong believe in gods, demons, evil spirits, and the spirits that reside in natural objects. They believe sickness is caused by the wrath of gods, so their healers are priests who negotiate with the gods to remove or alleviate sickness. These healer-priests, called shamans, are believed to have superhuman powers because of their ability to influence the gods (Muecke, 1983). The Hmong also use many herbal remedies.

Many Cambodians or Kampucheans also believe in the presence of spirits. Sickness may be the result of evil spells or spirit possession. Traditional healers, called "Kru Khmer," are called on to treat emotional disorders and any physical conditions thought to be caused by spirits. Like other Asian groups the Khmer believe in Yin-Yang, or "hot-cold," and also employ dermabrasive procedures to treat health problems (see p. 101) (Kemp, 1985).

Many Southeast Asians wear strings around their wrists and amulets on necklaces. The Laotians and Kampucheans believe wrist strings prevent soul loss, which is thought to cause illness. In a commonly practiced ritual, a soul-caller and respected elders bind the sick person's soul in his or her body by tying strings around the wrists (and, for infants, the neck, ankles, or waist). The strings thus signify both spiritual wholeness and social support of the sick person. This ritual is also performed when a person is going to face a major change, such as marriage or leaving home. If Western health care workers decide the strings must be removed for medical purposes, they should explain the need and obtain the patient's consent; some patients might want to keep the strings (Muecke, 1983).

Refugees may feel vulnerable and afraid in the United States. Access to other institutional sources, such as church and school, and to informal social groups may be limited for members of these cultures. Because the health care system may be one of the few culturally sanctioned sources of support, many immigrants may actually seek care and attention from health care providers. Nurses can use this to their advantage to promote prevention and early detection activities by planning traditional and nontraditional programs and services geared to these populations.

Physical Assessment and Cultural Implications

The cultural implications of physical assessment techniques identified for Vietnamese clients (see the box on p. 106) can also be applied to the Hmong of Laos and the Kampucheans.

Health care personnel should be aware that many Southeast Asians stigmatize mental illness. When these patients are in psychological distress they often complain about physical ailments without being able to specify the problem; indeed, there may be no clinical evidence of a physical problem (Kemp, 1985). This reaction called "somatization," is a culturally acceptable way of revealing an emotional illness.

Southeast Asian patients may fail to comply with the medical or nursing plan of care if their symptoms abate, the medical regimen is inconvenient, or there is no precedent for the regimen in their culture. The nurse needs to carefully explain the plan of care to the patient and incorporate cultural self-care practices to promote adherence to the regimen and to follow-up (Muecke, 1983). For example, the nurse might explain that the patient can continue to drink herbal tea to treat their stomach pain as long as they also take the medication that the doctor prescribed. This will help maintain the balance of "hot" and "cold" that many of these patients believe is necessary to restore their health. Trained interpreters, refugee advocates, or caseworkers who understand ethnic and cultural backgrounds of Laotians and Kampucheans can help ensure compliance with the plan of care.

KOREANS

According to the 1980 census, Koreans make up about 10% of the Asian-American population. Most members of this group have immigrated to this country since 1965, when a new U.S. immigration bill was passed that prohibited discrimination against Asian immigrants. By and large, Korean families have come to this country by their own choice, and they come with the intention of staying. Koreans are usually well educated (Pang, 1980); however, because of language barriers and professional licensure requirements, they have difficulty in finding jobs commensurate with those they held

in Korea, and must often accept a lowered socioeconomic status.

Epidemiology

Because the Korean American population is fairly small, few national statistics or other data exist documenting their health care needs. As with other Asian American groups, recent immigrants from Korea need to be screened for tuberculosis, parasitic infections, and hepatitis B.

Culture, Health Beliefs, and Practices

Many Koreans have adapted to Western culture without losing their ethnic identity. Traditional values center around a strict hierarchical society and the extended family. These values include respect for elders, family pride, respect for learning, and strict sex role differences, with women generally in a subservient position. However, as they assimilate Western values, Koreans have largely replaced the extended family with the nuclear family, and women are taking their place in society (Pang, 1980).

Today, most Koreans are Christian. However, Chinese philosophies of Confucianism, Taoism, and Buddhism have all influenced Korean culture. Since the beginning of the twentieth century, a number of religions have developed around various charismatic leaders, such as the church of Sun Myong Moon (Pang, 1980).

Koreans traditionally believe that to stay healthy, they must maintain a balance between the elements that make up a person: the mind and the body. Many

Koreans also feel that if there is discord in interpersonal relationships, illness will ensue. On the other hand, if the mind is at peace, the body is free to be healthy.

Some Korean patients with mental illnesses will present the problem as a somatic complaint. Koreans recognize psychosomatic complaints as legitimate illnesses.

Koreans may employ a number of alternative therapies. They may consult traditional medical practitioners, such as shamans or mudangs, who are herbalists and faith healers. For large problems, such as cancer or a condition that may require surgery, the Korean patient will go to a Western medical doctor first. If he does not get results, then he may turn to a herbalist or a shaman. For a small problem such as a headache, stomach ache, or high blood pressure, the patient will probably try a herbalist; this healer may recommend a diet change, drugs to "purify the blood," or poyak which is a general health supplement or tonic such as ginseng (Pang, 1980).

Most Korean immigrants adamantly believe that individuals know best about their own health, and they are accustomed to taking responsibility for their health care. Koreans also believe shots are more effective than pills, so they may demand them. Koreans may also become impatient with physicians who want to run lengthy diagnostic tests, and so seek Western health care only as a last resort.

Physical Assessment and Cultural Implications

Health care professionals should apply the same cultural sensitivity to the physical assessment of Korean patients as is recommended for other Asian Americans. Again, attention to the patients' modesty is essential in any exam, and clear explanations of all procedures are also necessary (see boxes on pp. 106 and 107).

Risk Factor Assessment Questions

Besides a thorough physical assessment, care providers should also perform a thorough cancer risk factor assessment (see box on pp. 87-89) and cultural assessment (see box on p. 107). Health care workers should note that each immigrant to the United States must be evaluated as an individual in order to determine the degree of their conformity to traditional American views, and the extent of their adaptation to American views and values.

RESOURCES FOR CANCER PREVENTION/EARLY DETECTION

Health care providers serving Asian Americans need to familiarize themselves with the special health problems and the ethnocultural barriers that limit the use of health services. Educational efforts must target Asian American community organizations, churches, grocery stores, and newspapers. Cancer education materials and outreach programs must be culturally sensitive, understandable, and relevant to the Asian/Pacific Islanders. "Sources for Cancer Prevention/Early Detection Materials," is a current listing of sources of health information for the Asian Pacific populations.

REFERENCES

1. American Cancer Society: *Cancer and the poor: A report to the nation*, Atlanta, 1989, American Cancer Society.
2. Anderson JN: Health and illness in Pilipino immigrants, *Western Journal of Medicine* 139:811-819, 1983.
3. Baquet CR: *Cancer data*. Paper presented at the meeting of the American Society of Clinical Oncologists, May 1990.
4. Baysa E, Cabrera E, Camilon F, Torres M: The Pilipinos. In Palafox N, Warren A, editors: *Cross-cultural caring: A handbook for health care professionals in Hawaii*, 197-231. Honolulu, 1980, Transcultural Health Care Forum.
5. Benoliel JQ: Implications for nursing interventions, *Cancer Nursing* 10 (Suppl):167-170, 1987.
6. Chao Y: Folk curing and caring activities concurrently practiced by Chinese patients receiving radiotherapy, *Cancer Nursing* 10 (Suppl 1):145-152, 1987.
7. Chiu L: *Heavy metal poisoning from Chinese medications*. Conference on health problems related to the Chinese in America: 64-67, San Francisco, 1986, Chinese Hospital.
8. Fitzpatrick S, et al: Health care needs of Indochinese refugee teenagers. *Pediatrics* 79:118-124, 1987.
9. Flaskerud JH, Soldevilla EQ: Pilipino and Vietnamese clients: Utilizing an Asian mental health center, *Journal of Psychosocial Nursing* 24:32-36, 1986.
10. Frank-Stromborg M: The epidemiology and primary prevention of gastric and esophageal cancer: A worldwide perspective, *Cancer Nursing* 12:53-64, 1989.
11. Frank-Stromborg M, Olsen SJ: Focus group interview data, National cancer prevention and screening workshops for minority nurses. 1988. Unpublished report.
12. Frogge MH: Gastrointestinal cancer: Esophagus, stomach, liver, and pancreas. In Groenwald SL, Frogge MH, Goodman M, Yarbro CH, editors: *Cancer nursing: Principles and practice*, 806-841. Boston, 1990, Jones and Bartlett.
13. Gayal R: *Disease of the esophagus*. In Petersdorf R, Adams R, Braunwald E, Isselbacher K, Martin J, Wilson J, editors: *Harrison's principles of internal medicine*, 1687-1697, New York, 1983, McGraw-Hill.
14. Gordon V, Matosek I, Lang T: Southeast Asian refugees: Life in America, *American Journal of Nursing* 80:2031-2036, 1980.
15. Harras Angela: Personal correspondence, 1991.
16. Hoang GN: Cultural barriers to effective medical care among Indochinese patients, *Annual Review of Medicine* 36:229-239, 1985.
17. Hoang G, Erickson R: Guidelines for providing medical care to southeast Asian refugees, *Journal of the American Medical Association* 248:710-714, 1982.
18. Jenkins C, McPhee S, Bird J, Bonilla N: Cancer risks and prevention practices among Vietnam refugees, *Western Journal of Medicine* 153:34-39, 1990.
19. Keehn D, Frank-Stromborg M: A worldwide perspective on the epidemiology and primary prevention of liver cancer, *Cancer Nursing* 14:163-174, 1991.
20. Kemp C: Cambodian refugee health care beliefs and practices, *Journal of Community Health Nursing* 2:41-52, 1985.
21. Kolonel LN: Cancer incidence among Filipinos in Hawaii and the Philippines, *National Cancer Institute Monographs* 69:93-98, 1984.
22. Kunz K, Lam C, Sui K, Yeung K: The Chinese. In Palafox N, Warren A, editors: *Cross-cultural caring: A handbook for health care professionals in Hawaii*, 26-50. Honolulu, 1980, Transcultural Health Forum.
23. Lee P, Takamura J: The Japanese. In Palafox N, Warren A, editors: *Cross-cultural caring: A handbook for health care professionals in Hawaii*, 105-135. Honolulu, 1980, Transcultural Health Care Forum.
24. Leininger GR: Cultural diversities of health and nursing care, *Nursing Clinics of North America* 12:5-18, 1977.
25. Lin-Fu JS: Population characteristics and health care needs of Asian Pacific Americans, *Public Health Reports* 103:18-25, 1988.
26. Locke B, King H: Cancer mortality risks among Japanese in the United States, *Journal of the National Cancer Institute* 65:1149-1156, 1980.
27. London WT, McGlynn KA: Hepatitis and the prevention of liver cancer. In DeVita Jr VT, Hellman S, Rosenberg SA, editors: *Cancer prevention*, Philadelphia, 1990, JB Lippincott.
28. Louie KB: Providing health care to Chinese clients, *Topics in Clinical Nursing* 10:18-25, 1985.
29. McGlynn K, London W, Hann H, Sharrar R: Prevention of primary hepatocellular carcinoma in Asian populations in the Delaware Valley, *Progress in Clinical and Biological Research* 216:237-246, 1986.
30. Muecke M: Caring for southeast Asian refugee patients in the USA, *American Journal of Public Health* 73:431-438, 1980.
31. Muecke MA: In search of healers—Southeast Asian refugees in the American health care system, *Western Journal of Medicine* 139:835-840, 1983.

32. Newell GR: Social characteristics of minorities and the underprivileged, *The Cancer Bulletin* 40:105-107, 1988.

33. Niederhauser V: Health care of immigrant children: Incorporating culture into practice, *Pediatric Nursing* 15:569-574, 1989.

34. Nguyen M: Culture shock: A review of Vietnamese culture and its concept of health and disease, *Western Journal of Medicine* 142:409-412, 1985.

35. Nomura A: Stomach cancer. In Schottenfeld D, Fraumeni J, editors: *Cancer epidemiology and prevention*, 624-637, Philadelphia, 1982, WB Saunders.

36. Office of Disease Prevention and Health Promotion: *Disease prevention/health promotion: The facts*, Bethesda, Md, 1986, U.S. Public Health Service.

37. Owan TC: *Southeast Asian mental health: Treatment, prevention, services, training, and research*, Rockville, Md, 1985, National Institute of Mental Health.

38. Pang C: The Koreans. In Palafox N, Warren A, editors: *Cross-cultural caring: A handbook for health care professionals in Hawaii*, 136-154. Honolulu, 1988, Transcultural Health Forum.

39. Shimizu H, Wu AH, Koo LC, Gao Y, Kolonel LN: Lung cancer in women living in the Pacific Basin area, *National Cancer Institute Monographs* 69:197-201, 1985.

40. Sirota H, Rubovits D, Cousins J, Weinberg A, Laufman L, Lane M: Cancer control: Special populations, *Health Values* 12:46-50, 1988.

41. Stoloff L: Aflatoxin is not probably a human carcinogen: The published evidence is sufficient, *Regul Toxicol Pharmacol* 10:272-283, 1989.

42. Sun Y: The role of traditional Chinese medicine in supportive care of cancer patients, *Recent Results in Cancer Research* 108:327-334, 1988.

43. Sutherland J, Avant R, Franz W, Monzon C, Stark N: Indochinese refugee health assessment and treatment, *Journal of Family Practice* 16:61-67, 1983.

44. Tominaga S: Cancer incidence in Japanese in Japan, Hawaii, and Western United States, *National Cancer Institute Monographs* 69:83-92, 1985.

45. Van Rensburg S: Esophageal cancer risk factors common to endemic regions, *South African Medicine* (Suppl):9-11, 1987.

46. Wanebo HJ, Falkson G, Order SE: Cancer of the hepatobiliary system. In DeVita VT, Hellman S, Rosenberg SA, editors: *Cancer: Principles and practice of oncology*, 836-874, Philadelphia, 1989, JB Lippincott.

47. Warren A, Lam T: The Vietnamese. In Palafox N, Warren A, editors: *Cross-cultural caring: A handbook for health care professionals in Hawaii*, 289-302, Honolulu, 1980, Transcultural Health Care Forum.

48. World Health Organization: *World health statistics annual*, 381-382, Geneva, 1989.

49. Whittemore AS, Zheng S, Wu A, Wu ML, Fingar T, Jiao D, Ling C, Bao J, Henderson BE, Paffenbarger Jr RS: Colorectal cancer in Chinese-Americans, *National Cancer Institute Monographs* 69:43-46, 1985.

50. Wu AH: Epidemiology of lung cancer in Chinese females, *Conference on health problems related to the Chinese in America*, San Francisco, 1982, Chinese Hospital.

51. Yu ES: Health of the Chinese elderly in America. *Research on Aging* 8:84-109, 1986.

Cancer Prevention and Early Detection in Native Hawaiians

This chapter takes a critical look at the alarming health profile of the Native Hawaiian, the indigenous people of Hawai'i, and gives focus to the particular vulnerability of this population to cancer mortality. While this disease is a leading cause of death nationwide. Native Hawaiians suffer a death rate for cancer that is 39% greater than their American counterparts. They also suffer disproportionately from other significant chronic diseases which underlie premature disability and early mortality, such as diabetes mellitus, heart disease, stroke and hypertension.

Among the multicultures who live in Hawai'i, Native Hawaiians have been singled out to be at greatest health risk. In a state that can boast a longer life span than any other state, Native Hawaiians experience the shortest life expectancy and have earlier onset, poorer survival, and higher rates of occurrence in every major disease category.

Adding to this dilemma are evidences of psychosocial-cultural decline as seen in the overrepresentation of Native Hawaiian children in special education classes, the overrepresentation of the Native Hawaiians on Medicaid roles and as incarcerated adults and in youth correctional facilities.

This chapter recalls the skill and sophistication of the Native Hawaiian culture prior to Captain Cook's arrival in 1778, when health, or ola, included a consciousness of spiritual and psychological well-being, as well as physical well-being.

Time passage and acculturation influenced the systematic suppression of this sophisticated past and has impacted profound changes in the lifestyle of present day Native Hawaiians.

The challenge to change this dismal situation is before us. Success will come in the ability of health care providers to understand and empathize the tremendous impact acculturation has made on the Native Hawaiian population. The strengths of their rich history, should be recalled and acknowledged as the health care system reaches out to engage them in creative ways. Pride of heritage can be the stimulus for a powerful awakening and can provide the sustaining motivation necessary to bring about the needed positive change.

This chapter provides the impetus for planning such change.

3

Cancer Prevention and Early Detection in Native Hawaiians

LORETTA OBEDLYN LEINANI HUSSEY
JOANNE K. ITANO
KAREN N. TAOKA
YVONNE C. YOUNG

Native Hawaiians are often classified with other Asian/Pacific Islander groups such as the Japanese, Chinese, and Pilipinos because of their common geographic origins. However, the culture, historic background, and cancer statistics of Native Hawaiians differ from those of the other ethnic groups classified as Asian/Pacific Islanders.

As an ethnic group indigenous to the United States, Native Hawaiians are, technically speaking, Native Americans, but are more specifically referred to as Native Hawaiians since they originate exclusively from the state of Hawai'i. In fact, approximately 66% of all Native Hawaiians in the U.S. live in Hawai'i, and studies and surveys of this population deal only with Hawaiian residents.

However, like Native Americans from the continental United States, Native Hawaiians have experienced an invasion of their homeland by Westerners, deculturation, and subsequent attempts by the government to provide reparation. Today, Native Hawaiians are experiencing a cultural resurgence and renewed pride in their heritage and identity.

Under Title VIII of the Native American Programs Act of 1975, the term Native Hawaiian refers to all descendants of the population of Hawai'i before 1778, i.e., before Western contact (Wegner, 1989c). However, people residing outside Hawai'i frequently misapply the term "Native Hawaiian" to any non-white ethnic group living in Hawai'i. This is an affront to the true indigenous people of Hawai'i, who have their own unique culture. Native Hawaiians are divided into two categories, pure Hawaiians of un-mixed ancestry and part-Hawaiians (progeny of interracial marriages/alliances); each has certain distinct characteristics.

GENERAL DEMOGRAPHIC CHARACTERISTICS

Within the Native Hawaiian population a certain amount of diversity exists in lifestyles, socioeconomic status, and degree of assimilation of mainstream American culture. However, the majority of the Native Hawaiians share certain cultural and demographic characteristics. Unless otherwise noted, the demographic information in this section is based on figures from the 1980 U.S. Census report.

Population Statistics

According to the 1990 U.S. Census, 211,014 Native Hawaiians reside in the U.S. with 138,742 living in the state of Hawai'i (U.S. Bureau of the Census, 1991). This census did not distinguish between pure Hawaiians and part Hawaiians. However, the majority of Native Hawaiians are part-Hawaiian due to marriages across ethnic boundaries.

Before contact with Westerners in 1778, Native Hawaiians numbered 1 million and were all pure Hawaiian. By 1893, their numbers had dropped to 40,000 and the race had been "diluted" by intermarriage to the extent that only about 45% were pure Hawaiian. In 1985, this group comprised 19% of the state's population. However, of this number, less than 5% could be considered pure Hawaiian (Blaisdell, 1989; Native Hawaiian Health Care Improvement Act, 1988).

Native Hawaiians live on all seven inhabited islands of the state of Hawai'i, that is, O'ahu, the Big Island of Hawai'i, Maui, Kaua'i, Molokai, Lānai, and Ni'ihau. The majority, over 50%, live in the urban and rural areas of O'ahu (Goodman, La Croix, and Goodman, 1987). Approximately 10% of the Native Hawaiian population in the state lives on government-designated Hawaiian homestead lands concentrated in the rural areas (Goodman et al., 1987). In addition, an estimated 200 to 300 Native Hawaiians live in an unmixed community on the privately-owned, somewhat secluded, island of Ni'ihau (D'Amato, 1986).

Approximately 32% of the state population is under age 20; however, approximately 45% of Native Hawaiians are below this age. Fewer Native Hawaiians than other residents of the state are over age 60, however, the subgroup of pure Native Hawaiians is older, overall, than the larger group classified as part-Hawaiian. In addition, overall mortality and morbidity rates for pure Hawaiians are higher than those for part-Hawaiians, which more closely resemble those of the general population (Native Hawaiian Health Research Consortium, 1985b).

Household and Employment Characteristics

Native Hawaiian households tend to have more members than the state average, with 33% of Native Hawaiian households having five or more persons, compared to the statewide figure of 20%. In addition, more Native Hawaiian families have a female head of household (22% as compared to 13% statewide) (Goodman et al., 1987).

The percentage of Native Hawaiians completing high school, 68%, is comparable to the nationwide figure of 66% but lower than the state figure of 74%. Only 7.7% of Native Hawaiians complete a college education, compared to 9.5% in the state of Hawai'i and 16.2% nationwide (Goodman et al., 1987).

In 1980, Native Hawaiians earned an average of almost $3,000 less per capita than other state residents ($7,740 compared to $10,140). Also, 15% of Native Hawaiian families in Hawaii lived below the poverty level, compared to 7% of state residents overall. A comparison of median household incomes in 1980 also revealed a lower figure for Native Hawaiians ($16,326) when compared to overall state ($22,750) and nationwide ($19,917) figures (Goodman et al., 1987).

Native Hawaiians are consistently underrepresented in white collar, professional, technical, and managerial occupations: 24.5% of Native Hawaiian men and 18.3% of women are employed in white collar occupations, compared to 31.5% of men and 25.7% of women in such occupations statewide (Goodman et al., 1987). The unemployment rate for this group was slightly higher than those for the state and the nation: 6.9%, 6.5%, and 4.7%, respectively (Goodman et al., 1987).

GENERAL HEALTH

Vital statistics collected on Native Hawaiians since 1900 show that this group has the worst health profile in the state of Hawai'i, including the highest rates for most chronic diseases, the highest overall mortality rates, and shortest life

expectancy (Blaisdell, 1983; Blaisdell, 1987). This group's health profile is also poorer than that for the nation overall. More specifically, Native Hawaiians face a disproportionate risk of heart disease, cancer, cerebrovascular disease, and diabetes—acute and chronic conditions that contribute significantly to disability and mortality in this group (Native Hawaiian Health Research Consortium, 1985b; Native Hawaiian Health Care Improvement Act, 1988).

Life Expectancy and Causes of Death

The average life expectancy for Native Hawaiians is approximately 5 to 10 years less than that for the other ethnic groups in Hawai'i (Hammond, 1988). Some of the factors contributing to this group's lower life expectancy are high rates of accidental death and high incidence of chronic and life-threatening illnesses.

According to the Native Hawaiian Health Care Improvement Act of 1988, the overall death rate for Native Hawaiians from 1980 to 1985 was 34% higher than the death rate nationwide. In addition, further analysis of this 1980 to 1985 data revealed that the death rate of *pure* Hawaiians was 146% higher and part-Hawaiians 17% higher than national figures (Native Hawaiian Health Care Improvement Act, 1988).

This pattern also held true at the state level. The Native Hawaiian Health Research Consortium (NHHRC) (1985b), a group of individuals from the University of Hawai'i and community with a common interest in the health needs of Native Hawaiians, noted that since the early 1900s, "Native Hawaiians have experienced the highest age-sex standardized mortality rates of any major ethnic group in Hawai'i" (pp. III-3). In 1985, Native Hawaiians accounted for nearly one in three deaths among state residents between 45 and 54 years old. In addition, a comparison of mortality rates among the ethnic groups in Hawai'i showed that Native Hawaiians died at a younger age than any other ethnic group (Goodman et al., 1987).

The two leading causes of death for Native Hawaiians, heart disease and malignant neoplasms, are also the leading causes of death nationwide. However, the death rate from 1980 to 1985 among Native Hawaiians, compared to that for the rest of the U.S. population, was 44% greater for heart disease, 39% greater for cancer, 31% greater for cerebrovascular diseases, and 222% greater for diabetes mellitus (Native Hawaiian Health Care Improvement Act, 1988).

Because the majority of Native Hawaiians are only part Hawaiian, the true mortality rates for pure Hawaiians must be extracted from these figures. Disease-specific death rates for pure Hawaiians stand out in even starker contrast to national figures: 177% greater for heart disease; 126% greater for cancer, 145% greater for cerebrovascular disease, and 580% higher for diabetes mellitus (Native Hawaiian Health Care Improvement Act, 1988).

Incidence of Cancer and Other Diseases

Native Hawaiians experience the highest rate of hypertension and the highest age-adjusted rate of heart disease of any ethnic group in the U.S. From 1980 to

1984, they also had the highest prevalence of diabetes of any group. Since 1910, Native Hawaiians have had the highest mortality rates from diabetes (Native Hawaiian Health Research Consortium, 1985b). This group also exhibits significantly high rates of cancers of the stomach, lung, esophagus, female breast, and cervix (Native Hawaiian Health Research Consortium, 1985b).

The 1978-81 SEER data on average age-adjusted cancer rates indicate that Native Hawaiians have the second highest rate of cancer in the nation. Black Americans have the highest rate (see Table 4-2, p. 145) (Baquet and Ringen, 1986). Among the five major ethnic groups living in Hawai'i, Native Hawaiians of both genders rank second for cancer incidence in all sites (Table 3-1).

Data on different types of cancers that occur among the five ethnic groups in Hawai'i indicate that Native Hawaiian women are ranked first or second for the incidence of granulocytic leukemia and

TABLE 3-1 Age-Adjusted (World Population Standard) Cancer Incidence (per 100,000) by Ethnicity and Sex, Hawai'i, 1983-86)

Ethnic Group	Male	Female
Caucasian	370.8	339.7
Hawaiians	296.0	274.7
Japanese	251.3	203.0
Pilipino	204.9	212.0
Chinese	203.7	236.8

From unpublished data by the Cancer Research Center of Hawai'i, 1991, Honolulu, HI, University of Hawai'i.

cancers of the breast, lung, uterus, cervix, stomach, ovaries, pancreas, and esophagus (Table 3-2). Native Hawaiian men rank first or second for the incidence of granulocytic leukemia and cancers of the lung, stomach, esophagus, liver, larynx, and thyroid (Table 3-3).

Among the five ethnic groups in Hawai'i, Native Hawaiians also have the highest mortality rates from cancer (Table 3-4). Men and women of this group have the highest mortality rates in lung, stom-ach, rectal, and esophageal cancers, and the women also have the highest mortality rates of breast, uterine, and cervical cancers in the state (Tables 3-5 and 3-6).

Factors Contributing to Poor Health

Researchers have identified several factors that may contribute to Native Hawaiians' poor health profile. First on the list are certain high-risk behaviors, including a diet high in fat and salt, cigarette smoking, and heavy alcohol con-

TABLE 3-2 Age-Adjusted (1970 U.S. Census) Cancer Incidence Rates (per 100,000) for Females, Hawai'i, 1983-86

Cancer Site	Hawaiians	Caucasians	Japanese	Chinese	Pilipino
Breast	113.1	121.8	81.0	89.6	52.3
Lung	45.9	41.6	12.8	17.8	18.3
Uterine	22.1	23.1	18.6	19.3	12.7
Cervical	19.5	22.6	7.9	11.7	17.0
Stomach	14.1	5.6	16.6	6.9	7.7
Ovarian	12.7	14.6	8.4	9.6	12.4
Pancreas	8.8	8.3	6.5	9.6	5.0
Granulocytic leukemia	4.5	3.0	3.1	0.4	4.2
Esophagus	1.2	1.0	0.6	1.1	3.3

From unpublished data by the Cancer Research Center of Hawai'i, 1991, Honolulu, HI, University of Hawai'i.

TABLE 3-3 Age-Adjusted (1970 U.S. Census) Cancer Incidence Rates (per 100,000) for Males, Hawai'i, 1983-86

Cancer Site	Hawaiians	Caucasians	Japanese	Chinese	Pilipino
Lung	103.2	83.5	3.6	2.0	4.2
Stomach	30.6	14.4	35.0	13.7	11.2
Esophagus	11.4	4.6	5.6	1.3	3.5
Liver	9.8	3.2	6.5	6.6	7.5
Larynx	6.1	14.1	3.6	2.0	4.2
Thyroid	6.3	2.8	5.4	7.6	7.6
Granulocytic leukemia	5.3	3.8	3.7	4.8	6.7

From unpublished data by the Cancer Research Center of Hawai'i, 1991, Honolulu, HI, University of Hawai'i.

sumption. In addition, many Hawaiians do not exercise sufficiently or are overweight (Native Hawaiian Health Research Consortium, 1985b). Native Hawaiians also have a relatively high intake of some foods, such as dry or salted fish and **kālua** pig, that have high concentrations of mutagens (Ichinotsubo and Mower, 1982).

However, frequent exposure to suspected carcinogens and high-risk behaviors do not completely explain the increased incidence of certain cancers. For

TABLE 3-4 Age-Adjusted (World Population Standard) Mortality Rates (per 100,000) by Ethnicity, Hawai'i, 1983-86 for all Cancer Sites

Ethnic Group	Male	Female
Hawaiians	178.6	138.5
Caucasians	165.0	115.3
Japanese	120.5	66.8
Pilipino	110.7	70.9
Chinese	98.8	70.2

From unpublished data by the Cancer Research Center of Hawai'i, 1991, Honolulu, HI, University of Hawai'i.

TABLE 3-5 Age-Adjusted (World Population Standard) Mortality Rates (per 100,000) for Females, Hawai'i, 1983-86

Cancer Site	Hawaiians	Caucasians	Japanese	Chinese	Pilipino
Breast	31.1	21.4	11.5	11.1	10.1
Lung	30.4	26.6	7.7	14.6	11.2
Stomach	9.7	2.7	8.7	2.3	3.8
Uterine	3.3	1.6	0.8*	0.2*	0.7*
Cervix	3.4	2.6	0.7*	1.5*	2.6*
Rectum	2.6*	1.6	2.0	1.1*	0.3*
Esophagus	1.6*	0.6*	0.2*	0.4*	1.1*

*Based on fewer than 10 cases.
From unpublished data by the Cancer Research Center of Hawai'i, 1991, Honolulu, HI, University of Hawai'i.

TABLE 3-6 Age-Adjusted (World Population Standard) Mortality Rates (per 100,000) for Males, Hawai'i, 1983-86

Cancer Site	Hawaiians	Caucasians	Japanese	Chinese	Pilipino
Lung	64.3	53.0	28.2	23.7	24.4
Stomach	21.5	10.5	15.9	5.3	5.1
Pancreas	9.8	8.8	7.8	6.4	5.4
Liver	6.2	2.6	5.9	5.8	5.5
Esophagus	6.2	3.3	3.0*	1.7*	1.7
Rectum	4.4	3.4	4.4	1.2*	3.8

*Based on fewer than 10 cases.
From unpublished data by the Cancer Research Center of Hawai'i, 1991, Honolulu, HI, University of Hawai'i.

example, although alcohol consumption among Native Hawaiians is similar to that among Caucasians, the esophageal cancer rate among Native Hawaiian males is three times higher. In addition, the increase in lung cancer mortality occurred much earlier among Native Hawaiians than other ethnic groups in Hawai'i, suggesting the influence of genetic or other lifestyle factors.

In addition to high-risk behaviors, Native Hawaiians receive fewer health services and tend to seek Western medical treatment at a later stage of disease, only after attempting self-care and traditional practices. The Native Hawaiian Health Research Consortium (1985b) also reported that "Native Hawaiians appear to participate less than other groups in health education, health promotion, and screening and referral programs, even when these programs have been intentionally made available to communities where a high proportion of Native Hawaiians live and are offered free of charge" (p. M-16).

This underutilization of health services is due not so much to a lack of available health service resources, but to a "lack of accessibility due to financial barriers, and even more importantly, . . . [to a] lack of acceptability of services to Native Hawaiians due to cultural differences" (Native Hawaiian Health Research Consortium, 1985b, pp. M-6, 7).

Furthermore, Native Hawaiians' infrequent use of services may also be attributed to their low level of cancer knowledge. In three surveys conducted between 1978 and 1982 by the Community Cancer Program of Hawai'i, Native Ha-

waiians ranked next-to-last in their knowledge of cancer risk factors, signs and symptoms, and early detection methods (Community Cancer Program of Hawai'i, 1982).

CULTURE AND BELIEFS
Historical Perspectives

The ancient Hawaiians were greatly skilled, known for their fishing, navigation, astronomy, agricultural skills (as evidenced by their taro patches), and engineering (as evidenced by their thatched houses and weaving). They were a peaceful people who placed high value on harmony between themselves and nature (Maney and Schultz, 1991).

The traditional Hawaiians did not view themselves just as individuals, but rather as a part of a continuum that included their ancestors, all of their living family, those who will succeed them, and nature. An individual without relationships was unthinkable. Each Hawaiian was linked physically and in a mystical sense with the ancestors and with the descendants to come. This was the **'ohana,** or family.

For the Hawaiian, the head, considered the first body center, was the site of communication between one's own spirit and the departed **kūpuna** (elders), ancestors. These ancestors were now deified family spirits, or **'aumakua.** The second body center, the navel, represented the person's link with the parents, or **mākua.** This body center also included the gut which was synonymous with the mind and was the seat of learning and knowledge. The third body center, the genitals, linked the living person with current offspring and those to come (Native Hawaiian Health Research Consortium, 1985a).

Just as everything in the universe was living, conscious, and communicating, each part of a person's body was endowed with a special spirit capable of thinking, sensing, and relating on its own. Thus the Hawaiian was a collective self that encompassed not only a physical body, but also spiritual sources.

To the Hawaiian, the family, or 'ohana was the center of all relationships. The word 'ohana comes from the word "oha," which means the root of the taro plant, and "na," a word for plural or many. The taro root was a mainstay of the Hawaiian diet and also closely linked with the origin of the Hawaiian people. Legend describes the progenitor of the Hawaiians as a mystic man-and-taro named "Hāloa" (Pukui, Haertig, and Lee, 1972).

Figure 3-1 shows the taro shoots, or lateral **keiki** (representing children), from the **ka makua** (representing the central parent) of the taro corm. This signifies how the 'ohana all comes from the same root.

Another part of the 'ohana was the extended family, from which any member could expect warmth and support. The true meaning of **aloha,** the love of one member for another, was found. Members of the 'ohana were interdependent, and each had prescribed tasks. Elders taught youngsters to fish, raise taro, weave, and build (Pukui et al., 1972b). Parents or adults taught certain skills and crafts used in fishing, navigation, and farming through demonstration, chants, rituals, or sacred restricting taboos called **kapu.**

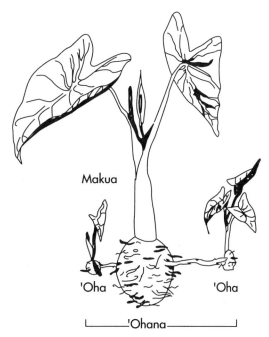

Makua

'Oha   'Oha

'Ohana

Figure 3-1 He mau lā'au kalo (taro plants) showing ka makua (central parent), with its parts, and two 'ohā (lateral keiki) collectively forming 'ohana.

From Blaisdell K: Taro as Kāne and Hiapo of Hāloa, Ka Wai Ola O Oha 5(12):23, 1988. Copyright 1988 by Office of Hawaiian Affairs. Adapted by permission.

Native Hawaiians also used rituals and kapus to teach their children proper behavior. Such behavior included keeping the eyes down and recognizing the authority of one's seniors (or other persons) by never looking directly at them during conversations. Children were also taught not to brag, boast, or act like the equal of their elders or superiors in rank (Pukui et al., 1972b). However, Native Hawaiians did feel that human physical contact was important, including touching, embracing, and **honi,** a Hawaiian way of kissing, when greeting family or friends.

From these precepts, the child learned a Hawaiian ideal for social relationships, that of humility, or **ha'aha'a.** Hawaiians expended great effort to maintain harmony within themselves, with others, and with nature. They did not condone confrontation or the public resolution of conflicts, but felt it was better to deny and suppress conflicts because of their potential to harm relationships. This group also discouraged self-centered behaviors such as striving for individual success, competing for personal gains, or public displays to draw attention to oneself (Young, 1980). Proper social behavior was especially important, as it reflected on the honor of one's family. Ways to express and correct hostilities and injustices were established with **ho'oponopono,** "to make right; to correct; to restore and maintain good relationships among family, and family-and-supernatural powers" (Pukui et al., 1972a) further defined ho'oponopono as regular family therapy, "the specific family conference in which relationships were 'set right' through prayer, discussion, confession, repentance, and mutual restitution and forgiveness" (p. 60).

In addition to strong family ties, Native Hawaiians also felt close links with the **'āina,** a term that refers not only to land, but which is also inclusive of air, plants, birds, and all of nature. Since Hawaiians depended on the **'āina** for existence, they paid homage to and respected nature. They believed in taking only what they needed from the land, thus allowing natural resources on their isolated islands to replenish themselves (Chang,

Durante, Nahulu, and Wong, 1980).

The health beliefs of Native Hawaiians were based on the concept of **lōkahi,** or harmony of the mind, body, and spirit. Individuals achieved wellness if they maintained inner harmony and harmonious relationships with their families, other people, nature, and deified family spirits and other gods. Compliance with kapu and frequent communications with the spirit realm were also necessary. Aloha, or an unconditional love for family, nature, and spirit also promoted wellness.

Hawaiians followed many favorable health practices. They ate a high-fiber, high-starch, low-fat, low-sugar, nutritious diet. Vigorous physical fitness was part of daily living in enjoyable recreation and in hard work to provide food and shelter for their families. In addition, they buried their waste in designated areas in the village and only bathed downstream from their sources of drinking water.

Treatment for illnesses began with "self-healing." If this was unsuccessful, the individual sought the assistance of the **kūpuna 'ohana,** or elder member of the family. If still unsuccessful, a **kahuna lapa'au,** or medical practitioner, provided treatment at the **heiau hō'ola,** or healing temple. The Hawaiians integrated psycho-spiritual healing methods such as prayer, revelation, suggestion, and extrasensory perception with physical methods such as observation, palpation, body molding, **lomi-lomi,** or massage, hydro-thermo-heliotherapy, fracture setting, and pharmacological therapies using various herbs (Native Hawaiian Health Research Consortium, 1985a). Among the native herbs used were 'awa, a mild narcotic; **kukui** nut, a cathartic; and **pōpolo** berries and/or young guava shoots, antidiarrheal agents.

Consequences of Western Contact

Captain Cook's arrival in Hawai'i had profound effects upon the Hawaiian people, marking the beginning of the decline of the Hawaiian race and its culture.

Because the Hawaiians lived in isolation from the rest of the world for more than 500 years, they lacked immunity and were highly susceptible to the new infectious diseases brought by Cook and subsequent explorers and traders. Therefore, thousands of Hawaiians died during epidemics of venereal diseases, cholera, tuberculosis, measles, infectious coughs, diarrhea, smallpox, Hansen's disease, diphtheria, and bubonic plague (Native Hawaiian Health Research Consortium, 1985a). Hansen's disease was particularly psychologically destructive because in an effort to control the rising incidence of this disease, afflicted individuals were removed from their 'ohana and banished to an isolated village on the island of Moloka'i (Young, 1980).

The people lost confidence in their elders and their medical practitioners, because they were unable to cure, heal, or control any of the new illnesses.

Before the arrival of Cook and other Westerners, the Hawaiians believed they knew their whole world. With Western contact, many questions arose about these foreigners regarding their pale skin, their origin, and their possession of

clothing and metal. Metal, in particular, astounded the Hawaiians because they could not manufacture it and because it could be used to make valuable items such as nails, fishhooks, tools, mirrors, ornaments, and especially weapons and firearms (Young, 1980).

The introduction of metals catalyzed a shift of the Hawaiians' economic base from one of subsistence to one based on trade between foreigners and natives. This change had immense effects on a people whose economy had been based not on acquisition of material goods but on supplying daily needs. The development of the whaling and sugar industries also promoted the profit motive, a concept very foreign to the Hawaiians (Young, 1980).

With the introduction of new ideas, and unanswered questions, the Hawaiians realized their knowledge was no longer adequate. They began to see themselves as inferior to European settlers.

The Western influence upon Native Hawaiians was so tremendous that by 1893, when the Republic of Hawai'i was established, virtually all public schools in Hawai'i used English as the language of instruction. "Perhaps no other country has ever permitted such a cultural invasion of their schools unaccompanied by military or political domination" (Kamehameha Schools, 1971, p. 47).

In the area of government, the eradication of the kapu system, or body of laws established by the **kahuna**, or priest specialist and sanctioned by the **ali'i**, or ruling chiefs, eroded the Hawaiians' sense of being. No longer were men and women certain about their roles in the 'ohana and society (Kamehameha Schools, 1971; Young, 1980).

The year 1819 brought the death of Kamehameha I, who had united the Hawaiian Islands and established himself as the first ruler of the Kingdom of Hawaii. What followed was a quick and dramatic evolution of government. Hawaii changed from an individual monarchy to a constitutional monarchy, and finally to a government of the people, or democracy. To Native Hawaiians, "people" had actually referred to "a few men of wisdom and prudence," or those who could read and who owned property. By 1852, the constitution was basically identical to that of the U.S., and completely alien to traditional Hawaiian laws (Kamehameha Schools, 1971; Wang, 1982).

All these changes, coupled with differences between traditional Hawaiian and newly introduced Western values, confused Native Hawaiians and had a devastating effect on their concept of self. The box at the bottom of this page summarizes some of these differences in values.

The Christian missionaries who arrived in 1820 added to this denigration of Hawaiian society by making Hawaiians ashamed of their culture. The missionaries viewed practically every aspect of the Hawaiian culture as sinful. They condemned the traditional dance, **hula,** the songs and music, or **mele,** and the native wood carvings as sexual; they also felt that the Hawaiians exposed too much of their bodies. The missionaries also decried the worship of native gods and other native religious practices (Gray, 1972; Kamehameha Schools, 1971).

The Hawaiian population, which numbered approximately 1 million in 1778, had declined to about 40,000 by 1893, a decrease of 96% in 155 years (Blaisdell, 1989).

Disease alone cannot account for this rapid decline. Many Hawaiians felt such tremendous guilt and shame that they chose suicide to heal the split in their

---

A COMPARISON OF HAWAIIAN AND WESTERN VALUES

HAWAIIAN VALUES	WESTERN VALUES
Love of the land; harmony between people and nature	Control of nature by humans
Protection and conservation of nature	Continual consumption of natural resources
Use and sharing among the 'ohana (extended family) of resources	Focus on individual ownership and benefit
Harmonious working relationships	Competition
Lōkāhi: unity	Confrontation

souls. Others, confused and weakened, lost their will to live. As the Hawaiians expressed it themselves, **"Nā kānaka 'ōku'u wale aku no i kau 'uhane,** the people dismissed freely their souls and died" (Young, 1980, p. 10). Furthermore, in their findings related to the poor health profile of this group, the Native Hawaiians Study Commission (1983) reported that "the psychological despair and sense of being a conquered people in their own homeland **['āina]** is a factor in the health conditions of Native Hawaiians" (p. 149) today.

MAJOR CULTURAL IMPLICATIONS FOR HEALTH CARE

The Native Hawaiians' current health problems largely reflect their social situation and the impact of the traumatic social changes they have experienced over the past 200 years. Although these changes have resulted in the loss of many traditions, including the loss of traditional healers and healing methods, many Native Hawaiian values persist. Some of these values and attitudes now may prevent Native Hawaiians from seeking help from Western healers.

General Barriers to Western Health Care

Many Native Hawaiians avoid Western medical services, except when experiencing the most severe conditions or advanced stages of illness, because the manner in which services are provided is so alien to their culture.

Hawaiians view Western medicine as an autocratic style of medicine that conflicts with their own holistic approach. In the traditional Hawaiian system, health practices were integrated with daily religious and social practices. Hawaiians also emphasized the "spiritual unity of the individual with the environment and the spiritual significance of events such as illness" (Native Hawaiian Health Research Consortium, 1985b, pp. VIII-7). In addition, health promotion and disease prevention were generally the responsibility of the extended family. Even today, many native Hawaiians still rely on their own comprehensive system of rituals, health practices, and the work of traditional healers (Native Hawaiian Health Research Consortium, 1985b). So it is not surprising that the Native Hawaiian Health Research Consortium (1985b) found that "Native Hawaiians are reported to enter medical treatment at the late stages of disease, only when self-care and traditional practices have not brought sufficient relief" (pp. VIII-5).

Wegner (1989a) noted that Native Hawaiians often feel uncomfortable and threatened in hospitals, clinics, doctors' offices, and other medical settings or situations. Because there are few Native Hawaiian health care professionals, these patients often cannot identify with their caregivers. They often perceive that non-Hawaiian medical professionals lack an understanding of and appreciation for the Hawaiian culture, views on illness, and style of interaction.

In addition, Native Hawaiians may avoid public agencies and impersonal authority figures such as those found in medical settings because they fear the possibility of embarrassment or confrontation. The Native Hawaiian Health Research Consortium (1985b) noted that

Hawaiians' desire to avoid such interpersonal conflicts can have negative implications for their health care because "individuals who avoid confrontation were also found less likely to have had a recent physical examination from a physician" (pp. I-15).

The desire to avoid confrontation also leads Native Hawaiians to accept decisions without raising questions. In the medical setting, these patients may not feel that the health care professional's advice is satisfactory but may be unwilling to challenge this advice, ask questions, or ask for clarification (Wegner, 1989a).

The Hawaiian culture also emphasizes the importance of preserving harmony and minimizing risk-taking behaviors. Native Hawaiians tend to minimize the importance of experiences ("ain't no big thing") that may set them apart from others or threaten to disrupt the group. The result of this coping strategy is that Native Hawaiians may accept symptoms of illness, adjust to these symptoms, and postpone seeking professional health (Native Hawaiian Health Research Consortium, 1985b).

Native Hawaiians usually have an external, rather than internal, locus of control; that is, they tend to view events as beyond the control or influence of the individual. Generally, people with lower levels of education or lower socioeconomic status, or those who feel powerless possess an external locus of control; these characteristics describe many Native Hawaiians today. Individuals with an external locus of control may accept symptoms of illness fatalistically, rather than taking the initiative to seek medical

help (Native Hawaiian Health Research Consortium, 1985b).

Native Hawaiians' preference for relying on those close to them to resolve problems may create another barrier to the effective use of modern health services. For these individuals, the experience of social intimacy and acceptance among family and peers is more important than individual achievement or individual self-sufficiency; thus, they frequently rely on family members or upon trusted individuals in their community to handle health problems. As Wegner (1989a) explained, Native Hawaiians may feel "a distrust of impersonal, bureaucratic services, and a discomfort in unequal authority relationships based on scientific expertise rather than spiritual knowledge and personal relationships" (p. 41).

Health education programs now used by most medical institutions in the U.S. have been developed for the American population as a whole and do not reflect a sensitivity to the values, world views, and languages of groups such as the Native Hawaiians. Because Native Hawaiians are generally less educated than Caucasians in the U.S., many health education programs may be inaccessible to them. Hawaiians also prefer to learn from, and participate in group activities with, people with whom they have a personal affiliation. These factors may become dual obstacles to the effectiveness of communication through written materials or impersonal presentations in large groups (Wegner, 1989a). Health information disseminated through the news media is also less likely to reach segments of the population with a low level of formal education, including most Native Hawaiians.

Some research has suggested that Native Hawaiians do not participate in health promotion programs as actively as other ethnic groups. However, this is not necessarily because they lack interest in preventive health care. Instead, Native Hawaiians may be facing many more pressing concerns in their lives, such as immediate financial and survival problems (Native Hawaiian Health Research Consortium, 1985b). Native Hawaiians may see promoting "wellness," then, as a luxury affordable only by the affluent.

Native Hawaiians of low socioeconomic status may also be reluctant to participate in screening programs because these programs are usually not reimbursed by insurance companies. The out-of-pocket expense is a very real barrier for low-income Native Hawaiians who have other more pressing financial concerns (Native Hawaiian Health Research Consortium, 1985b).

As discussed earlier in this chapter, research also suggests that Native Hawaiians engage in behaviors that place them at high risk for developing cancer. These behaviors, such as cigarette smoking, excessive drinking, and overeating, may be viewed as coping mechanisms to manage socially-based stress (Native Hawaiian Health Research Consortium, 1985b).

Health care workers also need to be sensitive to issues of cultural conflict and domination when presenting health education programs to Native Hawaiians. Because of the traumatic consequences of Western contact, Native Hawaiians may resent outside "missionaries" who try to dictate their behavior. Health care providers cannot assume that their credentials and expertise will be enough to convince Native Hawaiians to abandon their existing health practices or lifestyles (Native Hawaiian Health Research Consortium, 1985b).

Native Hawaiians need role models to advocate and to adopt these practices themselves. However, few Native Hawaiians who have survived cancer are willing to share their experiences and teach because of their strong preference for keeping family matters private and their unwillingness to speak out and volunteer (Pukui et al., 1972b).

Working Effectively with Native Hawaiians

In order to improve the overall health status of Native Hawaiians in the long term, social changes that would improve their life situation are necessary. As the Native Hawaiian Health Research Consortium (1985b) put it, "any steps taken to empower this group, to increase the level of self-efficacy, and to improve their economic situation, must be regarded as important to the promotion of health" (pp. I-3).

However, Native Hawaiians' current health crises cannot wait for general socioeconomic change; immediate strategies for promoting this group's use of health services are required. Such strategies must be based on three general principles: "the necessity for the empowerment of Native Hawaiians in the health care system, . . . the obligation to develop targeted programs for Native Hawaiians, and . . . the need to adapt health care services to Native Hawaiian cultural beliefs and practices" (Wegner, 1989b, p. 152).

One key strategy health care professionals can employ is to involve respected Native Hawaiian individuals in the planning and delivery of effective health services (Native Hawaiian Health Research Consortium, 1985b).

In addition, because Native Hawaiians highly value personal affiliations, health care workers should try to take advantage of the natural social relationships among Native Hawaiians when planning the delivery of health care services or information. For example, Native Hawaiian community leaders could be asked to endorse new community-based programs.

Specifically, "rather than providing health education through impersonal presentations and in settings with large groups of unacquainted individuals, programs are more likely to be effective with Native Hawaiians if they are provided in the context of natural groups and by individuals with whom they have close personal contact" (Native Hawaiian Health Research Consortium, 1985b, p. VIII-17). Health care providers could work with canoe clubs, Hawaiian churches, neighborhood groups, and other organizations in the Hawaiian community, including Hawaiian civic clubs. In addition, the providers of the health information should be Native Hawaiians, such as the leaders of these groups, other respected public figures such as entertainers or athletes, or Native Hawaiian health care workers. These community-based programs could then serve as part of a system of active outreach, because

relying on individual initiative is not an effective means of providing health care to Native Hawaiians (Native Hawaiian Health Research Consortium, 1985b).

The support and involvement of respected Native Hawaiian community leaders is also essential to changing or modifying high-risk behaviors. Success will be more likely if these leaders and respected role models advocate and adopt these changes themselves (Native Hawaiian Health Research Consortium, 1985b). Also, because of the value of affiliation, "individuals are likely to undertake new behaviors only insofar as those behaviors are adopted and supported by their friends and families" (Native Hawaiian Health Research Consortium, 1985b, p. VIII-20).

In addition to adopting these general strategies for providing health care to Native Hawaiians, health care workers should also consider more specific interventions to increase the effectiveness of their interactions with these patients.

Health care professionals can help to build these patients' self-esteem and pride in their heritage by encouraging their participation in cultural activities such as weaving, dance, song, language, and canoe paddling. By fostering interest and value for these activities, health professionals can facilitate the reconnection of Native Hawaiians to their cultural identity.

Medical professionals should also integrate the concept of 'ohana into the patient's plan of care. Since a significant number of Hawaiians lack a home—that is, a place of comfort, consistency, safety, and nurturing—health professionals should address these needs during their interactions with their clients.

In addition, to facilitate communication with Native Hawaiians, health professionals should take an easy-going, low-key, but sincere approach to encourage familiarity and personal contact. This can often be achieved by "talking story," or starting an ordinary conversation in a relaxed, undirected exchange. During such a conversation, Native Hawaiians may view the health professional as being empathetic and open, and thus be more willing to share problems and concerns.

However, health professionals are also advised not to be **niele,** or nosy, and to avoid personal questions. Young (1980) noted that "sarcasm or humor which could be taken as insulting or critical, should never be directed at the client" (p. 20). Although most Native Hawaiians speak English, use of "pidgin," or Hawaiian Creole English, may also be helpful in effectively communicating with some Native Hawaiians (Palafox, 1980). A culturally specific cancer risk assessment for Native Hawaiians is provided on pp. 129-131.

NATIVE HAWAIIAN CANCER RISK ASSESSMENT TOOL

Note: The following *key areas* in which to obtain information are deliberately provided versus examples of direct questions because it is essential to keep in mind that in gathering data from a client of Hawaiin ancestry, direct questioning may be viewed as intrusive and should be avoided. Instead, it is valuable to c reate an easy-going, low-key, personal atmosphere by "talking story" or starting the assessment with a relaxed, undirected exchange. "Connecting" with the client through a mutual acquaintance or common interest also greatly enhances the interview process.

DEMOGRAPHIC DATA

Name _____ Age _____ Marital Status _____
Religious Preference _____ Height _____ Weight _____
Occupation _____
Pure Hawaiin _____   Part Hawaiin _____
Number of people and relationship living in household _____
_____

Languages spoken in the home _____
Explanation of illness (cause and meaning of illness)
_____
_____

Use of traditional healer _____
Use of traditional medicine/healing:
prayer _____   herbs or la'au _____   teas _____   foods _____   massage or lomi lomi _____
body molding _____   medicines _____   steam baths _____   enemas _____
other: _____
Typical diet (high salt, high fat?): _____
_____
Foods eaten or avoided during illness: _____

Continued.

NATIVE HAWAIIAN CANCER RISK ASSESSMENT TOOL—cont'd

GASTRIC CANCER

Previous problems with:
_____ indigestion _____ recent weight loss _____ abdominal pain _____ easy satiety
_____ nausea _____ vomiting _____ blood in stools _____ chronic ulcers
Prior stomach surgery: _____
Family history of gastric cancer: _____
Diet high in salt-cured foods: _____
Regular consumption of fresh fruits and vegetables: _____

LIVER CANCER

Previous problems with:
_____ abdominal pain   _____ yellowing of skin
_____ abdominal bloating   _____ yellowing of whites of eyes
_____ recent weight loss   _____ fever of unknown cause
_____ easy bruising   _____ hemochromatosis
Family history of liver cancer: _____
Prior blood test for hepatitis/liver infection: _____
    Date: _____
    Results: _____
Prior test for alpha-fetoprotein: _____
    Date: _____
    Results: _____
Alcohol consumption: _____
    Beer_____   Other alcohol _____
    Amount: _____
Recent change in color of stool: _____
Recent change in color of urine: _____
Recent change in energy level: _____

ESOPHAGEAL CANCER

Previous problems with:
_____ chronic esophagitis _____ indigestion _____ heartburn _____ difficulty swallowing
_____ regurgitation
Regular consumption of fresh fruits and vegetables: _____
Diet high in salt-cured foods: _____
Alcohol consumption: _____
    Beer_____   Other alcohol _____
    Amount: _____

LUNG CANCER

Previous problems with:
_____ cough _____ change in color, odor or amount of sputum _____ dull chest pain
_____ persistent cold _____ recent weight loss _____ loss of appetite
_____ shortness of breath _____ malaise _____ coughing up blood
_____ wheezing or difficulty breathing

NATIVE HAWAIIAN CANCER RISK ASSESSMENT TOOL—cont'd

Exposure to:
_____ passive smoke _____ asbestos _____ volcano haze _____ kerosene _____ Radon
_____ outdoor charcoal/wood cooking
History of smoking: _____
   Packs per day/years: _____
History of chronic lung disease:
_____ bronchitis _____ pneumonia _____ emphysema _____ asthma _____ tuberculosis
Regular consumption of fresh fruits and vegetables: _____
BREAST CANCER
Previous problems with:
_____ lump or thickening in breast or axilla
_____ discharge from nipple(s)   _____ nipple retraction
_____ dimpling, puckering or redness in breast
_____ change in size, contour or texture of breast
History of:
_____ breast cancer _____ ovarian, endometrial, or colong cancer
_____ relatives on maternal side with breast cancer
_____ no children or first child after 30 years of age
Menstrual history: Menarch _____ (year)
                  Menopause _____ (year)

UTERINE CANCER

Previous problems with:
_____ unusual vaginal bleeding or spotting
_____ use of female hormones
   # of years: _____
_____ pain or mass in abdomen/pelvis
High fat diet: _____
Number of children: _____

CERVICAL CANCER

Previous problems with:
_____ abnormal Pap smear results
_____ abnormal vaginal bleeding/discharge
_____ spotting after intercourse
History of:
_____ human papilloma virus (condyloma/genital warts) infection
_____ multiple sexual partners by patient and partner
_____ early age at first intercourse
_____ multiple pregnancies
_____ smoking

Treatment plans should also include allowances for traditional healing and alternative therapies. Health professionals can facilitate bringing Western and traditional healing together.

CULTURALLY SENSITIVE CANCER CONTROL PROJECTS

Public health officials at the federal and state levels have recognized the health crises that Native Hawaiians are facing. Experts are developing or already implementing various programs and studies in order to improve the health status of this group, several of which are cancer-related or deal directly with prevention, screening, and early detection of cancer. These programs incorporate cultural values and health beliefs and practices of Native Hawaiians to garner their support and participation. Three of these exploratory programs are briefly described here.

Wai'anae Diet Program

A group of health professionals in cooperation with community groups from the Wai'anae area (located on the western shores of O'ahu) developed the Wai'anae Diet Program in an attempt to reverse the high incidence of and mortality from diet-related illnesses such as heart disease, cancer, stroke, and diabetes among Native Hawaiians. This program was "designed as a culturally appropriate, community-based intervention model with special consideration to accessibility, reasonable cost, and ability to be propagated and sustained in the community" (Shintani, Hughes, Beckham, and O'Connor, 1991, p. 1647S).

The diet program was based on the fact that the traditional Hawaiian diet was healthy, composed, according to Shintani and Hughes (1991), of "approximately 7% to 12% fat and high in complex carbohydrates and bulk" (pp. 64-65). In contrast, the Native Hawaiians' current diet consists of high-fat, high-cholesterol, and high-calorie foods, including fast foods, canned foods, and local plate lunches.

Originally, 20 Native Hawaiians—ten men and ten women—aged 25 to 64 years enrolled in this special diet program. However, one participant was unable to complete the program due to a viral illness. The remaining 19 participants consumed exclusively Native Hawaiian foods that were available before Western contact for 21 days. These foods included "taro (a starchy rootlike potato), poi (a mashed form of taro), sweet potato, yams, breadfruit, greens (fern shoots and leaves of taro, sweet potato and yams), fruit, seaweed, fish and chicken" (Shintani et al., 1991, p. 1648S). All the foods except fish and chicken were available in unlimited quantities. The food was eaten raw or steamed, to closely model ancient styles of cooking. To promote adherence to this program, the participants were also taught how to make appropriate substitutions using modern foods and modern recipes.

The program did not focus strictly on nutrition, but also acknowledged the importance of ancient Hawaiian cultural values by including traditional Hawaiian healers who taught "spiritual, mental, emotional as well as physical health as an integral part of the program" (Shintani and Hughes, 1991, p. 65). The participants of the program were also encouraged to teach others in their 'ohana about this diet. This was an example of using the natural social relationships among Hawaiians to promote a healthy lifestyle.

The results were remarkable. The average weight loss among participants was 17.1 pounds over 21 days. The group also exhibited an average decrease in cholesterol levels of 14% (from 222.3 to 191 mg/dl) and an average decrease in triglyceride levels from 211.3 to 163 mg/dl. The seven individuals with diabetes also exhibited improvements in blood sugar levels, with an average decrease from 161.9 to 123.4 mg/dl. Blood pressure readings also fell an average of 10% (Shintani and Hughes, 1991).

The Wai'anae Diet Program was clearly a success among Native Hawaiians and has the potential to improve their health status. Much of the program's success has been attributed to its community-based, culturally sensitive interventions.

Ethnic Differences in Mammography Utilization in Hawai'i

"Ethnic Differences in Mammography Utilization in Hawai'i" was a study targeted specifically for Native Hawaiian women. The study stemmed from results of the Hawai'i Breast Cancer Detection Demonstration Project (BCDDP), in which 10,031 women were screened for breast cancer from 1974 to 1980 (Goodman, Gilbert, Mi, Grove, Catts, and Low, 1982).

The demonstration project used the standard media outlets (i.e., newspaper, radio, and television announcements) to encourage women to self-refer for mammograms. This project successfully increased the number of women who had screening mammograms. However, in analyzing the characteristics of the women who participated in the project, the researchers found that they were better educated, had higher household incomes, and were more likely to be Caucasian or Japanese than the average woman in Hawai'i (Cancer Research Center of Hawai'i, Queen's Medical Center, and American Cancer Society— Hawai'i Pacific Division, 1990). Furthermore, only 700 (7.3%) of the BCDDP participants were Native Hawaiian women, even though this group comprised 12.8% of the women between the ages of 35 and 74 years in the state (Goodman et al., 1982; Goodman, Gilbert, and Low, 1984).

Based on the low participation of Native Hawaiian women, an identified high-risk group, the primary objective of the study was to see whether a "culturally-focused cancer control program, utilizing social and professional networks to encourage participation in cancer screening, yields greater participation rates among Native Hawaiian women than conventional, media-based cancer control programs" (Cancer Research Center of Hawai'i et al., 1990, p. 2). In addition, the researchers sought to obtain information on knowledge and attitudinal variables related to breast cancer among Native Hawaiian women.

The first step of the study was the distribution to Native Hawaiian women of a survey instrument that included questions on general demographic characteristics and knowledge, attitudes, and practices related to breast cancer (e.g., regarding breast self-examination and mammograms).

The surveys were distributed at existing social and professional organizations such as churches with large Hawaiian congregations, Hawaiian dance studios, Hawaiian civic organizations (e.g., E Ola Mau, Alu Like, Professional Secretaries Association), Hawaiian Civic Clubs, and businesses that employed a significant number of Native Hawaiians (e.g., the Office of Hawaiian Affairs). For example, during the Hawaiian civic clubs' annual statewide convention in November 1989, 600 survey instruments were distributed to the female members. A health fair in a community with a large population of Native Hawaiians also served as a site for survey distribution. Along with the survey, education on breast self-examination and assistance with completing the survey were provided at these two distribution sites.

The researchers planned to give vouchers for a free mammogram to the first 600 women who completed and returned the survey and who met the American Cancer Society's screening guidelines. The women could redeem their vouchers at any of five providers on Oahu.

Out of 4,000 surveys distributed, 837 (20.9%) were returned; of 697 vouchers distributed between November 1989 and December 1990, 536 (76.9%) were redeemed.

The data from this program are still being analyzed; however, preliminary findings indicate that the study was successful in significantly increasing the number of Native Hawaiian women who ob-

tained mammograms. This success can be attributed to several of the techniques used in the program: (a) the elimination of barriers to participation by bringing the program to the women, (b) the provision of assistance to the women in filling out the survey, and (c) the acquisition of the support of Native Hawaiian women identified as the community leaders.

Wai'anae Coast Cancer Control Project

Native Hawaiian women have the highest age-adjusted breast cancer incidence and mortality rates of any group of women over the age of 40 in the U.S. In addition, their cervical cancer incidence and mortality are 1.6 times and 1.3 times, respectively, the rates for U.S. Caucasians (Baquet and Ringen, 1986).

The Wai'anae Coast Cancer Control Project, which began in 1990 with funding from the National Cancer Institute, tests the effectiveness of an integrated, community-driven cancer control intervention in increasing knowledge, positively affecting attitudes, and increasing the use of mammography and Pap screening among Native Hawaiian women. The project, which originated in the Native Hawaiian community located in Wai'anae, Hawai'i, emphasizes community-driven cancer control. A Native Hawaiian community resident serves as the community co-principal investigator, the community health center's medical director serves as the principal investigator, and a scientific consultant is co-principal investigator.

The project's community-based intervention takes advantage of the Native Hawaiian social and family networks and this group's sense of **kōkua,** a social concept that encourages mutual support of community members. Kōkua groups were formed to link health workers and Native Hawaiian women, and to encourage mutual support in addressing cancer issues among community members. These groups consist of 10 to 12 Native Hawaiian women organized by other women who tapped existing friendships and kinship groups. The groups link health workers and Native Hawaiian women and also validate and enhance the participants' sense of competence about and control over their health. These groups help build self-esteem among the participants by helping them to recognize the healthy behaviors they already practice and encouraging them to adopt other healthy behaviors. Finally, the groups provide means to reduce the psychological, social, and economic barriers that restrict access to adequate health care.

The project coordinators recruit peer leaders from the community to help organize meetings of friends and family. There are also navigators for each group who, like the ancient navigators who assisted the Hawaiian people to journey across uncharted waters, help participants find their way through the unfamiliar domain of the health care system. These navigators also come from the community and are trained in group facilitation, providing information on cancer, and scheduling clinic appointments and patient follow-up services.

When the project is completed in March, 1995, the researchers will determine whether the project was successful in improving breast and cervical cancer screening practices among Native Hawaiian women (The Wai'anae Coast Cancer Control Project, 1990).

RESOURCES

Papa Ola Lōkahi
Kawaiaha'o Plaza
567 South King Street
Honolulu, HI 96813
808-536-9453

This is a federally funded office under the Native Hawaiian Health Care Act. It is governed by a consortium board of public and private agencies concerned with Native Hawaiian health care and assists in the planning and development of Native Hawaiian health care systems statewide utilizing federal funding.

Office of Hawaiian Affairs
711 Kapi'olani Blvd., Suite 500
Honolulu, HI 96813
808-586-3777

This is a semiautonomous state agency dedicated to the betterment of the Hawaiian people. It is governed by an elected board of trustees and has several administrative priority programs including health and human services. It publishes a monthly newspaper, *Ka Wai Ola O OHA*, which contains monthly articles concerning Native Hawaiian health issues.

Alu Like, Inc.
1024 Māpunapuna Street
Honolulu, HI 96819
808-836-8940

This is a private service and training agency for Native Hawaiians. Among its various programs, Alu Like currently has a program on Substance Abuse Prevention and an Elderly Services Program for Native Hawaiians.

E Ola Mau, Inc.
1374 Nu'uanu Avenue, Suite 201
Honolulu, HI 96817
808-533-1628
This is a private, nonprofit consortium of Native Hawaiin health providers whose mission is to ensure that Native Hawaiians achieve lōkahi (healthful harmony of self with others and all of nature) and function effectively as citizens and leaders in their aina (homeland).

Office of Hawaiian Health
Hawai'i State Department of Health
50 Kukui Plaza, 208-B
Honolulu, HI 96817
808-586-4800
This is a government office located within the Department of Health to ensure that the health care system for the state is responsive to the health of Native Hawaiians. Its programs are developed to assist the improvement of services within the department to Native Hawaiians. This office publishes articles and other informational materials periodically on various subjects concerning Native Hawaiian health care.

State of Hawai'i Library System
478 South King Street
Honolulu, HI 96813
808-586-3500
This is a statewide public library system with a central library located in Honolulu. A reserve-reference collection on Hawaiian and Pacific Island materials is deposited at the central library with other lending materials.

University of Hawai'i at Mānoa
Center for Hawaiian Studies
1890 East-West Road
Moore Hall 428
Honolulu, HI 96822
808-956-6825
This is a multidisciplinary program offering a B.A. degree and emphasizing the study of both traditional and modern Hawaiian society, language, and culture.

University of Hawai'i at Mānoa
Hamilton Library
2550 The Mall
Honolulu, HI 96822
808-956-7203
This library has an extensive Hawaiian and Pacific Island collection that includes rare books, prints, and other materials not usually found at other repositories in the State.

Kamehameha Schools/Bernice Pauahi
Bishop Estate
Kapālama Heights
Honolulu, HI 96817
808-842-8211
This is a private 12-year school for Native Hawaiian children established under the estate of Priness Pauahi. The school offers classes in Hawaiian language, culture and history. It has a Hawaiian Studies Institute that produces materials and research on Hawaiian culture. The school also has a large Hawaiian collection of publications and other resource materials.

Native Hawaiian Culture and Arts Programs
650 Iwilei Road
Honolulu, HI 96817
808-532-5630

This is a federally funded program developed to assist in the research and perpetuation of Native Hawaiian culture. It has offered several grants to individuals and groups on a wide range of culturally related topics.

REFERENCES

1. Baquet CR, Ringen K: *Cancer among Blacks & other minorities: Statistical profiles,* Washington, DC, 1986, National Cancer Institute.
2. Blaisdell K: Health and social services— Historical and cultural background. In *Report on the culture, needs and concerns of native Hawaiians pursuant to public law 96-565, title III* vol 1:99-109, Washington, DC, 1983, The Native Hawaiians Study Commission.
3. Blaisdell K: *Historical and cultural aspects of native Hawaiians.* Panel Presentation, Hawai'i State Department of Health, Honolulu, December, 1987.
4. Blaisdell K: Historical and cultural aspects of native Hawaiian health. In Wegner EL, editor: *Social process in Hawaii: The health of native Hawaiians: A selective report on health status and health care,* 32:1-21, Honolulu, 1989, University of Hawai'i Press.
5. Cancer Research Center of Hawai'i: *Cancer Incidence and Mortality Data by Ethnicity and Sex,* unpublished data, University of Hawai'i, Honolulu, 1991.
6. Cancer Research Center of Hawai'i Queen's Medical Center, American Cancer Society—Hawai'i Pacific Division: *Ethnic differences in mammography utilization in Hawai'i: Media-based versus culturally focussed accrual,* Unpublished proposal, Honolulu, 1990.
7. Chang L, Durante K, Nahulu L, Wong R: The Hawaiians. In Palafox N, Warren A, editors: *Cross-cultural caring: A handbook for health care professionals in Hawaii,* Honolulu, 1980, University of Hawai'i.
8. Community Cancer Program of Hawai'i: *Final report of the National Cancer Institute of health awareness survey reports,* Honolulu, 1982, Cancer Research Center of Hawai'i.
9. D'Amato J: *We cool tha's why: A study of personhood and place in a class of Hawaiian second graders,* Unpublished dissertation, Honolulu, 1986, University of Hawai'i.
10. Goodman MJ, Gilbert FI, Low G: Screening for breast cancer in Hawai'i—further implications, *Hawai'i Medical Journal* 43:356-360, 1984.
11. Goodman MJ, Gilbert FI, Mi MP, Grove JS, Catts A, Low G: Breast cancer screening in Hawai'i 1974-80: Results of a six-year program, *Hawai'i Medical Journal* 41:150-155, 1982.
12. Goodman MJ, La Croix S, Goodman P: *Cancer prevention and control research in native Hawaiians,* Unpublished report, Special Populations Division Cancer Control Program, National Cancer Institute, Washington, DC, 1987.
13. Gray F.d.P. *Hawai'i: The Sugar-Coated Fortress,* New York, 1972, Random House.
14. Hammond O: Needs assessment and policy development: Native Hawaiians as native Americans, *American Psychologist* 43:383-387, 1988.
15. Ichinotsubo D, Mower FH: Mutagens in Hawaiian dried/salted fish, *Journal of Agriculture and Food and Chemistry* 30:937-939, 1982.
16. Kamehameha Schools: *Aspects of Hawaiian Life and Environment.* The Kamehameha Schools Press, Honolulu, 1971.
17. Maney M, Schultz MR: *Incidence, survival, mortality and risk factors of several prevalent cancer sites along with the cultural beliefs and health beliefs of Hawaiians.* Unpublished paper, DeKalb, Il. 1991, Northern Illinois University.
18. Native Hawaiian Health Care Improvement Act, 100th Congress, 2d session, Senate Report 100-580, 1988.
19. Native Hawaiian Health Research Consortium. Historical/Cultural Task Force: *E ola mau: the native Hawaiian health needs study: historical/cultural task force report/The native Hawaiian health research consortium, Alu Like, Inc.* Honolulu, 1985a, The Consortium.
20. Native Hawaiian Health Research Consortium. Medical Task Force: *E ola mau: the native Hawaiian health needs study: medical task force report/The native Hawaiian health research consortium, Alu Like, Inc.* Honolulu, 1985b, The Consortium.
21. Native Hawaiians Study Commission: *Report on the culture, needs and concerns of native Hawaiians pursuant to public law 96-565, title III,* vol 2:148-153, Washington, DC, 1983, The Commission.
22. Palafox N: Hawaiian pidgin English. In Palafox N, Warren A, editors: *Cross-cultural caring: A handbook for health care professionals in Hawaii.* Honolulu, 1980, University of Hawai'i.

23. Pukui MK, Haertig EW, Lee CA: *Nānā i ke kumu* [Look to the source], vol 1, Honolulu, 1972a, Queen Liliuokalani Children's Center.

24. Pukui MK, Haertig EW, Lee CA: *Nānā i ke kumu* [Look to the source], vol 2, Honolulu, 1972b, Queen Liliuokalani Children's Center.

25. Shintani TT, Hughes CK, editors: *The Wai'anae book of Hawaiian health: the Wai'anae diet program manual,* ed 2, Honolulu, 1991, Wai'anae Coast Comprehensive Health Center.

26. Shintani TT, Hughes CK, Beckham S, O'Connor HK: Obesity and cardiovascular risk intervention through the ad libitum feeding of traditional Hawaiian diet, *American Journal of Clinical Nutrition* 53:1647s-1651s, 1991.

27. U.S. Bureau of the Census: Race and Hispanic origin for the United States: 1990 and 1980, *Census and You* 26:3, 1991.

28. *Wai'anae Coast Cancer Control Project,* Washington DC, 1990, National Cancer Institute.

29. Wang JCF: *Hawai'i State and Local Politics,* Hilo, Hawaii, 1982, Wang Associates.

30. Wegner EL: A framework for assessing health needs. In Wegner EL, editor: *Social process in Hawai'i: The health of native Hawaiians: A selective report on health status and health care in the 1980's* 32:32-54, Honolulu, 1989a, University of Hawai'i Press.

31. Wegner EL: Recommendations for more effective healthcare. In Wegner EL, editor: *Social process in Hawai'i: The health of native Hawaiians: A selective report on health status and health care in the 1980's* 32:149-167, Honolulu, 1989b, University of Hawai'i Press.

32. Wegner EL: *Social process in Hawai'i: The health of native Hawaiians: A selective report on health status and health care in the 1980's,* vol 32, Honolulu, 1989c, University of Hawai'i Press.

33. Young BBC: The Hawaiians. In McDermott JF Jr., Tseng W-S, Maretzki TW, editors: *People and cultures of Hawaii: A psychocultural profile,* Honolulu, 1980, University Press of Hawai'i.

Cancer Prevention and Early Detection in African Americans

Until the early 1950s, reported rates for cancer mortality in the United States were higher for whites than for ethnic minority populations. However, since that time, statistics show that African Americans experience higher cancer incidence and mortality rates as well as substantially lower cancer survival rates than whites. Despite recent advances in the prevention, diagnosis, and treatment of cancer, these disproportionately unfavorable cancer rates among African Americans have persisted. In fact, the disparities between the cancer experiences of African Americans and whites appear to be increasing.

For example, the age-adjusted cancer incidence rates for African Americans are 6% to 10% higher than for whites, depending on the time period and geographic area. Trends in these rates from 1982 through 1986 indicate that African Americans experienced higher increases in cancer incidence rates than whites. The disparity between African Americans and whites is more striking for cancer mortality. Not only do African Americans have age-adjusted cancer mortality rates that are 20% to 40% higher than those for whites, but mortality rates also are increasing faster among African Americans for certain cancer sites. Furthermore, mortality rates that are decreasing for whites are either still increasing for African Americans or not decreasing as fast as for whites. Statistics also show an overall difference in patient survival between African Americans and whites. For the period 1981 to 1987, the 5-year relative survival rate for all cancer sites combined for both sexes was only 38.4% for African Americans compared to 52.5% for whites. These figures indicate that African Americans were more likely than whites to die from causes associated specifically with their cancer within 5 years following their diagnosis.

The disproportionately unfavorable cancer rates experienced by African Americans and other ethnic minority populations have been targeted for improvement by the national health promotion and disease prevention objectives outlined in *Healthy People 2000*. Strategies to meet these objectives and to reduce the cancer burden among African Americans and other high-risk groups include the development of specifically targeted and culturally sensitive intervention programs. These programs must be based on an understanding of the factors that influence cancer incidence and mortality rates in the target groups.

This chapter provides an overview of risk factors and other considerations that are essential for planning and implementing effective cancer prevention and early detection programs aimed at African Americans. A sociocultural profile of this group provides information on the demographics, health and socioeconomic status, and cultural characteristics that establish a context for intervention activities in African American populations. Several of these characteristics constitute established or emerging risk factors that contribute to cancer incidence and mortality rates among African Americans.

For example, African Americans have been more likely than whites to be employed in less skilled jobs, where occupational exposures to carcinogenic agents may be greater. This chapter reviews studies that have linked these exposures to disproportionately high cancer incidence rates in African American workers. The marked disparities in the cancer experience of African Americans and whites have been attributed in part to differences in socioeconomic status (SES). Findings from a recent analysis of data from the National Cancer Institute's Surveillance, Epidemiology, and End Results (SEER) Program and the U.S. Bureau of the Census suggest that the disproportionate distribution of African Americans at lower SES levels accounts for some of the excess cancer burden among African Americans. This chapter describes the effect of SES on the health status of African Americans and on their use of health care services.

Although African Americans suffer a disproportionate share of the cancer burden, they are less likely to have access to and use health care services, including preventive care and cancer screenings. This chapter discusses institutional, socioeconomic, and educational barriers that limit African Americans' access to health care. Culturally specific perspectives on health and health-care-seeking behaviors also influence access to and use of health care services. This chapter provides an overview of African Americans' beliefs about the causes of illness and the relationship between faith and healing as well as their reliance on folk healers and a lay referral system for health care providers.

A lack of knowledge about cancer may contribute to nonparticipation in cancer screening programs, failure to recognize early warning signs of cancer, and delays in seeking cancer diagnosis or treatment. Data concerning the cancer-related knowledge, attitudes, and practices of African Americans are presented. These limited studies indicate that African Americans have lower levels of cancer knowledge than whites, are more likely than whites to have pessimistic attitudes regarding cancer, and are less likely than whites to use certain cancer screening procedures.

Because there may be a long latency period between exposure to a cancer risk factor and cancer onset, screening for premalignant and early malignant disease can lead to improved mortality and survival rates for many types of cancer. This chapter provides detailed information on assessing the cancer risk of African Americans based on their unique cultural and physical attributes. It summarizes available data on the relationship between risk factors in the African American population and cancers that are more prevalent in this group. In addition, the chapter includes an example of a comprehensive medical history questionnaire and guidelines for conducting a physical examination to detect cancer in African American patients.

African Americans face many obstacles to reducing the burden of cancer in their communities. Health care providers can become valuable allies in this effort by increasing their awareness, respect, and appreciation of the cultural qualities that affect the health status and practices of their African American patients. Health care professionals and program planners can provide tools to help African Americans fight cancer by adopting culturally specific strategies to improve access to health care, to increase knowledge about cancer, and to encourage the adoption and continuation of cancer prevention and control practices in African American communities. The risk factors and sociocultural characteristics described in this chapter are important considerations in designing interventions that seek to improve cancer rates among African Americans. As we learn more about the factors that contribute to the development and control of cancer in African Americans, we will be able to apply this knowledge to the development and implementation of more effective interventions for this group as well as for other populations.

Claudia R. Baquet, M.D., M.P.H.

Associate Director
Cancer Control Science Program
Division of Cancer Prevention and Control
National Cancer Institute

4

Cancer Prevention and Early Detection in African Americans

VERONICA A. CLARKE-TASKER

Although recent advances in the therapeutic approach to cancer have benefited all Americans, gross disparities in cancer incidence and survival rates between African Americans and Caucasian Americans still exist (see Figures 4-1 and 4-2). Cancer statistics for 17 of the 24 sites in the United States studied by the National Cancer Institute's Surveillance, Epidemiology, and End Results Program (SEER) indicate that African Americans have lower rates of survival than Caucasians. Data reported in *Cancer Statistics Review: 1973-1988* (USDHHS, 1991) show that both African Americans and Caucasians have experienced significant increases in the overall incidence of cancer between 1973 and 1988. However, cancer mortality rates for several individual sites (i.e., larynx, oral cavity, pancreas, colon/rectum, and leukemia) are increasing in African Americans while decreasing in Caucasians. Because of these disparities, cancer prevention and detection for African Americans have become major health issues in the United States.

SOCIOCULTURAL CHARACTERISTICS

African Americans have been variously defined and described in the literature. The term "African American" is used in this chapter to describe an individual born in the United States of African parentage. This includes individuals of mixed parentage, such as Native American and African-American or white American and African-American parentage. Individuals of West Indian, Bahamian, Haitian, and Jamaican heritage have contributed to the diversity of the African-American ethnic group and to the considerable variations in skin color and appearance among its members.

Demographics

Before the mid 1800s, the majority of African Americans resided in the southern states. After slavery ended, many stayed in the South; however, a significant percentage migrated North to seek a better way of life for themselves and their families (United States Department

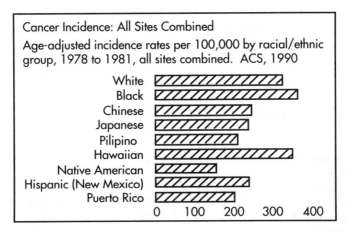

Figure 4-1 Graph shows disparities in cancer incidence among racial/ethnic groups.

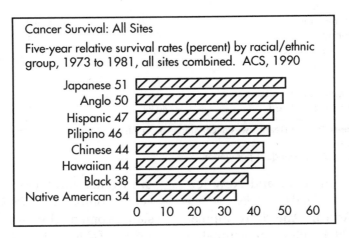

Figure 4-2 Graph shows disparities in cancer survival among racial/ethnic groups.

of Health and Human Services, 1985). In recent years, however, many African Americans relocated to the South, and now, most African Americans (56%) live in the South. In 1988, they made up 20% of the Southern population; 10% of the Northeastern population; 9% of the Midwest; and only 5% of the West. In 1988, 57% of African Americans lived in central cities of metropolitan areas, more than twice the proportion of the Caucasian population (27%). In contrast, in 1988, 50% of the Caucasian population but only 25% of the African American population lived in suburban areas (Bureau of the Census, 1989). States and metropolitan areas with the largest African American populations are: New York State (3.2 million), California (2.1 million), Chicago (1.6 million), Los Angeles (1.2 million),

TABLE 4-1 Mortality for Leading Causes of Death Among African Americans—1988

Rank	Causes of Death	Number of Deaths	Death Rate per 100,000 Population*	Percent of Total Deaths
	All Causes	**264,019**	**998.1**	**100.0**
1	Heart Diseases	79,466	313.4	30.1
2	Cancer	53,968	216.5	20.4
3	Cerebrovascular Diseases	18,479	72.5	7.0
4	Accidents	13,487	45.0	5.1
5	Homicide	10,403	30.6	3.9
6	Pneumonia & Influenza	7,191	27.1	2.7
7	Diabetes	6,972	27.7	2.6
8	Diseases of Infancy	6,614	19.9	2.5
9	Chronic Obstructive Lung Disease	5,476	21.7	2.1
10	HIV Infection	5,197	14.9	2.0
11	Nephritis	4,157	16.1	1.6
12	Cirrhosis of Liver	3,903	14.8	1.5
13	Septicemia	3,740	14.4	1.4
14	Suicide	2,022	6.2	0.8
15	Congenital Anomalies	2,019	6.3	0.8
	Other & Ill-defined	40,925	151.0	15.5

From Boring CC, Squires TS, and Heath CW: Cancer statistics for African Americans CA *Cancer J Clin* 42(1):16, 1992. Reprinted by permission.
*Age-adjusted to the 1970 U.S. standard population.

Philadelphia (1.1 million), and New Jersey (1.0 million) (USDHHS, 1986a).

In 1988 the African American population numbered 29.3 million, an estimated 12.2% of the U.S. population and by far this nation's largest minority group. Since 1980 the African American population has grown 12.7%, more than twice the growth rate for Caucasians (6.2%); U.S. Census Bureau projections indicate that this trend will continue through the 1990s (Bureau of the Census, 1989).

Life Expectancy and Causes of Death

African American men can expect to live to about 65.2 years, compared to 72.0 years for Caucasian men; African American women have a life expectancy of 73.5 years, compared to 78.8 years for Caucasian women (Bureau of the Census, 1989). Table 4-1 outlines the leading causes of death for African Americans.

Between 1977 and 1983, the most recent dates for which data are available, cancer was the fifth most common cause of death for African Americans under age 45; accidents and homicide were the top two causes of death for this age group. For the group aged 46 to 70, cancer was the third leading cause of death, behind heart disease and stroke. African Americans exhibit the highest overall age-adjusted cancer incidence and mortality rates of minority groups in the United

TABLE 4-2 Age-Adjusted (1970 U.S. Standard) Cancer Incidence Rates Per 100,000 Population by Race and Cancer Site, Both Sexes 1977-1983.

Cancer Site/Type	African American	Chinese	Japanese	Pilipino	Native American	Mexican American	Native Hawaiian	Alaska Native	Caucasian
All Sites	382.8‡	247.6	242.5	212.4	137.6	245.1	346.5	314.3	358.5
Oral cavity	15.0	15.4	4.8	8.9	2.1	6.6	9.0	16.5‡	11.7
Esophagus	11.6‡	3.3	2.8	3.4	1.0	1.6	7.3	6.1	3.4
Stomach	14.5	10.5	26.6	7.8	15.1	15.3	27.0‡	15.5	8.9
Colon & rectum	50.3	40.4	48.8	30.3	9.6	26.2	31.7	62.6‡	52.8
Liver	3.6	9.6‡	3.6	5.4	2.1	3.1	5.5	6.4	2.1
Gallbladder	1.0	1.0	1.5	1.4	10.0	4.6	1.3	10.6‡	1.3
Pancreas	13.8‡	6.3	7.1	4.9	3.7	11.0	8.0	9.9	9.5
Lung	69.8‡	40.6	27.1	27.3	6.3	23.4	66.9	46.9	56.4
Melanoma (skin)	0.8	0.7	1.2	1.0	1.9	1.9	1.1	na	9.4‡
Breast*	75.2	57.8	55.0	41.3	21.3	52.1	106.1‡	44.2	92.9
Cervix uteri*	19.7	10.3	5.9	8.6	19.9	16.1	15.2	28.0‡	8.6
Corpus uteri*	15.0	18.0	17.7	11.3	7.2	11.3	28.2‡	na	26.6
Ovary*	10.2	9.2	8.8	9.7	7.5	11.3	14.4‡	9.5	14.1
Prostate gland†	125.5‡	29.6	43.8	44.0	31.0	76.3	56.1	34.5	73.2
Urinary bladder	9.6	9.0	8.0	4.4	1.4	7.9	8.5	6.1	18.0‡
Kidney & renal	6.8	3.5	3.6	3.1	5.7	6.4	4.2	11.2‡	7.2
Brain & CNS	3.4	2.4	2.4	1.9	1.2	3.7	3.0	2.1	6.3‡
Hodgkin's disease	1.8	0.6	0.5	1.2	0.2	2.6	1.0	na	3.2‡
Non-Hodgkin's	7.2	8.5	7.2	8.3	2.8	6.7	8.4	na	11.1‡
Leukemia	9.1	4.8	5.7	7.1	4.6	6.9	8.2	na	10.4‡

Data source: African American, Caucasian—San Francisco-Oakland, Atlanta, Detroit, Connecticut;
Chinese, Japanese, Pilipino—San Francisco-Oakland, Hawaii;
Native Hawaiian—Hawaii;
American Indian—New Mexico, Arizona;
Mexican American—New Mexico;
Alaska Native—State of Alaska, 1969-83.
From SEER, The National Cancer Institute Surveillance Program, Cancer Statistics Branch: Bethesda, Md, 1991, National Cancer Institute. Reprinted by permission. Contains no copyrighted information.
*Females only.
†Males only.
‡Indicates the racial group with the highest rate for the cancer.

States for which statistics are available (Tables 4-2 and 4-3) (SEER, 1991).

Occupation and Disease Risk

Many African Americans have worked and continue to work in occupations that place them at risk for certain cancers. Data suggest (U.S. Bureau of Census, 1978) that there are significantly more Af-

rican American men and women than Caucasians in blue collar and service jobs. The three major areas of employment for African American men and women are: service occupations, 23%; administrative support personnel, 24%; and fabricators, laborers, and operators, 27%. Occupational exposures to nickel, chromium, radioisotopes, petroleum

TABLE 4-3   Age-Adjusted (1970 U.S. Standard) Cancer Mortality Rates Per 100,000 Population by Race and Cancer Site, Both Sexes 1977-83.

Cancer Site/Type	African American	Chinese	Japanese	Pilipino	Native American	Mexican American	Native Hawaiian	Alaska Native	Caucasian
All Sites	209.8	125.0	108.0	72.0	89.3	132.0	207.2	182.1	164.2
Oral cavity	5.7	5.4	1.7	2.4	1.8	1.9	3.9	5.9‡	3.3
Esophagus	9.1‡	2.8	2.1	1.8	2.0	1.7	7.2	3.2	
Stomach	10.0	7.6	17.9	3.5	5.8	11.8	21.8‡	10.8	5.2
Colon & rectum	22.4	17.9	16.8	7.9	8.9	13.2	14.6	26.6‡	21.4
Liver	3.6	10.1‡	3.4	3.5	2.0	3.9	5.2	6.9	1.9
Gallbladder	0.7	0.7	1.1	0.6	2.6	3.2	0.5	3.6‡	0.9
Pancreas	11.2‡	6.4	7.0	3.5	4.6	10.2	10.0	8.7	8.4
Lung	51.3	31.7	19.8	14.5	18.1	9.5	56.5‡	32.1	41.6
Melanoma (skin)	0.4‡	0.2	0.2	0.3	0.3	0.4	0.3	—	2.2‡
Breast*	26.9	12.0	10.2	7.8	9.0	19.4	37.2‡	14.0	26.8
Cervix uteri*	8.7	3.3	2.2	1.9	5.5	.2	5.6	11.1‡	3.2
Corpus uteri*	6.5‡	2.7	2.4	1.7	1.8	2.3	6.3	1.1	3.9
Ovary*	6.4	3.8	4.4	2.6	3.2	5.9	8.2‡	4.0	8.1
Prostate gland†	43.9‡	7.4	8.4	8.7	11.7	19.4	15.8	10.7	21.1
Urinary bladder	3.8‡	1.7	1.8	1.4	1.0	2.3	2.9	1.7	3.8‡
Kidney & renal	2.7	1.7	1.6	0.8	2.7	2.6	2.3	5.2‡	3.2
Brain & CNS	2.4	1.3	1.3	1.1	1.3	3.2	2.0	2.4	4.2‡
Hodgkin's disease	0.6	0.3	0.1	0.3	0.3	1.0‡	0.2	0.3	0.9
Non-Hodgkin's	3.3	2.8	3.5	3.4	2.1	3.1	5.6‡	3.1	5.2
Leukemia	5.8	4.1	3.5	4.1	2.9	4.8	6.8‡	3.8	6.7

Data source: African American, Caucasian, Chinese, Japanese, Pilipino, Native American—United States;
Native Hawaiian—Hawaii;
Mexican American—New Mexico;
Alaska Natives—Alaska, 1969-83.
From SEER, The National Cancer Institute Surveillance Program, Cancer Statistics Branch: Bethesda, Md, 1991 National Cancer Institute. Reprinted by permission. Contains no copyrighted information.
*Females only.
†Males only.
‡Indicates the racial group with the highest rate for the cancer.

chemicals, asbestos, nitrosamines, coal and tar fumes, and arsenic in such jobs have been associated with the development of cancers of the lung, bladder, and head and neck (Doll and Peto, 1981). In addition, historical and recent data confirm that African Americans are assigned to hazardous worksites more often than Caucasians are; they also endure greater occupational exposure to cancer-causing agents compared to Caucasians (Pottern, Morris, Blot, Ziegler and Fraumeni, 1981; Miller and Cooper, 1982; Rogers, Goldkind, and Goldkind, 1982; Michaels, 1983; USDHHS, 1986a).

Although researchers have studied the cancer rates among African Americans in only a few industries, the results of these investigations are startling. A 1953 study noted that of all ethnic groups, African

Americans were most likely to be employed in the most dangerous jobs in the steel industry (Michaels, 1983). They were disproportionately employed in jobs involving the coke ovens and therefore received the greatest exposure to benzo-(a)-pyrene and several other carcinogens. Years later these workers exhibited 10 times the lung cancer rate, 7 times the kidney cancer rate, elevated skin cancer rates, and increased nonmalignant lung disease rates when compared to other co-workers who were employed farther away from the coke ovens and in less dangerous jobs and locations (Michaels, 1983).

Workers in the most hazardous segment of the rubber industry, the tire-making process, have elevated rates of stomach, lung, blood, bladder, lymphatic, and prostate cancer, indicating that they have been exposed to high levels of carcinogens. African Americans are more often employed in this segment of the industry than other ethnic groups. In addition, African American workers in this industry suffer almost twice the lung cancer and prostate cancer rates of Caucasians performing the same tasks (Michaels, 1983).

Socioeconomic Status and Education

Research has shown that African Americans are disproportionately represented among the poor, constituting one-third of the U.S. population below the poverty line and one-fourth of the unemployed, but only about one-tenth of the total U.S. population. The African American family earns a median income of $13,270 a year, compared to $23,520 for a Caucasian family (U.S. Bureau of Census, 1990). In general, when compared to Caucasians, African Americans are more likely to live in the central city, have a higher proportion of families headed by women only, and, among married couples, have wives who work a greater number of weeks on average. All these characteristics, according to economists Blau and Graham (1990), are associated with lower wealth.

From 1939 to 1969, African Americans made steady gains in per capita incomes, family incomes, and male workers' earnings compared to Caucasians; however, since the mid-1970s measures of relative socioeconomic status (SES) among African Americans have remained stagnant or declined (Blau and Graham, 1990). Today, 35.7% of African American families live below the poverty level, while only 12.1% of Caucasian families live below that level. Between 1970 and 1988, the proportion of African Americans in the category "female head of house, no spouse present," rose from 28.3% to 42.8%. It is among such families that the incidence of poverty is greatest (U.S. Bureau of Census, 1990).

Health care workers must remember that impoverished individuals are at greater risk for illness than those with a higher SES; in addition, few of these clients visit doctors' offices or clinics for preventive care. Values of the poor are no different from those of the rest of society; however, health care may not be a top priority for those struggling for day-to-day survival.

The proportion of African Americans completing a given level of education is consistently much smaller than the proportion of Caucasians, according to the Census Bureau's 1989 report. Of African

Americans age 25 or over, 63% had completed high school and 11% had four or more years of post-secondary education, compared to 77% and 21%, respectively, for Caucasians.

Diet

Before migrating to the North, most African Americans consumed a diet that included many freshly grown vegetables. However, as they have become more urbanized, African Americans have tended to include less fresh produce in their diet. Currently, most foods in the typical African American diet are highly seasoned. This group's frequent use of smoked and fatty meats as seasoning for vegetables and soups may contribute to stomach cancer; the high levels of saturated fat in their diet may also be a risk factor for colorectal cancer.

Pork has always been a staple of the African American diet because it is inexpensive and can be prepared in a variety of ways. In the early 1960s, many younger African Americans eliminated pork from their diet for religious reasons, but the majority of the population continues to eat pork. Fried and broiled meats, poultry, fish, and a variety of wild game (depending on location) are also part of the African American diet.

Food is an important aspect of African American society, as it is with most cultures. Branch and Paxton (1976) noted that:

Food is the focus of emotional association, a mechanism for interpersonal relations, and is used in the communication of love and affection. This is especially true for many people of color. Food practices among ethnic people of color play an important role in their lives. Attempting to change food preferences is likened to attempting to change the individual. (p. 177)

Researchers and epidemiologists consider obesity a risk factor that can contribute to an increased incidence of breast, ovarian, uterine, colorectal, and prostate cancer; but in African American culture obesity is viewed as "having some meat on the bones" to fight illness. In this culture, a person of "normal" weight and stature by modern health standards may be considered too thin.

Family

In African American culture, the extended family plays an important role in child rearing, and the elderly are highly respected. In some families, the oldest member (grandmother or grandfather) serves as the authoritarian and historian.

Children are valued, and learn at an early age the rules governing a strong family bond. The oldest child is often responsible for the younger children and expected to act as a role model. To those not familiar with the culture, it may appear that the children assume adult roles at an early age. In reality, children are taught survival skills at an early stage.

African American parents tend to be very strict with their children, believing strongly that "spare the rod and spoil the child" and "children should be seen not heard." Female children are often raised more strictly than male children; women are expected to manage their homes and children and work at the same time. Men are expected to work and are usually viewed as the authority figure. Young men are also taught the importance of being able to provide for their families. The "man" of the house is expected to put food on the table and provide a roof over his family's head whether the woman works or not.

Religion

The church has played an important role in the lives of poor people in the United States, particularly African Americans, by championing their interests and offering tangible assistance during periods of economic and social instability. As a long-standing tradition, African American churches have met not only the spiritual, but also the educational, physical, and social needs of their members (Eng, Hatch, and Callan, 1985; Askey, Parker, Alexander, and White, 1983). The church, more than any other institution, has been in a position to help African Americans to cope with and sometimes overcome the social and political barriers of unequal access to resources. When necessary, the church serves to link the rural African American community to the more powerful societal systems that control resources.

The church has also functioned as a source of social identity; it is one of the few formal institutions within which African Americans have been able to confer titles of honor and respect on their own people (Eng, Hatch, and Callan, 1985). This has encouraged the maintenance of a dual system of identity among African Americans: identities ascribed by the dominant society, in which African Americans may hold low-paying, unskilled jobs, and the alternative, prestigious identities earned within their ethnic community. The sense of achievement and self-worth that many African Americans gain through involvement in their church can counteract the negative self-images often imposed upon this group by the dominant society (Eng, Hatch, and Callan, 1985).

Given the importance of the church in the African American community, Smith (1976) advocates a role for its clergy as allied health professionals. Pastors have participated in history taking, diagnosis, treatment, follow-up, and evaluation (Westburg, 1973). Levin (1984) cites several examples of the use of the African American church as a locus for health promotion and disease prevention, including programs dealing with the control of hypertension and diabetes, and pre-natal and infant care.

EPIDEMIOLOGY OF CANCER IN AFRICAN AMERICANS

During the past 30 years a number of descriptive studies have shown that the incidence of and mortality from cancer are greater among African Americans (Baquet, 1990; American Cancer Society, 1986; Pollack and Horn, 1980; Devesa and Silverman, 1978; Young, Devesa, and Cutler, 1975; Henschke, et al., 1973). Beardsley (1987) noted that even as early as 1930, cancer was among the top eight killers of African Americans in most southern states.

Researchers have attributed the excessive incidence of and mortality from cancer experienced by African Americans to such diverse variables as lack of access to medical care, low socioeconomic status, improvements in case-finding, underrepresentation in census data, smoking, alcohol consumption, diet, negative social behavior, employment in hazardous occupations, a failure of early detection, low-quality treatment, and urban living. To date, however, few analytic studies have been conducted to sort through these subjective and ill-defined variables.

Wilson (1989) contends it is clear that many or all of the above factors are related to cancer etiology, but that the precise association between each one and an increased risk of cancer among African Americans needs to be delineated.

Social and Biological Influences

Baquet (1990) suggested that selective personal, cultural, and sociohistorical factors may partly account for the higher incidence of and mortality from cancer among African Americans. For example, some studies suggest that immune function and nutritional status in poor individuals may differ from those of more affluent persons, and such differences have been known to influence carcinogenesis. There are 34 million poor in the United States; this accounts for approximately 15% of our population. One-third of these poor are African American, the remaining two-thirds are Caucasian, Hispanic, Native American and other ethnic groups.

Hargreaves, et al. (1989) compared data on African Americans to that on Caucasians from diet and nutritional status surveys conducted in 1972 and 1979 by the Centers for Disease Control and the National Center for Health Statistics (NCHS), respectively. Their review indicated that, compared with Caucasians, African Americans eat more animal fat, less fiber, and fewer fruits and vegetables; they obtain lower levels of thiamine, riboflavin, vitamins A and C, and iron. In addition, compared to Caucasians, African American women are more likely to be obese, and men of this ethnic group more likely to be underweight. The researchers concluded that the eating habits and compromised nutritional status of African Americans could contribute to higher incidence and mortality rates from cancer.

Studies of cancer in African Americans have documented evidence for differences in histology, or tissue structure, when compared to Caucasians. Although little is known on this subject, histologic patterns may be related to survival and prognosis, and contribute in part to poor survival and prognosis in African Americans for some cancer sites. Baquet, Ringen, and Pollack (1986), suggest African Americans have a higher distribution of aggressive histologic tumors than Caucasians for certain cancers, especially esophageal cancer. For cancers of the bladder and corpus uteri, differences in cell type and grade have been noted in African Americans (Baquet and Ringen, 1986).

Table 4-4 summarizes the histologic types for the three more aggressive cancers among African Americans.

Finally, Bang (1987) suggests that the rapid increases in reported incidence of and mortality from cancer among African Americans may, in part, be a reflection of improvements in diagnosis and medical care that permit more accurate diagnoses and certification of death.

Cancer Incidence

The cancer incidence data on African Americans and Caucasians are summarized in Table 4-5 (U.S. Department of Health and Human Services, 1991). In general, the incidence of cancer (all sites combined) in African Americans is about 6% higher than that of Caucasians. In addition, racial disparities are even more

TABLE 4-4 Percent Distribution of Cases by Histologic Type of Cancer for African Americans and Caucasians, SEER Program 1978-81

Number of Cases and Histologic Type	Caucasians	African Americans
BLADDER		
Total number of cancer cases	12,018	520
Number and percent of cases microscopically confirmed	11,826 (98.4%)	508 (97.7%)
Carcinoma, NOS*	1.8%	3.9%
Papillary adenocarcinoma	3.6	1.6
Squamous cell carcinoma	2.1	9.1
Transitional cell	36.0	41.4
Papillary transitional cell	54.5	36.2
All others	2.0	7.9
	100.0%	100.1%
ESOPHAGUS		
Total number of cancer cases	2,262	734
Number and percent of cases microscopically confirmed	2,099 (92.8%)	708 (96.5%)
Squamous cell carcinoma	72.8%	91.1%
Adenocarcinoma, NOS*	16.6	1.1
Carcinoma, NOS*	6.1	5.8
All others	4.5	2.0
	100.0%	100.0%
CORPUS UTERI		
Total number of cancer cases	10,323	475
Number and percent of cases microscopically confirmed	10,261 (99.4%)	470 (98.9%)
Carcinoma, NOS*	2.1%	1.9%
Papillary adenocarcinoma	6.6	14.0
Adenocarcinoma, NOS*	73.4	52.8
Adenosquamous carcinoma	10.8	8.7
Mullerian mixec tumor	1.9	7.0
Leiomyosarcoma	1.2	6.0
All others	4.0	9.6
	100.0%	100.0%

From U.S. Department of Health and Human Services: *Cancer Among Blacks and Other Minorities: Statistical Profiles*, March 1986, pp. 216, 223, 224. Contains no copyrighted material.
*NOS = not otherwise specified.

TABLE 4-5   Age-Adjusted Cancer Incidence Rates* By Race, Primary Cancer Site, Gender and Time Period

Site	African Americans SEER Incidence (1984-88)			Caucasians SEER Incidence (1984-88)		
	Total	Male	Female	Total	Male	Female
All sites	405.4	522.7	324.9	373.6	433.1	339.8
Oral Cavity & Pharynx:	14.7	24.1	7.2	10.8	16.3	6.4
Lip	0.1	0.1	0.1	1.4	2.8	0.3
Tongue	2.9	4.7	1.5	2.2	3.2	1.4
Salivary gland	0.8	0.8	0.7	1.0	1.3	0.8
Floor of mouth	1.8	3.1	0.9	1.2	1.8	0.7
Gum & other mouth	2.4	3.7	1.4	2.0	2.5	1.5
Nasopharynx	0.6	1.1	0.3	0.4	0.6	0.3
Tonsil	2.3	4.1	0.9	1.0	1.5	0.6
Oropharynx	0.5	0.8	0.2	0.3	0.5	0.2
Hypopharynx	2.3	4.3	0.7	1.1	1.8	0.5
Other buccal cavity & pharynx	0.9	1.5	0.4	0.4	0.5	0.2
Digestive System:	99.1	124.1	80.7	77.2	96.5	63.1
Esophagus	10.9	18.3	5.1	3.2	5.2	1.6
Stomach	12.9	18.9	8.5	7.1	10.6	4.5
Small intestine	1.8	2.3	1.4	1.1	1.3	0.9
Colon/Rectum	51.0	57.7	46.4	50.6	61.6	42.7
Anus, anal cancal & anorectum	1.2	1.0	1.3	0.8	0.7	0.9
Liver & Intrahep.	3.9	6.4	1.9	2.1	3.2	1.4
Liver	3.6	5.9	1.8	1.9	2.9	1.2
Gallbladder	1.0	0.7	1.2	1.1	0.8	1.4
Other biliary	1.0	1.3	0.8	1.1	1.4	1.0
Pancreas	14.6	16.4	13.2	9.1	10.7	7.9
Retroperitoneum	0.5	0.5	0.5	0.4	0.5	0.3
Peritoneum, omentum & mesentery	0.1	0.2	0.1	0.2	0.2	0.2
Other digestive organs	0.3	0.5	0.2	0.3	0.3	0.2
Respiratory System:	86.2	142.8	44.1	62.9	93.3	40.3
Nose, nasal cavity & middle ear	0.6	0.8	0.5	0.6	0.8	0.5
Larynx	7.2	13.1	2.6	4.6	8.3	1.6
Lung & bronchus	77.8	127.8	40.7	56.8	82.5	37.8
Pleura	0.4	0.7	0.1	0.7	1.4	0.2
Trachea, mediastinum & other resp organs	0.2	0.3	0.2	0.3	0.4	0.2
Bones & Joints	0.6	0.7	0.6	0.9	1.0	0.7
Soft Tissue (incl Heart)	2.5	2.8	2.4	2.1	2.5	1.8
Skin (exc Basal & Squam)	2.9	4.4	1.7	13.9	17.9	10.5
Melanoma of skin	0.7	0.7	0.8	10.9	12.6	9.7
Other non-epithelial skin	2.2	3.8	0.9	3.0	5.2	0.8
Breast	52.1	1.4	91.7	59.5	0.8	108.8

TABLE 4-5 Age-Adjusted Cancer Incidence Rates* By Race, Primary Cancer Site, Gender and Time Period—cont'd.

Site	African Americans SEER Incidence (1984-88)			Caucasians SEER Incidence (1984-88)		
	Total	Male	Female	Total	Male	Female
Female Genital System:	24.4	—	43.1	26.0	—	48.0
Cervix Uteri	8.9	—	15.8	4.0	—	7.8
Corpus Uteri	7.7	—	13.6	12.3	—	22.4
Uterus, NOS	0.3	—	0.4	0.2	—	0.3
Ovary	5.5	—	9.8	7.9	—	14.6
Vagina	0.8	—	1.4	0.3	—	0.6
Vulva	0.7	—	1.2	1.0	—	1.7
Other female genital organ	0.5	—	0.9	0.4	—	0.7
Male Genital System:	55.0	135.7	—	40.2	97.9	—
Prostate gland	54.2	134.0	—	37.4	92.2	—
Testis	0.3	0.7	—	2.3	4.7	—
Penis	0.3	0.8	—	0.3	0.8	—
Other male genital organ	0.1	0.2	—	0.1	0.3	—
Urinary System:	19.1	28.8	12.0	27.1	45.0	13.8
Urinary bladder	9.8	16.0	5.3	18.0	32.1	7.8
Kidney & renal pelvis	8.5	11.8	6.1	8.2	11.6	5.6
Ureter	0.2	0.3	0.1	0.5	0.9	0.3
Other urinary organ	0.6	0.7	0.5	0.3	0.4	0.1
Eye & Orbit	0.2	0.3	0.2	0.7	0.8	0.6
Brain & Nervous System:	4.0	4.5	3.6	6.5	7.6	5.5
Brain	3.7	4.2	3.3	6.2	7.3	5.3
Cranial nerves & other nervous system	0.3	0.3	0.3	0.3	0.4	0.3
Endocrine System:	3.0	2.0	3.9	4.8	3.1	6.5
Thyroid gland	2.4	1.3	3.4	4.3	2.5	6.0
Other endocrine (incl. Thymus)	0.6	0.7	0.5	0.5	0.6	0.5
Lymphomas:	10.4	12.9	8.3	16.7	20.1	13.8
Hodgkin's disease	1.8	2.3	1.4	3.1	3.5	2.7
Non-Hodgkin's lymphoma	8.6	10.5	6.9	13.7	16.6	11.2
Multiple myeloma	8.2	10.2	6.7	3.9	4.7	3.2
Leukemias:	8.7	11.2	7.0	10.1	13.3	7.8
Lymphocytic:	3.4	4.6	2.5	4.5	6.1	3.3
Acute lymphocytic	0.9	0.9	0.8	1.5	1.8	1.2
Chronic lymphocytic	2.5	3.5	1.6	2.9	4.2	2.0
Other lymphocytic	0.1	0.1	0.1	0.1	0.1	0.1
Myeloid:	4.0	4.8	3.4	3.9	4.9	3.1
Acute myeloid	2.1	2.6	1.8	2.3	2.8	1.9
Chronic myeloid	1.6	1.9	1.4	1.3	1.7	1.0
Other myeloid	0.3	0.3	0.2	0.3	0.4	0.2
Monocytic:	0.2	0.2	0.2	0.3	0.3	0.3
Acute monocytic	0.1	0.1	0.2	0.2	0.2	0.2
Chronic monocytic	0.0	0.0	0.0	0.0	0.0	0.0
Other monocytic	0.0	0.1	0.0	0.0	0.0	0.0

Continued.

TABLE 4-5 Age-Adjusted Cancer Incidence Rates* By Race, Primary Cancer Site, Gender and Time Period—cont'd.

Site	African Americans SEER Incidence (1984-88)			Caucasians SEER Incidence (1984-88)		
	Total	Male	Female	Total	Male	Female
Other:	1.1	1.5	0.9	1.4	2.0	1.0
Other acute	0.4	0.6	0.3	0.7	0.8	0.5
Other chronic	0.0	0.0	0.0	0.0	0.0	0.0
Aleukemic, subleuk, & NOS	0.7	0.9	0.6	0.7	1.1	0.5
Ill-defined & Unspecified Sites	14.1	16.8	11.8	10.3	12.2	9.0

*Incidence rates are per 100,000 and are age adjusted to the 1970 U.S. standard population.
From U.S. Department of Health and Human Services: *Cancer Statistics Review* 1973-1988 Bethesda, Md, 1991, National Institutes of Health. Contains no copyrighted material.

evident for certain cancers: for instance, the incidence of prostate cancer in African American men is significantly greater than that in Caucasian men, as is the incidence of lung and bronchus cancers. African American women experience significantly more cervical and early-age breast cancers than Caucasians. African Americans also experience multiple myeloma at a rate higher than that for Caucasians.

Bang (1987) noted that the high incidence of cancers of the lung, esophagus, and oral cavity among African Americans are to be expected, as these are associated with cigarette smoking or with cigarette smoking combined with alcohol intake. Studies have consistently documented that African American men report heavier alcohol use, poorer nutritional habits, and higher smoking rates. Bang also suggests these high cancer rates may be related to increased exposure to industrial and environmental pollutants associated with changes in occupation and lifestyle.

Cancer Mortality and Survival Rates

Mortality figures, based on 1984-1987 rates, are more disconcerting (Table 4-6). In general, African Americans experience significantly higher death rates from cancer than Caucasians. Several types of cancer account for this higher death rate: oral, esophageal, stomach, liver, pancreas, cervical, prostate, lung and bronchus, colon/rectum, breast cancers, and multiple myeloma. These findings are particularly troublesome because, with the exception of multiple myeloma, most of these deaths can be prevented with changes in lifestyle and early detection.

Table 4-7 demonstrates that the five-year survival rate for African Americans diagnosed with cancer is approximately 30% lower than that for Caucasian Americans. The minority group's survival rates for colon/rectum, lung, prostate, and cer-

TABLE 4-6 Age-Adjusted Cancer Mortality Rates* By Race, Primary Cancer Site, Gender and Time Period

Site	African Americans SEER Mortality (1984-88)			Caucasians SEER Mortality (1984-88)		
	Total	Male	Female	Total	Male	Female
All Sites	221.5	301.6	165.8	165.3	206.0	139.0
Oral Cavity & Pharynx:	5.5	9.5	2.2	3.0	4.5	1.9
Lip	0.0	0.0	0.0	0.0	0.1	0.0
Tongue	1.1	2.0	0.5	0.7	1.0	0.5
Salivary gland	0.1	0.2	0.1	0.2	0.4	0.2
Floor of mouth	0.3	0.7	0.1	0.2	0.2	0.1
Gum & other mouth	0.9	1.5	0.4	0.5	0.7	0.3
Nasopharynx	0.6	0.8	0.3	0.2	0.3	0.1
Tonsil	0.4	0.6	0.2	0.2	0.3	0.1
Oropharynx	0.3	0.6	0.1	0.2	0.3	0.1
Hypopharynx	0.5	0.9	0.2	0.3	0.5	0.1
Other buccal cavity & pharynx	1.2	2.2	0.3	0.5	0.8	0.3
Digestive System:	59.9	79.5	45.4	40.2	51.3	32.3
Esophagus	8.9	15.5	3.8	2.9	4.9	1.4
Stomach	8.9	13.7	5.3	4.8	7.1	3.1
Small intestine	0.7	0.8	0.6	0.3	0.4	0.2
Colon/Rectum	23.1	27.3	20.2	19.7	23.9	16.8
Anus, anal canal & anorectum	0.3	0.2	0.4	0.1	0.1	0.2
Liver & Intrahep.	4.0	6.2	2.3	2.2	3.1	1.4
Liver	3.6	5.7	1.9	1.8	2.7	1.1
Gallbladder	0.6	0.5	0.7	0.8	0.5	0.9
Other biliary	0.5	0.6	0.5	0.7	0.8	0.6
Pancreas	12.6	14.3	11.4	8.4	9.8	7.3
Retroperitoneum	0.1	0.1	0.1	0.1	0.1	0.1
Peritoneum, omentum & mesentery	0.1	0.1	0.0	0.1	0.1	0.1
Other digestive organs	0.2	0.3	0.2	0.2	0.2	0.2
Respiratory System:	62.1	104.4	30.9	45.1	68.2	28.3
Nose, nasal cavity & middle ear	0.3	0.5	0.1	0.2	0.2	0.1
Larynx	2.6	4.8	0.9	1.2	2.2	0.4
Lung & bronchus	58.9	98.8	29.7	43.4	65.3	27.5
Pleura	0.1	0.1	0.1	0.2	0.4	0.1
Trachea, mediastinum & other resp organs	0.1	0.3	0.0	0.1	0.2	0.1
Bones & Joints	0.4	0.5	0.2	0.4	0.5	0.3
Soft Tissue (incl Heart)	1.6	1.3	1.9	1.1	1.2	1.0
Skin (exc Basal & Squam)	1.0	1.6	0.5	3.1	4.4	1.9
Melanoma of skin	0.3	0.3	0.3	2.3	3.2	1.7
Other non-epithelial skin	0.7	1.3	0.1	0.7	1.3	0.3
Breast	18.7	0.5	32.8	15.7	0.3	28.1

Continued.

TABLE 4-6 Age-Adjusted Cancer Mortality Rates* By Race, Primary Cancer Site, Gender and Time Period—cont'd

Site	African Americans SEER Mortality (1984-88)			Caucasians SEER Mortality (1984-88)		
	Total	Male	Female	Total	Male	Female
Female Genital System:	10.3	—	17.9	8.3	—	14.8
Cervix Uteri	3.4	—	6.1	1.2	—	2.2
Corpus Uteri	1.5	—	2.6	1.1	—	1.9
Uterus, NOS	1.4	—	2.4	1.0	—	1.7
Ovary	3.4	—	5.9	4.6	—	8.3
Vagina	0.3	—	0.4	0.1	—	0.2
Vulva	0.1	—	0.2	0.2	—	0.3
Other female genital organ	0.2	—	0.3	0.1	—	0.2
Male Genital System:	18.5	47.7	—	9.0	23.8	—
Prostate gland	18.4	47.4	—	8.8	23.3	—
Testis	0.0	0.1	—	0.1	0.3	—
Penis	0.1	0.1	—	0.1	0.1	—
Other male genital organ	0.0	0.0	—	0.0	0.0	—
Urinary System:	6.2	8.5	4.5	6.8	11.1	3.9
Urinary bladder	3.3	4.6	2.4	3.4	6.1	1.6
Kidney & renal pelvis	2.7	3.8	1.9	3.2	4.7	2.1
Ureter	0.0	0.1	0.0	0.1	0.1	0.1
Other urinary organ	0.1	0.2	0.1	0.1	0.1	0.0
Eye & Orbit	0.1	0.1	0.1	0.1	0.1	0.1
Brain & Nervous System:	2.5	2.9	2.1	4.5	5.4	3.7
Brain	2.3	2.7	2.0	4.4	5.3	3.6
Cranial nerves & other nervous system	0.1	0.1	0.1	0.1	0.1	0.1
Endocrine System:	0.7	0.8	0.7	0.7	0.7	0.7
Thyroid gland	0.2	0.2	0.2	0.4	0.3	0.4
Other endocrine (incl. Thymus)	0.5	0.6	0.5	0.3	0.4	0.3
Lymphomas:	4.7	6.1	3.5	7.0	8.7	5.6
Hodgkin's disease	0.5	0.6	0.4	0.7	0.9	0.5
Non-Hodgkin's lymphoma	4.1	5.5	3.1	6.3	7.8	5.1
Multiple myeloma	5.3	6.7	4.3	2.6	3.3	2.2
Leukemias:	6.6	8.6	5.2	6.5	8.6	4.9
Lymphocytic:	1.9	2.7	1.4	1.9	2.7	1.2
Acute lymphocytic	0.6	0.6	0.6	0.7	0.9	0.5
Chronic lymphocytic	1.2	2.0	0.7	1.1	1.6	0.7
Other lymphocytic	0.1	0.1	0.1	0.1	0.2	0.1
Myeloid:	2.9	3.7	2.3	2.6	3.3	2.1
Acute myeloid	1.6	2.0	1.4	1.6	2.1	1.3
Chronic myeloid	1.2	1.6	0.9	0.8	1.0	0.7
Other myeloid	0.0	0.1	0.0	0.1	0.1	0.1

TABLE 4-6   Age-Adjusted Cancer Mortality Rates* By Race, Primary Cancer Site, Gender and Time Period—cont'd.

Site	African Americans SEER Mortality (1984-88)			Caucasians SEER Mortality (1984-88)		
	Total	Male	Female	Total	Male	Female
Monocytic:	0.1	0.1	0.0	0.1	0.1	0.2
Acute monocytic	0.0	0.1	0.0	0.1	0.1	0.1
Chronic monocytic	0.0	0.0	0.0	0.0	0.0	0.0
Other monocytic	0.0	0.0	0.0	0.0	0.0	0.0
Other:	1.8	2.1	1.5	1.9	2.6	1.4
Other acute	0.9	1.0	0.9	1.1	1.5	0.9
Other chronic	0.0	0.1	0.0	0.1	0.1	0.0
Aleukemic, subleuk, & NOS	0.8	1.0	0.6	0.7	1.0	0.5
Ill-defined & Unspecified Sites	17.5	22.8	13.6	11.2	13.8	9.4

*Mortality rates are per 100,000 and are age adjusted to the 1970 U.S. standard population.
From U.S. Department of Health and Human Services, *Cancer Statisticvs Review* 1973-1988, Bethesda, Md, 1991, National Institutes of Health. Contains no copyrighted material.

vical cancers lag behind whites by 15% to 20%.

HEALTH BELIEFS AND PRACTICES
Definition of Health, Illness, and Disease Causation

African Americans may differ from Caucasians in their definitions of health and illness and in their beliefs about the causes of illness. Winslow and Bishop (1969) found that among African Americans:

There is a tendency to lump events as to whether they are desirable or undesirable, resulting in a mixture of conceptual domains confusing to the science-oriented professional. Good health is classed with any kind of good luck, success, money, a good job, a peaceful home. Illness, on the other hand, may be looked upon as just another undesirable event, along with bad luck, poverty, unemployment, domestic turmoil, and so on. The attempted manipulation of events therefore covers a broad range of practices that are carried out to attract good, including good health, or to repel bad, including bad health. (p. 81)

Some African Americans believe that illness may be due to their failure to live according to or to accept God's will. Illness may also be characterized as natural or unnatural; influenced by harmony with God or disharmony; and indicative of balance or imbalance in some area of the individual's life. Jacques (1976) interprets the African American view of illness as:

a loss of self, a sense of disharmony with one's soul, or being 'the only one,' lost, and lacking communion with others. This may be expressed physically, socially, emotionally, spiritually, and culturally. From this perspective, one's illness can be perceived as ill-at-ease, a state of disease without being functionally incapacitated. Illness is not seen as individual deviancy that is measurable, but a state of being out of union, physically, emotionally, or spiritually. (p. 18)

TABLE 4-7 Age Adjusted 5-Year Relative Survival Rates* By Race, Primary Cancer Site, Gender and Time Period

Site	African Americans SEER Survival (1981-87)			Caucasians SEER Survival (1981-87)		
	Total	Male	Female	Total	Male	Female
All Sites	38.4	33.4	44.0	52.5	47.2	57.4
Oral Cavity & Pharynx:	31.2	26.1	44.9	53.6	52.0	56.9
Lip	—	—	—	90.9	91.7	84.8
Tongue	26.2	21.2	40.3	47.6	46.4	49.8
Salivary gland	67.2	68.8	65.8	70.0	60.1	80.4
Floor of mouth	35.3	31.6	52.6	55.8	52.8	61.6
Gum & other mouth	42.0	35.1	54.1	54.8	47.9	64.8
Nasopharynx	43.2	27.3	—	43.5	42.5	45.6
Tonsil	27.8	25.2	34.2	39.9	38.8	42.2
Oropharynx	17.6	16.6	—	26.7	22.2	36.1
Hypopharynx	17.1	18.2	12.5	27.1	24.7	33.6
Other buccal cavity & pharynx	9.8	4.6	—	27.0	23.3	34.3
Digestive System:	29.0	24.4	34.0	41.4	39.8	43.0
Esophagus	6.2	5.3	8.6	8.9	7.7	11.5
Stomach	17.4	16.8	18.3	16.0	14.7	18.0
Small intestine	40.3	34.1	45.6	42.5	40.5	44.7
Colon/Rectum	46.6	43.8	48.8	57.0	57.0	57.0
Anus, anal canal & anorectum	46.3	21.6	60.4	60.4	56.4	62.7
Liver & Intrahep.	4.5	3.1	7.3	5.4	3.3	9.1
Liver	4.5	3.1	7.3	5.4	3.3	9.1
Gallbladder	8.6	6.7	9.4	13.1	13.9	12.8
Other biliary	15.1	0.0	19.9	13.0	12.1	14.1
Pancreas	4.3	3.8	4.9	2.8	2.4	3.2
Retroperitoneum	32.5	—	32.7	38.7	37.4	40.1
Peritoneum, omentum & mesentery	—	—	—	22.3	21.0	23.0
Other digestive organs	14.3	14.6	—	1.5	1.2	1.8
Respiratory System:	14.7	14.4	15.6	18.1	17.6	19.0
Nose, nasal cavity & middle ear	29.5	26.3	36.1	54.9	56.9	52.4
Larynx	54.3	55.4	50.3	67.9	68.4	65.6
Lung & bronchus	10.8	9.9	13.0	13.4	11.8	16.3
Pleura	0.0	0.0	—	5.7	3.7	15.2
Trachea, mediastinum & other resp organs	—	—	—	44.4	44.1	45.2
Bones & Joints	50.8	52.0	49.0	53.8	51.2	57.5
Soft Tissue (incl Heart)	58.4	51.7	65.0	59.7	57.9	62.2
Skin (exc Basal & Squam)	60.6	44.5	89.7	73.6	63.8	86.5
Melanoma of skin	69.5	59.8	75.9	81.7	76.8	86.7
Other non-epithelial skin	57.9	41.6	100.0	38.4	29.5	83.8
Breast	63.3	82.1	63.1	78.1	74.7	78.2

Site	African Americans SEER Survival (1981-87)			Caucasians SEER Survival (1981-87)		
	Total	Male	Female	Total	Male	Female
Female Genital System:	51.8	—	51.8	67.2	—	67.2
Cervix Uteri	57.4	—	57.4	67.5	—	67.5
Corpus Uteri	55.5	—	55.5	84.4	—	84.4
Uterus, NOS	27.0	—	27.0	27.4	—	27.4
Ovary	36.1	—	36.1	38.7	—	38.7
Vagina	54.6	—	54.6	48.0	—	48.0
Vulva	71.3	—	71.3	74.7	—	74.7
Other female genital organ	49.4	—	49.4	54.2	—	54.2
Male Genital System:	63.4	63.4	—	76.9	76.9	—
Prostate gland	63.0	63.0	—	75.6	75.6	—
Testis	93.5	93.5	—	92.8	92.8	—
Penis	63.7	63.7	—	72.3	72.3	—
Other male genital organ	—	—	—	65.0	65.0	—
Urinary System:	54.7	58.3	48.5	70.8	73.1	65.6
Urinary bladder	59.2	65.3	47.0	79.0	80.2	75.4
Kidney & renal pelvis	52.1	51.5	53.1	53.2	54.1	51.6
Ureter	—	—	—	66.3	72.1	55.2
Other urinary organ	36.7	51.1	25.6	58.0	66.9	45.7
Eye & Orbit	79.1	—	—	76.7	77.0	76.4
Brain & Nervous System:	33.1	34.4	31.2	24.2	23.0	25.8
Brain	30.1	33.2	25.9	22.2	21.1	23.8
Cranial nerves & other nervous system	60.8	—	—	61.8	59.4	64.7
Endocrine System:	94.1	97.2	93.1	93.7	92.2	94.2
Thyroid gland	94.1	97.2	93.1	93.7	92.2	94.2
Other endocrine (incl. Thymus)	44.7	55.3	29.2	49.9	48.0	52.2
Lymphomas:	51.5	50.6	52.8	57.0	56.1	58.0
Hodgkin's disease	73.6	72.6	75.8	76.8	75.7	78.2
Non-Hodgkin's lymphoma	44.5	42.5	47.0	51.3	50.1	52.6
Multiple myeloma	28.3	27.5	29.3	26.3	25.0	27.5
Leukemias:	29.0	28.5	29.6	36.3	36.0	36.7
Lymphocytic:	48.9	46.8	51.6	59.4	57.7	61.7
Acute lymphocytic	39.1	36.7	42.0	52.5	49.1	57.0
Chronic lymphocytic	55.4	52.3	60.0	64.5	63.4	65.9
Other lymphocytic	—	—	—	32.1	29.7	34.2
Myeloid:	15.1	15.0	15.3	14.3	12.8	16.1
Acute myeloid	11.3	13.7	9.3	8.3	7.4	9.3
Chronic myeloid	20.4	17.3	24.5	25.4	22.5	29.2
Other myeloid	15.4	—	—	13.4	11.6	15.7

Continued.

TABLE 4-7 Age Adjusted 5-Year Relative Survival Rates* By Race, Primary Cancer Site, Gender and Time Period—cont'd.

Site	African Americans SEER Survival (1981-87)			Caucasians SEER Survival (1981-87)		
	Total	Male	Female	Total	Male	Female
Monocytic:	10.1	—	—	7.2	7.0	7.6
Acute monocytic	—	—	—	6.6	6.1	7.3
Chronic monocytic	—	—	—	—	—	—
Other monocytic	—	—	—	0.0	—	—
Other:	25.4	20.4	30.3	26.0	29.3	21.0
Other acute	8.0	0.0	—	7.3	6.7	8.6
Other chronic	—	—	—	41.0	—	—
Aleukemic, subleuk, & NOS	36.6	33.4	39.5	41.0	45.6	32.9
Ill-defined & Unspecified Sites	7.2	7.2	7.3	9.6	9.9	9.3

*Survival rates are expressed as percents.
From U.S. Department of Health and Human Services, *Cancer Statistics Review* 1973-1988, Bethesda Md, 1991, National Institutes of Health. Contains no copyrighted material.

A natural illness, for example, may result from failure to protect the body from exposure to dirt or the cold. An improper diet can have negative influences on the blood. Unnatural illness, on the other hand, may be caused by the supernatural: the Devil, witchcraft, hexing, rooting, evil forces, sorcery, cursing, demons or bad spirits. Sinful behavior can bring about divine punishment through illness.

Illness believed to be caused by unnatural means or by magic cannot be treated by traditional medicine. According to Snow (1983):

Reported symptoms of magical illness range from pseudocytis to headache, but most can be divided into two broad categories, gastrointestinal and behavioral. In most instances, it is believed that the fix or hex is administered in a victim's food or drink. It is often referred to as 'poison.' Snakes, frogs, or lizards may be introduced into the body in the form of eggs or powder, which hatch or reconstitute themselves and take up their abode in a victim's blood, stomach, or head. The thought of eating or drinking something evil that can literally exist in the body must be psychologically devastating. Many Blacks who believe in witchcraft are very careful about where and with whom they eat, and in extreme cases may eat no one's cooking but their own. Loss of appetite, nausea and vomiting, food that does not taste right, diarrhea or 'falling off' (weight loss, especially unexplained weight loss), or any sort of gastrointestinal problem that does not quickly respond to treatment, may be interpreted as unnatural, especially if there is conflict in a victim's personal relationships. (p. 826)

Roberson (1985) studied the spiritual or religious beliefs and health choices of 46 African American families and concluded that there was a strong relationship between faith and healing. Many African Americans believe strongly that all blessings come from God, and only God can heal the sick. For instance, as late as the 1930s many African Americans regarded tuberculosis as a form of divine retribution for sin, against which there was no defense (Beardsley, 1987). In addition, the devout African American considers prayer a very powerful tool in healing. The minister, family, and friends may all gather at the bedside of the sick and pray (Roberson, 1985).

A "today" or "present" health orientation is, according to Milio (1967), mirrored in social class. He describes the meaning of "health" for the middle class as a state of optimum capacity for the effective performance of valued tasks, a level of function that allows for occupational achievement and social mobility. For the lower classes "valued tasks" occur in the present and are related to physical activity. For them, optimum capacity means immediate satisfaction and comfort, and they deal with problems as they occur, rather than trying to prevent them.

African Americans use a variety of methods to stay "healthy" (Snow, 1983; Snow, 1978; Jacques, 1976; Winslow and Bishop, 1969). They believe that if you take care of yourself, you will stay healthy. African Americans, like most ethnic groups, believe that a body exposed to extreme temperatures, poorly nourished, or physically abused is prone to illness.

Many African Americans also believe that blood responds to external and internal stimuli. Blood is either good or bad; thick or thin; clean or dirty; sweet or bitter; high or low. In a healthy body, blood is balanced. Menses is one way the body gets rid of bad blood. During menstruation or immediately following childbirth, members of this group may avoid bathing and hair washing because they believe such activities open the pores and make one prone to illness.

Normally, blood naturally thickens in the winter and protects the body against cold and illness. In the spring, a tonic may be taken to thin the blood; this helps the body prepare for the hot summer months. Those with blood that is too thin are considered vulnerable to illness. Women, the elderly, and children fall into this group.

Traditional Medicine

African Americans may use a variety of folk healers. These individuals are a stable, respected, and powerful resource; they understand the beliefs and needs of the people they serve, who are often, but not solely, the poor.

In contrast to modern scientific medicine, which is clearly separated from religion, the folk system does not separate religion from therapy, or the means to a cure. Snow (1978) notes that in this system, "importance is placed on oppositions between good and evil [and] 'natural' and 'unnatural,' and all events, including illnesses can be classified along such lines" (p. 70).

Also in contrast to Western medicine, symptoms may be of minor import in the African American folk system. Snow (1983) found that among lower class African Americans, the natural or unnatural origin of the illness may be more important than whether it is somatically or mentally expressed. He found that in such situations, cure may involve self treatment or consultation with a neighbor knowledgeable in home remedies, a physician, or someone regarded to have unusual powers.

A lay referral system is inherent in the African American folk health system. This referral system accounts for the health needs of the community, investigates how western practitioners communicate with their people, and determines whether or not such practitioners can be trusted. If the report on a health care provider is positive, others from the community will use them; if the report is negative, many will stay away.

Some African Americans continue to practice voodoo, which combines African, Christian, and magical beliefs related to religion and health care (Jordan, 1975; Dorsan, 1967). A variety of names have been given to the men and women who have the voodoo "power": root doctor, spiritualist, voodoo priest, hougan, healer, fortune teller, root worker, herb doctor, conjure doctor, underworld man, and gooferdust man. Table 4-8 describes the services provided by these practitioners.

Powers (1982) discusses several guidelines for health care practitioners who counsel and care for African American clients: (a) do not assume that all African Americans use traditional folk medicine, as many may not; (b) investigate and accept clients' beliefs concerning the cause of their disease; (c) promote a trusting

and open relationship with the client to facilitate discussion about the use of alternative therapies (d) be open and willing to investigate possibilities for collaborating with folk healers; and (e) broaden one's own knowledge of the folk medicine system of care.

Cancer-Specific Beliefs and Practices: Results of National and Regional Surveys

In general, data on African Americans' cancer-related knowledge, attitudes, and practices are limited and dated. The most frequently cited source of this information is a national study of 780 African American men and women, age 18 years and older, conducted in 1980 by the African American owned evaluation organization EVAXX, Inc., and sponsored by the American Cancer Society (ACS) (EVAXX, 1981). EVAXX compared the attitudes of African Americans in 1980 to those of Caucasian Americans in 1978. Other studies of African Americans' beliefs, attitudes, and practices regarding cancer exist, but do not represent national samples.

Data from EVAXX (1981) and Cardwell and Collier (1981) indicate that African Americans tend to be less knowledgeable about cancer than Caucasians. Cancer is apparently the main health preoccupation of Caucasians, whereas high blood pressure and sickle cell anemia are the primary concerns of African Americans (EVAXX, 1981). Those compiling the data suggest that this is because the national and local media provide more information on high blood pressure and sickle cell anemia than on cancer.

TABLE 4-8 Common Descriptions of Voodoo Practitioners

Practitioner	Description
Fortune Teller (Dorson, 1967)	Solves personal problems and can "see" into the future.
Georgia Folk Practitioner (Stewart, 1971)	Person who, at a median age of 19 enters into practice to help others. Receives calling from God or possesses a supernatural gift. Uses ritualistic procedures along with natural and herbal remedies to remove hexes, spells, or illness.
Healer (Dorson, 1967)	Uses the "power" to remove unnatural symptoms, poison from the body, and the "magic snake" from the vein. Secret arts can cure illness of natural causes. Can cast or reverse a spell.
Hougan Priests or Mambo Priestess	Sorcerer used by Haitians.
Obeah Man	Sorcerer used by the Bahamians.
Older women	Grandmothers used in lay referral system to diagnose and treat a large variety of illnesses with home remedies. A spiritual component is part of the regimen especially if believed to be caused by someone evil.
Old Lady or granny woman (Jordan, 1975)	A local who is knowledgeable about herbs and remedies for treatment of common illness. Also advises and refers patients to other practitioners.
Root Doctor	A person born with the gift of healing.
Spiritualist (Jordan, 1975)	A diverse practitioner. Uses a combination of herbal medicines, ritual cures, and spiritual beliefs to treat client's emotional or physical needs.
Voodoo Doctor, Voodoo Priest or Hougan (Jordan, 1975; Dorson, 1967)	A specialist initiated and trained in the rites of divination. Has the greatest supernatural powers. Diagnoses and treats illnesses of supernatural origin.
Other titles include: Root worker, herb doctor conjure doctor, underworld man, and gooferdust man (referring to the graveyard dust such practitioners may sometimes use) (Powers, 1982).	These practitioners have different repertoires of folk knowledge and techniques related to a wide range of human problems.

Data also suggest African Americans tend to underestimate the prevalence of cancer and the significance of the common warning signs for cancer. They tend to be less apt to see a physician when they experience warning signs or symptoms (EVAXX, 1981) and less aware of the benefits of specific cancer screening or self-examination methods (Manfredi, et al., 1977). EVAXX (1981) reports that in comparison to Caucasians, African Americans are more fatalistic about cancer and less likely to believe that early detection or treatment can make a difference in the outcome of the disease. In fact, African Americans are much less likely than Caucasians to regard surgery, chemotherapy, and radiation as effective cancer treatments; this may explain why African Americans are less optimistic about the chances of surviving cancer.

African Americans are twice as likely as Caucasians to prefer to remain ignorant of their own cancer diagnosis; 33% of African Americans, compared with 16% of Caucasians, reported that "if I got cancer, I'd rather not know about it" (EVAXX, 1981, p. 18). Other experts have noted that these pessimistic attitudes influence African American cancer patients' medical care-seeking behavior and could account in part for the delays of 3 to 6 months in seeking diagnosis and treatment (Natarajan, et al., 1985).

In 1989, Bloom, Hayes, Saunders, and Hodge surveyed 1,137 African American adults in northern California and noted findings similar to those described above. A high percentage of individuals of all ages believed that cancer was a death sentence (64.3%), and that treatment was worse than the disease (65.3%); in addi-

tion 80% of the individuals in the study (all aged 50 or older) believed that cancer was spread by surgical treatment. Over 20% of the sample indicated they would rather not know that they had cancer.

EVAXX (1981) assessed the influence of income on health beliefs and behaviors. The researchers documented that lower-income African Americans (those with household incomes under $7,500 annually) were less likely than those with higher incomes ($15,000 or more annually) to see a doctor when they experienced symptoms or to obtain physician check-ups. In addition, African American women with lower incomes were less likely than those with higher incomes to obtain regular Pap tests and to perform monthly breast self-examination. They were also less likely to have heard of proctoscopic examination for colorectal cancer or mammography for breast cancer.

In 1987, the National Center for Health Statistics (NCHS) and the National Cancer Institute (NCI) collaborated on and published the results of a public knowledge survey that was part of a larger Centers for Disease Control study. Findings documented increased awareness about cancer tests and screening procedures. Table 4-9 shows the screening practices of African Americans compared to Caucasians in this study.

Recent studies of the cancer screening practices of African Americans support many of the findings of the NCHS/NCI study. Mitchell-Beren, Dodds, Choi and Waskerwitz (1989) implemented and evaluated a colorectal cancer screening program for African Americans in community churches in 1985. They distributed 1,488 colorectal cancer screening kits with

TABLE 4-9   Provisional Estimates of the Experience of Cancer Screening Procedures for the U.S. Population Aged 40 Years and Over for January-March 1987 based on the 1987 National Health Interview Survey Supplement on Cancer Control*

Procedure, race, and sex	Percent of population never having procedure		Percent of population having procedure for screening purposes			
	Never heard of procedure	Heard of but never had	For health problem	Total	<1 year ago	>1 year ago
Pap Smear†						
Total	3	6	10	81	50	31
White	2	6	10	82	50	32
Black	*	*	10	79	57	22
Breast Exam†						
Total	8	8	12	72	44	28
White	7	8	12	73	45	28
Black	*	*	*	63	43	20
Mammography†						
Total	17	45	6	31	17	14
White	15	46	7	32	17	15
Black	30	44	*	25	14	*
Digital Rectal						
Total	20	19	9	51	21	30
White	19	20	9	52	21	31
Male	20	19	10	51	18	33
Female	18	21	9	52	23	29
Black	28	17	7	48	22	26
Male	30	*	*	50	*	28
Female	26	20	*	48	23	25
Blood Stool						
Total	17	44	7	32	14	18
White	15	45	7	32	14	18
Male	17	42	7	34	15	19
Female	14	48	7	32	14	18
Black	25	39	6	31	12	19
Male	*	*	*	1	*	*
Female	20	44	*	31	14	17
Proctoscopy						
Total	32	44	7	18	3	15
White	29	45	7	19	3	16
Male	31	44	6	20	4	16
Female	28	47	8	17	3	14
Black	55	27	*	16	*	*
Male	59	*	*	*	*	*
Female	53	28	*	*	*	*

From U.S. Department of Health and Human Services, Centers for Disease Control: *Morbidity and Mortality Weekly Report*: Atlanta, 1988, Centers for Disease Control, p. 419. Reprinted by permission.
*Data are not included if the denominator is <100 or the cell size is <29.
†Females only. Pap smear data for women 18 and over.

specimen containers and dietary and procedural instruction for collecting the specimens. Only 17.5% of the participants returned the kits. Follow up interviews determined that this low return rate was due to the lack of compatibility of the diet with traditional foods and the perception that the diet was too expensive and not palatable (Bailey, 1981).

Burack and Liang (1989) conducted a study of the personal characteristics, knowledge, and beliefs associated with mammography utilization by African American women. Users were characterized as poor, inner city, age 50 or older, generally unemployed and poorly educated. The factor contributing most to positive mammography use was access to some form of third party payment. Users had limited knowledge of cancer control: 90% believed that early detection in general was useful; only one third believed cancer was curable if detected early; 30% identified mammography as a potentially useful early detection procedure, but only half of these could accurately define mammography. Older women without breast symptoms but with more frequent medical conditions were less likely to accept and complete mammography.

Burack and Liang (1989) were able to identify variables that favorably influenced mammography use. These included: the presence of breast symptoms, the lack of concern with expense, belief in the utility of cancer detection tests, and initial acceptance of the procedure.

Jacob, Penn and Brown (1989) assessed the knowledge, attitudes, and BSE performance of 180 African American women aged 18 years or older from two community churches in a large metropolitan area. In general, women who practiced BSE tended to be older than 40; have higher annual incomes; more often believed in the benefits of performing BSE and perceived social approval for BSE practice; had usually been taught to perform the exam; and were more likely to have had a Pap smear, a clinical breast exam, and a general physical exam within one year. Similar findings have been associated with studies of the BSE practice of Caucasian women of similar socioeconomic status. African American women who did not practice BSE were more likely to obtain their medical care from a hospital emergency room.

ACCESS TO HEALTH CARE
History of Health Care for African Americans

The health beliefs and practices of African Americans are grounded in their historical experiences with the health care system of the majority U.S. culture. During the period of slavery in the U.S., African Americans received inconsistent and often barbaric health care treatment (Savitt, 1978). Slaves felt a deep mistrust of the white master and his harsh remedies and prescriptions. Even after slavery was abolished African Americans received poor health care and inferior treatment in hospitals and clinics, which only served to reinforce their negative view of Western medicine. African Americans remaining in the South after abolition practiced self treatment, known today as folk medicine.

Until the early 20th century most white doctors believed, as had their ante-bellum counterparts, that African Americans were biologically inferior and subject to a different pathology than that governing whites (Beardsley, 1987). They regarded African Americans as psychologically unfit for freedom and for the most part "uneducable" in the practice of better hygiene. Even today, state-of-the-art health care resources are not equally distributed in the United States. The costs of health care services continue to rise and the U.S. health care system is so complex and confusing that it challenges even the most sophisticated, determined, and well-educated individuals. Barriers such as these result in limited access and, subsequently, inappropriate use or lack of use of health services. These barriers are compounded by the lack of convenient transportation, inability to pay for health care services, and negative perceptions about the degree of personal and social acceptance experienced with health care personnel.

In his scholarly review of health care for southern and some northern African Americans in the 20th century, Beardsley (1987) also described the influence of poverty and related variables, other than race, on health:

. . . poverty was surely the primary factor explaining ill health and excess death in the South [but] it was not the only one. Good health or its absence was the result of many variables, all interconnected and most related to economic status. Not only sanitary environment, but also nutrition, level of education, stress, the way one viewed and responded to illness, the availability and acceptability of medical care—all helped determine whether one was sick or well, lived or died. As for Blacks, especially those in the South, racism and institutionalized segregation heightened the effect of every other variable. (p. 28)

In 1984, the U.S. government made the health status of African Americans and other minorities a national priority. Secretary of health Margaret H. Heckler commissioned the *Report of the Secretary's Task Force on Black and Minority Health* to investigate and document the health status of minorities, and recommend strategies to ameliorate the problems found. The task force found what they termed a "persistent, distressing disparity" in key health indicators between African Americans and Caucasians. They documented six major causes of death that together accounted for more than 80% of the excess mortality observed among African Americans in comparison to that of the Caucasian population. These were heart disease and stroke, homicide and accidents, cancer, infant mortality, cirrhosis, and diabetes (USDHHS, 1985).

These findings mean that of the 140,000 African Americans who die each year before age 70, 42% would not have died if they had the same death rates as the Caucasian population. The task force also argued that a significant improvement in the health status of African Americans would depend on reducing health-damaging personal behaviors such as substance abuse, injuries (accidental and intentional), homicide, sexual activities leading to ill-timed pregnancy or infection with sexually transmitted diseases and AIDS, and tobacco use.

Today, despite expanded health services, poor African Americans who are on Medicaid or are uninsured continue to have unmet health care needs. In fact, the National Research Council (1989) suggests that since 1982, access to health care has been worsening for these groups. They also note that 22% of African Americans under age 65 are not covered by private health insurance or Medicaid. For many, health care is only available through a public clinic or the emergency room of a hospital, where the wait for medical attention may be extremely long.

The Office of Minority Health Resource Center was established by the U.S. Department of Health and Human Services' Office of Minority Health in October, 1987. This center maintains information on health-related resources available at the federal, state, and local levels that target Asian and Pacific Islanders, African Americans, Hispanics/Latinos, and Native Americans. In addition to serving as a central source of information on minority health, the center works with the Office of Minority Health to identify information gaps and stimulate the development of resources where none exist. The resource center concentrates on six priority health areas: cancer, chemical dependency, diabetes, heart disease/stroke, homicide/suicide/unintentional injury, and infant mortality.

Socioeconomic Status and Access to Care

In recent years, health professionals have begun to pay greater attention to the relationship between socioeconomic status (SES) and access to care. As early as 1933, African American activist and educator W. E. B. DuBois observed that the excessive rate of deaths in his ethnic group was due to nothing but poverty and discrimination (Beardsley, 1987).

In 1981, White, Enterline, Alan, and Moore concluded:

It appears that the major underlying factor contributing to the poor health status of U.S. Blacks (relative to U.S. whites) is their relatively low socio-economic status (SES). The low SES among Blacks not only makes it difficult for them to obtain the goods and services necessary for a high quality lifestyle, but [also] makes it difficult to concentrate on more future oriented goals such as regular medical checkups, preventive health practices, and entering the medical system at early states of disease. (p. 36)

African Americans may also fail to use health care services because of the costs involved in seeing a doctor, including transportation costs, child care costs, and pay lost when time is taken off from work. Even those with Medicaid coverage experience significant barriers, as outlined by Freeman (1981):

A poor person typically experiences great difficulty in entering the health care system. Not able to pay for a private physician in a medical system stressing fee-for-service, the poor patient with potential cancer is frequently seen first in an emergency room and referred to a clinic. Long waiting periods and complex registration procedures are common. The emergency room is geared toward treating apparently sick people. A minimally symptomatic patient is likely to be discouraged when faced by a process of diagnosis [that] may be perceived as being more disturbing than a painless lump. (p. 3)

Paxton (1976) also writes of the influence of poverty on the development of disease:

How a state of poverty influences one's level of wellness is related to the lifestyle of people in poverty. A survival lifestyle may be defined as a way of life which dictates actions directed toward meeting the most basic needs for the maintenance of life, rather than fulfilling it. Energy output is often greater than intake over an extended period of time. Constant energy output threatens the integrity of the organism. (p. 127)

Education and Access to Care

Knowledge about health care can also influence access to that care. As noted earlier, African Americans, as a group, have considerably significantly fewer years of education than Caucasians.

These lower levels of education may affect how much African Americans know about cancer risk, prevention, detection, and treatment. A national survey conducted for the American Cancer Society concluded that African Americans were less exposed to cancer information than whites (EVAXX, 1981).

Michielutte and Diseker's (1982) study of 42 African American and 98 Caucasian adults in North Carolina confirmed findings of the early ACS survey. Further analysis suggested that SES influenced knowledge, that is, middle- and upper-income African Americans and whites were more knowledgeable about cancer than lower income African Americans. SES did not, however, account completely for the differences between races in knowledge; sources of information, quality of education, and access to the medical system were also factors. The re-searchers found that African Americans more commonly received the kind of brief and simple health information broadcast on television and radio than the detailed information found in pamphlets, newspapers, and magazines. The researchers also found that the quality of education was lower for minority groups than for the white majority. Finally, the authors suggested that African Americans' relative lack of access to the health care system might dampen their motivation to acquire cancer information.

Patterns of Care-Seeking Behavior

Bailey (1987) noted that an individual's experience with access to health care can influence their pattern of care-seeking behavior. From a study of 203 African American men (39%) and women (61%), he documented a six step pattern of health care seeking behavior:

1. Illness appears (perceived symptoms associated with high blood pressure);
2. Individual waits for a certain period (delays days or weeks);
3. Allows body to heal itself (prayer or traditional regimens);
4. Evaluates daily activities (reduces work or stress);
5. Seeks advice from a family member or close friend (church leader and/or traditional healer included);
6. And finally, attends health clinic or sees family physician.

CANCER RISK ASSESSMENT

A risk factor can be defined as any behavioral, biological, or environmental factor that influences a person's chances of developing a disease such as cancer. An individual may or may not be able to alter a risk factor. For example, African American men over age 55 have been shown to be at risk for developing prostate cancer; this biological factor cannot be altered, as aging is inevitable. Alternatively, a smoker is at risk for developing lung cancer. This behavioral factor can be altered; one can stop smoking, and there is evidence that the damage done to the lungs can be reversed. It is also important to understand that exposures to risk factors can be significant when they are cumulative. For example, an individual's risk for developing lung cancer is increased by 90% if that person is both a smoker and has a historical exposure to asbestos. Again, one may not be able to alter a historical exposure to asbestos, but in this instance, quitting smoking is just as important.

Individuals will, inevitably, be exposed to a variety of cancer risk factors throughout their lives. Data suggest that long latency periods between exposure and cancer onset are common. For this reason, screening for premalignant and early malignant disease can lead to a decrease in mortality from many types of cancer, and an increase in patient survival time. Therefore, it is important that health care providers include questions about past exposures in routine risk assessments. Such questions should enable them to make comprehensive recommendations for risk factor reduction, screenings, and early detection examinations. Table 4-10 lists agents known to be carcinogenic in humans; Table 4-11 lists risk factors associated with cancers of specific sites; and Table 4-12 lists occupational exposures associated with specific cancer sites.

Risk Factors for Prevalent Cancers

Some data are available on the relationship between biological, behavioral, and environmental risk factors unique to the African American population and cancers that tend to occur more frequently with this group.

Lung cancer. When compared to Caucasian men, African American men experience lung cancer more frequently, are more likely to die from it, and survive with it for a shorter period of time. Research shows that the smoking habits of African American males differ from those of Caucasian males (Orleans, Strecher, Schoenbach, Salmon, and Blackmon, 1989). According to the 1985 Health Interview Survey, almost 40% of African American men now smoke, in contrast to 31.6% of Caucasian men. Smoking rates among African American women (31%) now exceed those among Caucasian women (28.1%) (Orleans, et al., 1989).

Although African Americans smoke fewer cigarettes, they tend to smoke brands with higher tar and nicotine yields, especially mentholated brands: Kools, Salem, and Newport account for 55%-60% of the brands smoked by African American smokers. Menthol additives may enable the smoker to tolerate deeper or more frequent inhalations, or to smoke the cigarette to a shorter length. As a result, low-rate smokers of high-nicotine, menthol cigarettes may achieve higher than assumed levels of nicotine intake and dependency and harmful smoke exposure.

TABLE 4-10 Established Human Carcinogenic Agents

Agent or Circumstance	Occupational	Medical	Social	Site of Cancer
Aflatoxin			+	Liver
Alcoholic drinks			+	Mouth, pharynx, larynx esophagus, liver
Alkylating agents:				
Cyclophosphamide		+		Bladder
Melphalan		+		Marrow
Aromatic amines:				
4-Aminodiphenyl	+			Bladder
Benzidine	+			Bladder
2-Naphthylamine	+			Bladder
Arsenic	+	+		Skin, lung
Asbestos	+			Lung, pleura, peritoneum
Benzene	+			Marrow
Bis(chloromethyl)ether	+			Lung
Busulphan		+		Marrow
Cadmium	+			Prostate
Chewing betel, tobacco, lime			+	Mouth
Chromium	+			Lung
Chlornaphazine		+		Bladder
Furniture manufacture (hardwood)	+			Nasal sinuses
Immunosuppressive drugs		+		Reticuloendothelial system
Ionizing radiations	+	+		Marrow and probably all other sites
Isopropyl alcohol manufacture	+			Nasal sinuses
Leather goods manufacture	+			Nasal sinuses
Mustard gas	+			Larynx, lung
Nickel	+			Nasal sinuses, lung
Estrogens:				
Unopposed		+		Endometrium
Transplacental (DES)		+		Vagina
Overnutrition (causing obesity)			+	Endometrium, gallbladder
Phenacetin		+		Kidney (pelvis)
Polycyclic hydrocarbons	+	+		Skin, scrotum, lung
Reproductive history:				
Late age at 1st pregnancy			+	Breast
Zero or low parity			+	Ovary
Parasites:				
Schistosoma haematobium			+	Bladder
Chlonorchis sinensis			+	Liver (cholangioma)

Continued.

TABLE 4-10 Established Human Carcinogenic Agents—cont'd

Agent or Circumstance	Occupational	Medical	Social	Site of Cancer
Sexual promiscuity			+	Cervix uteri
Steroids:				
Anabolic (oxymetholone)		+		Liver
Contraceptives		+		Liver (hamartoma)
Tobacco smoking			+	Mouth, pharynx, larynx, lung, esophagus, bladder
UV light	+		+	Skin, lip
Vinyl chloride	+		+	Liver (angiosarcoma)
Virus (hepatitis B)			+	Liver (hepatoma)

From Doll R, and Peto R: *The causes of cancer*, New York 1981, Oxford University Press. Reprinted by permission.
NOTE: Occupational exposure to phenoxyacid/chlorophenal herbicides (or their impurities) is a reasonably well-established cause of soft tissue sarcomas and perhaps lymphomas.

The sociodemographic correlates of smoking among African Americans are generally similar to those for the U.S. population as a whole, including: lower income, lower education levels, blue collar occupation, unemployment, being male, and being unmarried (Orleans, et al., 1989). Data suggest that African Americans are significantly less likely than Caucasians to quit smoking, less likely to report medical advice to stop smoking, and less likely to believe tobacco use increases cancer risks (Orleans, et al., 1989).

African Americans may also be more likely to be exposed in the workplace to substances that are associated with the development of lung cancer. For instance, African Americans were overrepresented among coke-oven workers in the Pittsburgh area, an occupational risk associated with increased risk for lung cancer (Wynder and Kabat, 1981).

Esophageal cancer. African Americans experience esophageal cancer three times more frequently than Caucasians (Table 4-5), and significantly more African Americans die of this cancer than any other ethnic group, including Caucasians. Research has shown that esophageal cancer is associated with both cigarette smoking and alcohol intake. Wynder and Kabat (1981) note that although total alcohol consumption may be similar among African Americans and Caucasians, there is evidence to suggest African Americans consume significantly more whiskey than Caucasians and are more likely to be heavy drinkers of hard liquor and wine. Correa (1981) noted that heavy drinking was twice as common among urban African Americans as among Caucasians of similar lower SES. Alcoholism among African American men, according to Correa (1981), is:

part of an intricate social complex involving poverty, broken homes, unemployment, poor performance in school, criminal activities, and high death rates for practically every disease affecting young and middle age Black males. Since some components of this complex can be found in Africa, not everything can be explained on the basis of postmigration conditions in America, but the interaction of social factors and disease patterns strongly suggests a conflict in the adaptation of man to the environment. According to Moyniham (1965), "this reflects the fact that three centuries of injustices have brought about deep-seated structural distortions in the life of the Negro American." (p. 203)

Bladder cancer. According to the most recent SEER data, Table 4-5, the bladder cancer incidence rate in African Americans (9.8) is exceeded only by the Caucasian rate (18.0). Bladder cancer mortality rates rank high for both African Americans and Caucasians. Bladder cancer has been associated with cigarette smoking and tobacco smoke; carcinogens are known to concentrate in and be excreted by the bladder.

Stomach Cancer. African Americans experience higher rates of stomach cancer than Caucasians. From 1937 to 1969, incidence and mortality rates for colon cancer increased in this ethnic group (Wynder and Kabat, 1981), suggesting that African Americans have become increasingly exposed to some factor to which Caucasians have been consistently exposed. Dietary factors have been implicated in the development of stomach and colon cancer; however, few comparisons of the dietary habits of African Ameri-

TABLE 4-11 Risk Factors for Specific Cancer Sites

Risk Factors	Cancer Sites
OCCUPATIONAL EXPOSURE	
Nickel, chromium, radiosotopes, petroleum, chemicals, asbestos, arsenic	Head and neck, lung
PREVIOUS HISTORY OF ILLNESS, INJURY, IRRITATION	
Ill-fitting dentures	Oropharynx
Chronic dermatitis, burn scars	Skin
Familial polyposis	Colon and rectum
Ulcerative colitis	Colon and rectum
Fibrocystic disease	Breast
Dyplasia of breast	Breast
Maldescent of testicle	Testicle
Herpes Type II infection	Cervix
Hormonal irregularities	Endometrium
BEHAVIORS/LIFESTYLE	
Smoking	Lung
Chewing tobacco, snuff	Head and neck
Heavy alcohol consumption	Head and neck
Excessive sun exposure	Skin
Obesity	Endometrium
Multiple sexual partners	Cervix
Early age of coitus	Cervix
Familial history	Breast, colon
DIETARY	
High fat, low fiber	Colon and rectum
High fat	Breast, prostate
ENVIRONMENTAL	
Air pollution	Lung
Wood smoke	Head and neck
Residence in sunbelt areas, and exposure to sun for extended periods of time	Skin

TABLE 4-12 Occupational Cancer Hazards

Agent	Cancer Site or Type	Type of Workers Exposed
Acrylonitrile	Lung, colon	Manufacturers of apparel, carpeting, blankets, draperies, synthetic furs, and wigs
4-aminobiphenyl	Bladder	Chemical workers
Arsenic and certain arsenic compounds	Lung, skin, scrotum, lymphatic system, hemangiosarcoma of the liver	Workers in the metallurgic industries, sheep-dip workers, copper smelter workers, vineyard workers, insecticide makers and sprayers, tanners, gold miners
Asbestos	Lung, larynx, GI tract, pleural and peritoneal mesothelioma	Asbestos factory workers, textile workers, rubber-tire manufacturing industry workers, miners, insulation workers, shipyard workers
Amuramine and the manufacture of auramine	Bladder	Dyestuffs manufacturers, rubber workers, textile dyers, paint manufacturers
Benzene	Leukemia	Rubber-tire manufacturing workers, painters, shoe manufacturing workers, rubber cement workers, glue and varnish workers, distillers, shoemakers, plastics workers, chemical workers
Benzidine	Bladder, pancreas	Dyeworkers, chemical workers
Beryllium and certain beryllium compounds	Lung	Beryllium workers, electronics workers, missle parts producers
Bis(chloromethyl)ether (BCME)	Lung	Workers in plants producing anion-exchange resins (chemical workers)
Cadmium and certain cadmium compounds	Lung, prostate	Cadmium production workers, metallurgical workers, electroplating industry workers, chemical workers, jewelry workers, nuclear workers, pigment workers, battery workers
Carbon tetrachloride	Liver	Plastic workers, dry cleaners
Chloromethyl methyl ether (CMME)	Lung	Chemical workers, workers in plants producing ion-exchange resin
Chromium and certain chromium compounds	Lung, nasal sinuses	Chromate-producing industry workers, acetylene and aniline workers, bleachers, glass, pottery, pigment, and linoleum workers
Coal tar pitch volatiles	Lung, scrotum	Steel industry workers, aluminum potroom workers, foundry workers
Coke oven emissions	Lung, kidney, prostate	Steel industry workers, coke plant workers
Dimethyl sulphate	Lung	Chemical workers, drug makers, dyemakers
Epichlorohydrin	Lung, leukemia	Chemical workers
Ethylene oxide	Leukemia, stomach	Hospital workers, research lab workers, beekeepers, fumigators

TABLE 4-12   Occupational Cancer Hazards—cont'd

Agent	Cancer Site or Type	Type of Workers Exposed
Hematite and underground hematite mining	Lung	Miners
Isopropyl oils and the manufacture of isopropyl oils	Paranasal sinuses	Isopropyl oil workers
Mustard gas	Respiratory tract	Production workers
2-naphthylamine	Bladder, pancreas	Dye workers, rubber-tire manufacturing workers, chemical workers, manufacturers of coal gas, nickel refiners, copper smelters, electrolysis workers
Nickel (certain compounds) and nickel refining	Nasal cavity, lung, larynx	Nickel refiners
Polychlorinated biphenyls (PCBs)	Melanoma	PCBs workers
Radiation, ionizing	Skin, pancreas, brain, stomach, breast, salivary glands, thyroid, GI tract, bronchus, lymphoid tissue, leukemia, multiple myeloma	Uranium miners, radiologists, radiographers, luminous dail painters
Radiation, ultraviolet	Skin	Farmers, sailors, arc welders
Soots, tars, mineral oils	Skin, lung, bladder, GI tract	Construction workers, roofers, chimney sweeps, machinists
Thorium dioxide	Liver, kidney, larynx, leukemia	Chemical workers, steelworkers, ceramic makers, incandescent lamp makers, nuclear reactor workers, gas mantle makers, metal refiners, vacuum tube makers
Vinyl chloride	Liver, brain, lung hematolymphopoietic system, breast	Plastic factory workers, vinyl chloride polymerization plant workers
Agent(s) not identified	Pancreas	Chemists
	Stomach	Coal miners
	Brain, stomach	Petrochemical industry workers
	Hematolymphopoietic system	Rubber industry workers
	Bladder	Printing pressmen
	Eye, kidney, lung	Chemical workers
	Leukemia, brain	Farmers
	Colon, brain	Pattern and model makers
	Esophagus, stomach, lung	Oil refinery workers

From Office of Technology Assessment: *Occupational cancer hazards*, Boulder, Colo., 1982, Westview Press. Contains no copyrighted material.

cans and Caucasians have been conducted. Correa (1981) suggests that the type of stomach cancer common in African Americans (the intestinal or epidemic type) differs from that commonly found in Caucasians. The epidemic form of gastric cancer is preceded by a type of chronic atrophic gastritis and this, says Correa, may indicate that this cancer is related to the African Americans' pattern of alcohol consumption.

Colon/Rectal cancers. African Americans have colon and rectal cancer incidence rates about equal to that of Caucasians. This does, however, represent an increasing trend for African Americans. Correa (1981) notes this increase may have begun around 1950 and is attributable to diet, especially the combination of high fat and low fiber. So far, no association between consumption of beef and colorectal cancer has been found among African Americans; Correa (1981) suggests this as an area for further study.

Gullatte (1989) suggests that in many instances, the problem lies not so much in the type of food in the traditional African American diet as in the manner of food preparation. Vegetables are boiled, usually using meat seasoning high in fat (e.g., fatback, streak-o-lean, or ham hocks). Meat seasoning is not only high in fat, it is usually cured with salt or nitrites. Fried and charcoal-cooked meats are often preferred over broiled or baked cuts.

Rectal cancers among African Americans seem to occur more commonly in the anus region and lower rectum, especially among African American women.

Although the etiology of this disease manifestation is poorly understood, some data exist to link perineal infections, which are common in African American women, with rectal cancer (Correa, 1981). However, health professionals should not rule out the importance of dietary factors, and these merit further study.

Pancreatic cancer. The incidence of pancreatic cancer is about 40% higher in African Americans than in Caucasians. Cigarette smoking has been linked with this cancer, and this could explain the increase in the incidence of the disease seen in African American men. This cancer has also been associated with diabetes in women but not in men, with alcohol consumption, and occupational exposure to chemicals (Wynder and Kabat, 1981).

Breast cancer. Among both African American and Caucasian women, breast cancer occurs more frequently than any other neoplasm. The incidence appears to be increasing in younger, premenopausal African American women. Breast cancer has traditionally been associated with reproductive factors including early age of menarche (before age 12), late menopause (after 55), and nulliparity. Women with a family history of breast cancer may be genetically predisposed to the development of the disease. Studies have also indicated a link between the disease and obesity, (perhaps related to dietary fat intake), or exposure to radiation.

Prostate cancer. Prostate cancer is a serious, leading cause of mortality among

African American men. Between 1930 and 1974, the prostate cancer mortality rate increased by 34% among Caucasians, but among other ethnic groups (primarily African Americans) the increase has been a striking 322% (Wynder and Kabat, 1981). African Americans have higher rates of benign prostatic hypertrophy than Caucasians; however, the link between this and prostate cancer is uncertain. Data (Wunder and Kabat, 1981; Gullatte, 1988) suggest that certain sexual factors, such as marital status, sexual experience (lower frequency of intercourse, lower sex drive, and greater use of prostitutes), and venereal disease could play a role in the etiology of prostate cancer. Dietary fat has also been associated with prostate cancer. Rubber workers, battery workers exposed to cadmium, and janitors exposed to cleaning fluids have been noted to have a higher incidence of prostate cancer.

Cervical cancer. Cervical cancer is fairly common and accounts for significant mortality among African American women. The disease is generally more common in lower socioeconomic groups, regardless of ethnicity. Risk factors include: early age of first intercourse, multiple sexual partners, and viral infections with herpes simplex virus II or human papilloma virus. More recently, cervical cancer has been associated with cigarette smoking.

Multiple myeloma. Multiple myeloma is the most common lymphoreticular neoplasm of African American men and women. It tends to occur around 40 years of age. Researchers are studying possible links between this disease and ionizing radiation, certain occupational exposures and certain viruses. Presenting signs and symptoms include back pain of insidious onset, anemia, pathological fractures, and repeated infections.

Risk Assessment Interview

Interview format. A comprehensive health history and thorough physical assessment is the initial and most vital tool for identification of an individual's risk. Valentine (1986, 1987) suggests that the history and physical should:

(1) be obtained from every person, (2) be complete, accurate, and documented, (3) take into account all body systems, present complaints, . . . personal and family history, as well as cultural, social, and economic factors, and (4) use risk factors identified to guide further screening, testing, and establishment of suggested prevention practices. (pp. 65-66)

When completing a comprehensive health history and physical assessment with clients of the African American culture, the health care professional should consider their cultural differences and unique physical attributes. Appendix 1 outlines a comprehensive medical history questionnaire covering vital statistics, present health, past health, family medical history and social and personal habits. The questionnaire also covers genetic and familial, personal, and group risk factors. Health professionals at the Employee Cancer Screening Clinic at The University of Texas M.D. Anderson Cancer Center have successfully used this tool with members of various minority groups. Clearly, no assessment tool is ideal for use in all settings or with all populations. The intent here is to provide practitioners with sufficient information to modify or develop an assessment tool that will meet the needs of their own institutions and clientele.

Two references (Frank-Stromborg, 1986, and University of Texas, 1988) provide step-by-step guidance for conducting a comprehensive, cancer-specific physical assessment. The following considerations and suggested exam techniques can enhance the cultural and racial specificity of the M.D. Anderson tool (Appendix A) and the clinician's comprehensive physical assessment.

The patient history. *Patient/Provider Communication:* Historically, the relationships between African Americans and Caucasians in the U.S. have resulted in deep mistrust and broad gaps in communication. Levy (1985) suggests people who share similar cultural patterns, values, experiences, and problems are more likely to trust, feel comfortable with, and understand each other. For these reasons, African American health care professionals should be given the opportunity to work with African American clients whenever possible. Data suggest that making African American health care professionals available to African American patients can improve accessibility and enhance the quality of health care delivery. These ethnic practitioners can also help to alleviate some of the apprehension their patients may have about health care; they can help African American patients feel they are accepted and they belong (Proctor and Rose, 1981; Miles and McDavis, 1982, Airhihenbuwa, 1989).

Health care providers often use medical terminology that can be confusing or misunderstood by patients with facility only in standard English. It is important for the practitioner to speak clearly and explain such terminology. Familiarity with lay medical terminology and its differences from scientific terminology can help avoid misunderstandings in communication and misinterpretation of symptoms described by the client. Although the dialect used by some African Americans is an integral part of their culture, health professionals should not try to adopt this dialect unnaturally, because the African American client may view this as both patronizing and inappropriate.

Occupation: Where do you work? What do you do there? How long have you been working there? If working in "high risk" areas (see Table 4-12), what is the air circulation like? Can you obtain protective clothing, and do you use it? Do you have difficulty breathing while at work? Is there "dust" in the air or on the furniture surfaces from the products you are making? Does your family come in contact with any of this "dust"? Do you shower and change clothes before leaving work? Where else have you worked? Have you noticed and/or experienced any changes in your health since working at your job(s)? Do you feel good when you go to work and then become unusually tired and weak, or regularly experience a headache and become nauseated?

Residence: Where do you live (inner city, rural, suburbs, urban area; high-rise apartment complex; private or public housing)? Are heat and hot water provided? Is the building well-kept or in need of repairs? What repairs are needed? How old is the building?

Weight and Diet: Note present and usual weight. Query regarding recent weight gain or loss without dieting and any loss of appetite. Snow (1978) notes that some African Americans perceive "falling off" (weight loss) to be particularly frightening, particularly if the usual amount of food is consumed. Such weight loss is deemed unnatural and may be interpreted as a sign of sorcery. Also ask about dietary habits and food preparation styles.

Performance Status: Assess present level of activity; involvement in regular exercise; presence of any unusual weakness, fatigue, malaise. Ascertain what, if anything, the client may be taking to feel stronger or better (include medications, herbal preparations, homemade tonics, etc.).

The physical assessment. *Examination Environment:* Lighting in the examination area should be bright (at least 60 watts) to facilitate evaluation of subtle changes in skin color. Over-bed lamps and flashlights are inadequate single-source light sources. Attempts to develop standardized skin color comparisons for use with African American patients have been unsuccessful due to the many variations in skin tone (Roach, 1987).

The temperature in the examination room should be comfortably warm. Extreme warmth can lead to superficial vasodilation that can increase redness; cold can contribute to a cyanosis of the lips and nailbeds, that masks any existing pallor.

The emotional status of the patient can also contribute to skin color changes such as pallor from fear and facial flushing from embarrassment.

Patient Positioning: The examiner should consider both the effects of gravity and the angle of light when deciding how to position the patient's extremities. An elevated or lowered limb can cause changes in skin color or enhance the subtle color change indicative of early pathology. Extremities should be examined at heart level, then elevated about 15 degrees (assuming no contraindications) for five minutes, and finally lowered to 30 to 90 degrees for at least five minutes. Any relationship between color, position, and contributing pathophysiology should be noted (Roach, 1981).

Normal and abnormal skin and mucous membrane. *Coloration:* Many African Americans with dark complexions are not aware they can become sunburned or develop skin cancer; they believe their dark skin protects them from burning. Some fair skinned African Americans sunbathe. These individuals should be asked about length and type of sun exposure, sunburn experiences, and changes in moles or freckles. Practitioners should ask about new moles or changes in moles on all body surfaces, including the palms and soles of the feet; they should also conduct a comprehensive skin examination. In addition, it is important to question the elderly who may have worked the fields, construction workers, longshoremen, or other outdoor laborers about sun exposure.

Darker-skinned African Americans have more melanin pigment in their skin.

Reddish tones (which tend to cause the skin to glow) may be noted in brown- to black-skinned persons. An absence of the reddish tone may indicate pallor.

In African American patients, the sclera of the eyes may normally contain small brown dots visible near the limbus. These should not be misinterpreted as petechiae.

The gums may vary in color from blue to a blotchy blue-purple; the lips may also appear blue, especially in darker-skinned African Americans. Brown spots may also be found on the palms, soles of the feet, nailbeds, and buccal mucosa. Fingernails and toenails of adolescents and adults may also be pigmented and have a bluish hue. African Americans commonly have brown freckle-like pigmentation on the gums, buccal cavity, border of the tongue, and nailbeds (Roach, 1981). Normal earwax secretions can be brown or black (Overfield, 1977; Malasanos, Barkauskas, Moss, and Stoltenberg-Allen, 1986).

African Americans frequently have hyperpigmented **Mongolian areas,** bluish patches usually found on the back. To determine whether jaundice, ecchymosis, or erythema are present, the examiner should assess areas of lighter melanin pigmentation such as the sclera, conjunctiva, soles of the feet, and palms of the hands. The abdomen, buttocks, and volar surface of the forearm may also be lighter in color. Petechiae may be very difficult to observe; the examiner should check the mouth and conjunctiva for reddish-purple pinpoints of color.

The presence of pallor in black-skinned persons is indicated by an ashen-gray skin tone. For brown-skinned persons, one should gently press an earlobe or nailbed and observe. A slowed blood return may indicate an underlying circulatory problem.

The examiner should check for cyanosis by examining areas of minimal pigmentation: the nailbeds, lips, buccal mucosa, tongue, sclera, palms, and soles. In African American individuals, observation of the nailbeds must always be supplemented by additional observations. Thick, colored, and lined nails can mask cyanosis or give a false impression of cyanosis (Roach, 1981). Edema can obscure true skin color or mask its intensity, causing darkly pigmented skin to become lighter (Roach, 1981).

Normal Skin and Hair Characteristics: As with Caucasians, the epidermis of African Americans is constantly shedding dead skin. This skin can appear as brown or black flakes. Facial *folliculitis* is a common problem among men who shave with hand or electric razors. The hair of African American individuals is usually different from that of Caucasians because of differences in the structure of the protein molecules that comprise the hair.

The nipples and areola of African American women will be darker than their skin color.

PROVIDING CULTURALLY APPROPRIATE CARE

Providing culturally sensitive health care to African Americans is a challenge. Health care providers must be alert to the needs of this population and the many variables that have an impact on their health beliefs and practices.

These patients' knowledge of cancer and cancer screening tests may be limited. Those who do practice prevention and early detection must be encouraged to continue these practices. All clinics should include cancer screening programs that use assessment and screening tools such as those mentioned in this chapter to gather as much information as possible about the patient. When health professionals do identify risk factors, they should outline a program of preventive care that includes education as well as ways to minimize additional exposure.

African Americans want to be healthy; when given the opportunity and the tools to fight cancer, many will do so. The barriers that prevent this population from receiving high-quality health care in hospitals and clinics must be lifted. Health care providers must be knowledgeable and willing to work hard to eradicate African Americans' negative beliefs about cancer and its treatments. Health professionals must send the message that early cancer prevention and detection do work.

When a patient does have cancer, the care provider must be careful to include the patient's beliefs and practices in the treatment protocol when at all possible. As stated in the literature, many African Americans fear cancer treatments and their side effects. Therefore, health professionals should, when at all possible, provide education and opportunities for these patients to speak with those who have been treated successfully for cancer.

When planning cancer screening programs, clinics, and health care programs in general, professionals should consider the following:

- socioeconomic status of the population to be served;
- health care beliefs and practices;
- the use of minority health care providers;
- distance to the care facility and transportation costs;
- education level of the community;
- religious beliefs and practices;
- including clergy in the planning and implementation of the program;
- establishing hours of operations that include early mornings and evenings for those clients who work; and
- having on-site child care.

The report of the Secretary's Task Force on Black and Minority Health demonstrates the needs of this population and the commitment made to close existing gaps in the quality and consistency of care. Everyone who cares for minority patients is well aware of their needs; now, however, health professionals have the backing of larger health care organizations to help change the care received by the poor.

REFERENCES

1. Airhihenbuwa CO: Health education for African Americans: a neglected task, *Health Educ* 20(5):9-14, 1989.
2. American Cancer Society: Black Americans' attitudes toward cancer and cancer tests: Highlights of a study, *Cancer* 31:212-218, July-Aug 1981.
3. American Cancer Society: Special Report on Cancer in the Economically Disadvantaged prepared by the American Cancer Society Subcommittee on Cancer in the Economically Disadvantaged. New York, 1986, The Society.
4. Adams M, Kerner JF: Evaluation of promotional strategies to solve the problem of underutilization of a breast examination/education center in a New York Black community. In Mettlin C, Murphy GP, eds, *Issues in cancer screening and communications*, New York, 1982, Alan R. Liss, pp 151-161.
5. Askey DG, Parker D, Alexander D, White JE: Clergy as intermediary—an approach to cancer control. In Mettlin C, Murphy GP, eds: *Progress In cancer control IV: Research in The Cancer Center*, New York, 1983, Alan R. Liss, pp 417-424.
6. Bailey EJ: Sociocultural factors and health care-seeking behavior among Black Americans, *J Natl Black Med Assoc* 79:388-392, 1987.
7. Bang KM: Increased cancer risk in Blacks: A look at the factors, *J Natl Med Assoc* 79(4):383-388, 1987.
8. Baquet CR: *Cancer epidemiology of American minorities*. American Society of Clinical Oncology Conference, Washington, DC, May 1990.
9. Baquet CR, Clayton LA, Robinson RG: Cancer prevention and control. In Jones LA, ed: *Minorities and cancer*, New York, 1989, Springer-Verlag Publishers, pp 67-76.
10. Baquet C, Ringen K: Cancer control in blacks: Epidemiology and NCI program plans. In Mettlin C, Murphy GP, eds: *Advances in cancer control: Health care financing and research*, New York, 1986. Alan R. Liss, pp 215-227.
11. Baquet C, Ringen K, Pollack E: *Cancer among Blacks and other minorities: A statistical profile*, Washington, DC, 1986, National Cancer Institute, Division of Cancer Prevention and Control.
12. Beardsley EH: *A history of neglect: Health care for Blacks and mill workers in the twentieth-century South*, Knoxville, 1987, The University of Tennessee Press.
12a. Blau FD Graham JW: Black-White differences in wealth and asset composition, *The Quarterly Journal of Economics*, CV, 421(2):321-339, 1990.
13. Bloom JR, Hayes WA, Saunders, F. Hodge F: Physician induced and patient induced utilization of early cancer detection practices among Black Americans, *Advances in Cancer Control: Innovations and Research* 293:279-296, 1989.
14. Branch MF, Paxton PP: *Providing safe nursing care for ethnic people of color*, New York, 1976, Appleton-Century-Crofts.
15. Burack, RC, Liang J: The acceptance and completion of mammography by older Black women, *Am J Public Health* 79(6):721-726, 1989.
16. Bureau of the Census: *America's Black population: A statistical view (1990)*, Washington DC, 1989. US Department of Commerce.
17. Bureau of the Census: *America's Black population, 1970 to 1982: A statistical view*, Washington, DC, 1989, US Department of Commerce.
18. Cardwell J, Collier W. Racial differences in cancer awareness: What Black Americans need to know about cancer, *Urban Health* 29-32, Oct 1981.
19. Correa, P. Gastrointestinal cancer among Black populations. In Mettlin C, Murphy GP, eds: *Cancer among Black populations*, pp 197-211, New York, 1981, Alan R. Liss.
20. DeVesa SS, Silverman DT: Cancer incidence and mortality trends in the United States: 1935-74. *J Natl Cancer Inst* 60:545-571, 1978.
21. DeVita V, ed: Cancer prevention awareness program targeting Black Americans, *Public Health Rep* 100(3):253-254, 1985.
22. Doll R, Peto R: The causes of cancer: Quantitative estimates of avoidable risk of cancer in the United States today, *J Natl Cancer Inst* 66:1191-1308, 1981.
23. Dorson RM: *American Negro folk tales*, New York, 1967, Fawcett Publishers.
24. Earles LC: Cancer epidemic in the Black community, *J Natl Med Assoc* 76(2):93-94, 1984.
25. Eng E, Hatch J, Callan A. Institutionalizing social support through the church and into the community, *Health Educ Q* 12(1):81-91, 1985.
26. EVAXX: *A study of Black Americans' attitudes toward cancer tests—highlights*. New York, 1981, EVAXX.
27. Fong CM: Ethnicity and nursing practice, *Topics In Clinical Nursing* 2:1-9, 1985.
28. Freeman H: Cancer in the socioeconomically disadvantaged, *CA Cancer J Clin* 39(5):266-288, 1989.
29. Freeman HP: Cancer mortality a socioeconomic phenomenon, Paper presented at the Twenty-Third Science Writers Seminar of the American Cancer Society, Daytona Beach, Fla., 1981.
30. Frank-Stromborg J: The role of the nurse in can-

cer detection and screening, *Semin Oncol Nurs* 2:191-199, 1986.

31. Grover PL, Kulpa B, Samson BT, Engstrom PF: Role of education in screening for cancer control: Results of follow up in two screening programs. In Mettlin C, Murphy GP, eds: *Issues In Cancer Screening And Communications,* New York, 1982, Alan R. Liss, pp 231-247.

32. Gregorio DI, Cummings KM, Michalek A: Delay, stage of disease, and survival among White and Black women with breast cancer, *Am J Public Health* 7(5):590-593, 1983.

33. Guillory J: Ethnic perspective of cancer nursing: The Black American, *Oncol Nurs Forum* 14(3):66-69, 1987.

34. Gullater AO: The role of life styles, *Proceedings of the American Cancer Society National Conference on Meeting the Challenge of Cancer Among Black Americans,* New York, Feb, 1979, American Cancer Society.

35. Gullatte MM: Cancer prevention and early detection in Black Americans: Colon and rectum, *Journal of the National Black Nurses' Association* 3(2):49-56, 1989.

36. Gullatte MM: Cancer prevention and early detection: Prostate, *In Touch* 9(1):4-5, 1988.

37. Hargreaves MK, Ahmed OI, Semenya KA, Pearson L, Sheth N, Hardy RE, Bernard LJ: Nutrition and cancer risk: Assessment and preventive program strategies for Black Americans. In Jones LA, ed: *Minorities and cancer,* pp 77-94, New York, 1989, Springer-Verlag Publishers.

38. Hautman MA: Folk health and illness beliefs, *Nurse Pract* 4:23-32, 1979.

39. Henschke UK, Leffall LD, Mason CH, Reinhold AW, Schneider RL, White JE: Alarming increase of the cancer mortality in the U.S. Black population (1950-1967), *Cancer* 31:763-768, 1973.

40. Jacob TC, Penn NE, Brown M: Breast self-examination: Knowledge, attitudes, and performance among Black women, *J Natl Med Assoc* 81(7):769-775, 1989.

41. Jacques G: Cultural health traditions: A Black perspective. In Branch MF, Perry-Paxton P, eds: *Providing Safe Nursing Care for Ethnic People of Color,* New York, 1976, Appleton-Century-Crofts, pp 115-124.

42. Jones EI: Preventing disease and promoting health in the minority community, *J Natl Med Assoc* 78(1):18-20, 1986.

43. Jordan WC: Voodoo medicine. In Williams RA, ed: *Textbook of Black-related diseases,* New York, 1975. McGraw Hill, pp 715-738.

44. Levin JS: The role of the Black church in community medicine, *J Natl Med Assoc* 76(5):477-483, 1984.

45. Levy DR: White doctors and Black patients: Influence of race on the doctor-patient relationship. *Pediatrics* 75(4):639-643, 1985.

46. Lightfoot OB: Preventive issues and the Black elderly: A biopsychosocial perspective, *J Natl Med Assoc* 75(10):957-963, 1983.

47. Malasanos L, Barkauskas V, Moss M, Stoltenberg-Allen K: *Health assessment,* St. Louis, 1986, CV Mosby.

48. Manfredi C, Warnecke R, Graham S, Rosenthal S: Social psychological correlates of health behavior: Knowledge of breast self-examination techniques among black women, *Soc Sci Med* 11:433-440, 1977.

49. Michielutte R, Diseker RA: Racial differences in knowledge of cancer: A pilot study, *Soc Sci Med* 16:245-252, 1982.

50. Michaels D: Occupational cancer in the Black population: The health effects of job discrimination, *J Natl Med Assoc* 75(10):1014-1018, 1983.

51. Miles GB, McDavis RJ: Effects of four orientation approaches on disadvantaged Black freshmen student's attitudes toward the counseling center, *Journal of College Student Personnel* 23(5):413-418, 1982.

52. Miller W, Cooper R: Rising lung cancer death rates among Black men: The importance of occupation and social class, *J Natl Med Assoc* 74(3):253-258, 1982.

53. Milio N: Values, social class, and community health services. *Nurs Res* 16:26-31, Winter 1967.

54. Milio N: Project in a Negro ghetto American. *J Nurs* 67:1006-1009, May 1967.

55. Mitchell-Beren ME, Dodds ME, Choi KL, Waskerwitz RR: A colorectal cancer prevention, screening, and evaluation program in community black churches, *CA Cancer J Clin* 39(2):115-118, 1989.

56. Mortenson LE, Engstrom PF, Anderson PN, eds: Advances in cancer control health care financing and research, *Proceedings of the Association of Community Cancer Centers 11th National Meeting. Oncology: Surviving the 80's,* New York, 1985, Alan R Liss, pp 215-226.

57. Natarajan N, Nemoto NJ, Mettlin C et al: Race related differences in breast cancer patients: Results of the 1982 national survey of breast cancer by the American College of Surgeons, *Cancer* 56(7):1704-1709, 1985.

58. National Cancer Institute: "Partners in preven-

tion" update, 1988. *National Cancer Institute/Office of Cancer Communications.*

59. National Research Council: *A common destiny: Blacks and American society,* Washington, DC, 1989, National Academy Press.

60. Newell GR: Lifestyles and cancer prevention. In Mettlin C, Murphy GP, eds: *Progress in cancer control IV: Research in the cancer center,* New York, 1983, Alan R Liss, pp 55-66.

61. Orleans CT, Strecher VJ, Schoenbach VJ, Salmon MA, Blackmon C: Smoking cessation initiatives for Black Americans: Recommendations for research and intervention, *Health Educ Res* 4(1):13-25, 1989.

62. Overfield T: Biological variation: Concepts from physical anthropology, *Nurs Clin North Am* 12:19-26, 1977.

63. Paxton PP: Epidemiology in health and disease. In Branch MF, Paxton PP, eds: *Providing safe nursing care for ethnic people of color,* New York, 1976, Appleton-Century-Crofts, p 127.

64. Pollack ES, Horm JW: Trends in cancer incidence and mortality in the United States, 1969-71, *J Natl Cancer Inst* 64:1091-1103, 1980.

65. Pottern LM, Morris LE, Blot WJ, Ziegler RG, Fraumeni JF: Esophageal cancer among Black men in Washington, D.C. I. Alcohol, tobacco, and other risk factors, *J Natl Cancer Inst* 67:777-783, 1981.

66. Powers BA: The use of orthodox and Black American folk medicine, *Adv Nurs Sci* 4:35-47, 1982.

67. Proctor E, Rose A: Expectations and preferences for counselor race and their relation to intermediate treatment outcomes, *J Counseling Psych* 28(1):40-46, 1981.

68. Roach LB: Color changes in dark skin. In Henderson G, Primeaux M, eds: *Transcultural Health Care,* Menlo Park, 1987, Addison-Wesley Publishing, pp 287-291.

69. Roberson MHB: The influence of religious beliefs on health choices of Afro-Americans, *Top Clin Nurs* 7(3):57-63, 1985.

70. Rogers EL, Goldkind L, Goldkind SF: Increasing frequency of esophageal cancer among Black male veterans, *Cancer* 49(3):610-617, 1982.

71. Rubin P: *Clinical oncology for medical studies and physicians,* ed 6, New York, 1983, American Cancer Society.

72. Sagalowsky AI, Admire RC: Increasing incidence of testicular cancer in Blacks, *Urology* 26:558-560, 1985.

73. Savitt TL: *Medicine and slavery: The diseases and health care of Blacks in antebellum Virginia,* Urbana, 1978, University of Illinois Press.

74. Smith JA: The role of the black clergy as allied health care professional in working with black patients. In Luckraft D, ed: *Black awareness,* New York, 1976, Am J Nurs.

75. Smith S, Greenblatt J, Darby C: *Cancer prevention awareness survey wave II. Black Americans and cancer prevention,* Bethesda, Md, 1987, National Institutes of Health.

76. Snow LF: I was born just exactly with the gift: An interview with a voodoo practitioner, *J of Am Folklore* 86:272-281, 1973.

77. Snow LF: Folk medical beliefs and their implications for care of patients, *Ann Intern Med* 81:82-96, 1974.

78. Snow LF: Popular medicine in a Black neighborhood. In Speece EH, ed: *Ethnic Medicine in the Southwest,* Tucson, 1977a. University of Arizona Press, pp 19-95.

79. Snow LF, Johnson SM: Modern day menstrual folklore: Some clinical implications, *J Am Med Assoc* 237:2736-2739, 1977b.

80. Snow L: Sorcerers, saints and charlatans: Black folk healers in urban America, *Cult Med Psychiatry* 2:69-106, 1978.

81. Snow LF: Traditional health beliefs and practices among lower class Black Americans, *West J Med* vol 8:820-828, 1983.

82. Spector RE: Health and illness among ethnic people of color, *Nurs Ed* 2:10-13, 1977.

83. Spitz MR, Sider JG, Pollack ES, Lynch HK, Newell GR Incidence and descriptive features of testicular cancer among United States Whites, Blacks, and Hispanics, 1973-1982, *Cancer* 58:1785-1790, 1986.

84. Stewart H: Kindling of hope in the disadvantaged: A study of the Afro-American healer, *Mental Hygiene* 55:96-100, 1971.

85. US Bureau of the Census: A statistical analysis, women in the United States, Series P-23, No. 100, Washington, DC, 1978, US Government Printing Office.

86. US Bureau of the Census: A statistical analysis, women in the United States, Series P-23, No. 100. Washington, DC, 1978. US Government Printing Office.

87. US Bureau of the Census: Statistical abstract of the United States, 1989, edition 109, Washington, DC, 1989, US Government Printing Office.

88. US Department of Health and Human Services: Cancer among Blacks and other minorities: Statistical profiles, Bethesda, Md, 1986a, National Institutes of Health.

89. US Department of Health and Human Services: *Cancer Statistics Review 1973-1988*, Bethesda, Md, 1991, National Institutes of Health.

90. US Department of Health and Human Services: *Report of the secretary's task force on Black and minority health*, Vol I, Executive summary, Bethesda, Md, 1985, National Institutes of Health,

91. US Department of Health and Human Services: *Report of the secretary's task force on Black and minority health*, Vol III, Cancer Bethesda, Md, 1986b, National Institutes of Health.

92. University of Texas: Medical history questionnaire. In *Cancer prevention and detection in the cancer screening clinic*, Houston, 1988, The University of Texas M.D. Anderson Cancer Center, pp 158-177.

93. Valentine AS: Behavioral dimensions in cancer prevention and detection, *Semin Oncol Nurs* 2:200-205, 1986.

94. Valentine A: Early detection measures. In Ziegfeld CR, ed: *Core curriculum for oncology nursing*, p 65, Philadelphia, 1987, WB Saunders.

95. Westberg GE: Can the clergy help overworked physicians? *Postgrad Med* 53:165-169, 1973.

96. White EH: Giving health care to minority patients, *Nurs Clin North Am* 12(1):27-40, 1977.

97. White JE, Enterline JP, Alan Z, Moore R: Cancer among Blacks in the U.S.: Recognizing the problem. In Mettlin C, Murphy GP, eds: *Cancer among Black populations*, New York, 1981. Alan R. Liss, pp 35-58.

98. Wilson J: Cancer incidence and mortality differences of Black and White Americans: A role for biomarkers. In Jones LA, ed: *Minorities and cancer*, New York, 1989. Springer-Verlag, pp 5-20.

99. Winslow DJ, Bishop EE: Everett and some aspects of occultism and folk religion in Negroes, *Keystone Folklore Quarterly* 14:81, 1969.

100. Wynder EL, Kabat GC: Opportunities for prevention of cancer in Blacks. In Mettlin C, Murphy GP, eds: *Cancer among Black populations*, New York, 1981, Alan R. Liss, pp 237-252.

101. Young JL, Devesa SS, Cutler SJ: Incidence of cancer in United States Blacks, *Cancer Research* 35:3523-3536, 1975.

Medical History Questionnaire

IDENTIFYING INFORMATION
For Office Use Only:

1. Case number_____
2. Date of examination_____
3. Number of visit_____

Please complete the following questionnaire. All responses will be held in strict confidence.

4. Name (Last-First-Middle initial)

    _____

5. Social security number___/___/___
6. Street address_____
7. City, state, and zip code

    _____

8. Home phone_____
9. Employer_____
10. Job title_____
11. Date of birth_____
12. Age_____
13. Sex
    ( ) Male
    ( ) Female
14. Race
    ( ) Caucasian
    ( ) African American
    ( ) Asian/Pacific Islander
    ( ) Hispanic/Latino
    ( ) Native American
    ( ) Other
15. Marital status
    ( ) Single/never married
    ( ) Divorced
    ( ) Separated

    ( ) Widowed
16. Highest education completed (check one):
    ( ) Grade school
    ( ) High school
    ( ) Some college
    ( ) College degree
    ( ) Some postgraduate
    ( ) Masters/Ph.D.
17. Would you like the reports of this screening examination sent to your personal physician?
    ( ) Yes
    ( ) No
    If yes, please give below the full name and address of your physician.

    _____

    _____

18. How did you hear about the screening program?
    ( ) Other employee
    ( ) Brochure
    ( ) Nurse from screening clinic
    ( ) Employee publication
    ( ) Memo
    ( ) Bulletin board
    ( ) Personnel orientation
    ( ) Check stub
    ( ) Other (Please specify)_____
19. What is your most important reason for coming for a screening examination? (Check only one.)
    ( ) To have an exam. I do not have a problem.

( ) To have an exam. I do have a problem.
(Please specify)

_____

( ) To learn about self-examinations.

( ) To learn about cancer prevention.

( ) Other (Please specify.)

20. Please list name, dosage, and duration of all medications you are currently taking.

_____

_____

_____

_____

21. Please list all surgeries you have undergone, giving type of surgery and year it was performed.

_____

_____

_____

HEALTH CARE PRACTICES

22. How often do you have a complete physical examination by your physician? (Women, please do not include examinations by your gynecologist or obstetrician.)
( ) More than once a year
( ) Every 13 months to 2 years
( ) Less than every 2 years
( ) Never

23. How often do you have checkups with your dentist?
( ) Every 6 months
( ) Every year
( ) Every 13 months to 2 years
( ) Less often than every 2 years
( ) Never

24. How often do you have chest X-ray films made?
( ) Every year
( ) Every 13 months to 2 years
( ) Every 2 to 5 years
( ) Less than every 5 years

25. Have you ever had a proctoscopic examination?
( ) Yes
( ) No
If yes, when?
_____ years ago

26. Have you ever had stool tests for hidden blood in stool?
( ) Yes
( ) No
If yes, when was your last test?
_____ years ago

Women, please answer questions 27-31. Men can skip to the next section.

27. How often do you have a pelvic examination and Pap smear?
( ) Every 6 months
( ) Every 12 months
( ) Every 13 months to 2 years
( ) Less often than every 2 years
( ) Never

28. When was your last Pap smear?
_____ years ago

29. Have you ever had abnormal results on a Pap smear?
( ) Yes
( ) No

30. Have you ever had a mammogram?
( ) Yes
( ) No
If yes, when was your last mammogram?
_____ years ago

31. How often do you have your breasts examined by a medical practitioner?
    ( ) More than once a year
    ( ) Once a year
    ( ) Every 2 years
    ( ) Less often than every 2 years

PAST MEDICAL HISTORY

32. Have you ever been diagnosed as having any of the medical conditions listed below? (Check all that apply).
    ( ) Cirrhosis of the liver
    ( ) Crohn's disease
    ( ) Diabetes
    ( ) Gardner's syndrome
    ( ) Herpes type II
    ( ) Polyps of the colon
    ( ) Hypertension
    ( ) Recurrent bronchitis
    ( ) Recurrent pneumonia
    ( ) Stomach ulcers
    ( ) Tuberculosis
    ( ) Ulcerative colitis
    ( ) Venereal disease or venereal warts
    ( ) Fibrocystic disease of the breasts

33. Have you ever undergone radiotherapy (cobalt, radium, etc.)?
    ( ) Yes
    ( ) No
    If yes, what year?

    ———————

    Treated for————————————————

    ————————————————————————

SELF-EXAMINATIONS

34. Have you ever been taught how to perform any of the following self-examinations?
    Skin   ( ) Yes   ( ) No
    Oral   ( ) Yes   ( ) No
    Breast   ( ) Yes   ( ) No
    Testicular (men only) ( ) Yes ( ) No
    Vulva (women only) ( ) Yes ( ) No

35. Do you now practice skin self-examination?
    ( ) Yes
    ( ) No

36. If yes, how often?
    ( ) At least once a month
    ( ) Every 2 months
    ( ) Every 3 to 6 months
    ( ) Less than every 6 months

37. Do you now practice oral self-examination?
    ( ) Yes
    ( ) No

38. If yes, how often?
    ( ) At least once a month
    ( ) Every 2 months
    ( ) Every 3 to 6 months

39. Do you now practice breast self-examination?
    ( ) Yes
    ( ) No

40. If yes, how often?
    ( ) At least once a month
    ( ) Every 2 months
    ( ) Every 3 to 6 months
    ( ) Less than every 6 months
    Men, please answer questions 41 and 42. Women, please skip to question 43.

41. Do you now practice testicular self-examination?
    ( ) Yes
    ( ) No

42. If yes, how often?
    ( ) At least once a month
    ( ) Every 2 months
    ( ) Every 3 to 6 months
    ( ) Less than every 6 months
    Men, please skip to the next section.
43. Do you now practice vulva self-examination?
    ( ) Yes
    ( ) No
44. If yes, how often?
    ( ) At least once a month
    ( ) Every 2 months
    ( ) Every 3 to 6 months
    ( ) Less than every 6 months

CANCER HISTORY

45. Have you ever had any type of cancer?
    ( ) Yes
    ( ) No
    If yes, list type of cancer, treatment received, and year of diagnosis.

    _____
    _____
    _____

46. How many of your blood relatives have had cancer?
    By blood relatives we mean:
    daughters
    sons
    sisters
    brothers
    mother
    father
    aunts (mother's sisters or father's sisters)
    uncles (mother's brothers or father's brothers)
    grandmothers (mother's mother or father's mother)
    grandfathers (mother's father or father's father)
    Number of relatives who have ever had cancer

    _____
47. Below please list any relatives who have ever had cancer. Give the relation the relative is to you, identify the kind of cancer the relative had, and give each relative's age at diagnosis.

    _____
    _____
    _____
    _____

Tobacco Use

48. Have you ever used any tobacco products on a daily basis for at least 6 months?
    ( ) Yes
    ( ) No
    If no, please skip to question 56.
49. Cigarettes
    ( ) Yes
    ( ) No
    _____ packs smoked per day
    _____ years used
50. Chewing tobacco
    ( ) Yes
    ( ) No
    _____ chews per day
    _____ years used
51. Snuff
    ( ) Yes
    ( ) No
    _____ chews per day
    _____ years used

52. Pipe
    ( ) Yes
    ( ) No
    _____ pipefuls smoked per day
    _____ years used
53. Cigars
    ( ) Yes
    ( ) No
    _____ cigars smoked per day
    _____ years used
54. At what age did you begin smoking?
    _____ years of age
55. If you are now a nonsmoker, how many years ago did you stop smoking?
    _____ years ago

Alcohol Use

56. Have you ever drunk alcoholic beverages?
    ( ) Yes
    ( ) No
    If no, skip to question 60. If yes, how often do you or did you drink?
57. Beer (cans/bottles)
    _____ per day
    _____ per week
    _____ years used
58. Wine (4 oz.)
    _____ per day
    _____ per week
    _____ years used
59. Liquor (shots)
    _____ per day
    _____ per week
    _____ years used

Diet and Nutrition

To indicate how often you eat the foods listed below, choose a number from the following scale:
    1 = one or more times per day
    2 = four to six times per week
    3 = two to three times per week
    4 = once a week
    5 = less than once a week
60. _____ fried foods
61. _____ charcoaled or barbecued foods
62. _____ pickled foods
63. _____ beef
64. _____ bacon/pork
65. _____ smoked or salted meat or fish
66. _____ non-low-fat dairy products (cheeses, milk, ice cream, etc.)
67. _____ butter
68. _____ fats on meat
69. _____ skin on chicken
70. _____ nuts and seeds, peanut butter
71. _____ fiber or bran foods
72. _____ cauliflower, brussel sprouts, cabbage, turnips, broccoli
73. _____ fresh fruits
74. _____ vegetables

PRESENT HEALTH
Skin

75. Do you now have any problems with
    Persistent skin rashes ( ) Yes ( ) No
    Sores that do not heal ( ) Yes ( ) No
    Moles that have changed in color, sensation, size, or shape ( ) Yes ( ) No
    Elevated, rough, scaly areas
76. What is your eye color?
    ( ) Blue/hazel

( ) Brown

77. What is your skin's response to the sun?
    ( ) Always burns, rarely tans
    ( ) Burns easily, tans minimally
    ( ) Burns moderately, tans gradually
    ( ) Burns minimally, tans easily
    ( ) Rarely burns, always tans
    ( ) Never burns, tans deeply

78. Have you had a history of painful or blistering sunburns before the age of 20?
    ( ) Yes
    ( ) No

79. If yes, approximately how many?
    ( ) 1-5
    ( ) 6-10
    ( ) 11-15
    ( ) Over 15

80. Over the past few years, how many times per year have you sunburned?
    ( ) 0-1
    ( ) 2-3
    ( ) More than 4

81. To which of the following is your sun exposure mainly owed?
    ( ) Occupation—you work outdoors
    ( ) Leisure activities and hobbies only—you work indoors

82. Have you used sunlamps or tanning salons for tanning?
    ( ) Yes
    ( ) No
    If yes, how many years?
    _____ years

83. Have you ever had a severe burn from fire or chemicals resulting in scar formation?

( ) Yes
( ) No

84. Do you use sunscreen regularly?
    ( ) Yes
    ( ) No
    If yes, what is the sunscreen's sun protection factor (SPF) number?
    _____ (SPF number)

Head and Neck

85. Do you now have problems with the following:
    Facial swelling ( ) Yes ( ) No
    Facial numbness or tingling
    ( ) Yes ( ) No
    Change in vision ( ) Yes ( ) No
    Persistent headaches ( ) Yes ( ) No
    Earaches ( ) Yes ( ) No
    Change in hearing ( ) Yes ( ) No
    Continuous nasal obstruction (stuffiness) ( ) Yes ( ) No
    Loss of smell ( ) Yes ( ) No
    Bleeding from nose or mouth
    ( ) Yes ( ) No
    Persistent color change(s) or sore(s) in nose, mouth, or lip( ) Yes ( ) No
    Dentures that do not fit
    ( ) Yes ( ) No
    Difficulty in chewing ( ) Yes ( ) No
    Hoarseness, voice change
    ( ) Yes ( ) No
    Repeated sore throats( ) Yes ( ) No
    Trouble swallowing, clearing throats
    ( ) Yes ( ) No
    Lump(s) in neck ( ) Yes ( ) No

Lumps

86. Do you now have problems with the following:
    Persistent cough or change in cough ( ) Yes ( ) No

Coughing up blood ( ) Yes ( ) No
Change in amount, color, or odor of sputum (phlegm, mucous)
( ) Yes ( ) No
Shortness of breath not caused by heavy exercise ( ) Yes ( ) No
Dull pains in chest ( ) Yes ( ) No
Wheezing or difficult breathing
( ) Yes ( ) No

Stomach, Intestines, Rectum

87. Do you now have problems with the following:
Frequent unexplained indigestion
( ) Yes ( ) No
Stomach pain ( ) Yes ( ) No
Frequent nausea or vomiting
( ) Yes( ) No
Vomiting of blood ( ) Yes ( ) No
Recent change in bowel movement or habits ( ) Yes ( ) No
Blood in bowel movements
( ) Yes ( ) No
Black, tarlike stools ( ) Yes ( ) No
Mucous in your stools
( ) Yes ( ) No
A feeling of pressure on your rectum or of not being able to complete a bowel movement ( ) Yes ( ) No

Kidney, Bladder

88. Do you now have problems with the following:
Burning on urination ( ) Yes ( ) No
Difficulty in urination( ) Yes ( ) No
Blood in urine ( ) Yes ( ) No
Need to get up more than twice during the night to urinate
( ) Yes ( ) No

Other

89. Do you now have problems with the following:
Enlarged lymph nodes/glands
( ) Yes ( ) No
Fever from unexplained causes
( ) Yes ( ) No
Unexplained weight loss of more than 10 pounds( ) Yes ( ) No
Loss of appetite( ) Yes ( ) No
Unexplained, unusual fatigue
( ) Yes ( ) No
Men, please skip to question 101.

Women Only

90. How old were you when you began having monthly periods?
_____ years old
When did your most recent menstrual period begin?
_____ (date)

91. Would you say that during most of your life your periods were regular (when not on birth control pills)?
( ) Yes
( ) No

92. At what age did you have sexual intercourse for the first time?
_____ years old

93. How many sex partners have you had in your lifetime?
( ) None
( ) 1-4
( ) 5-10
( ) More than 10

94. How many full-term pregnancies have you had?
( ) None
( ) One

( ) Two
( ) Three
( ) Four
( ) Five
( ) More than five

95. How old were you during your first full-term pregnancy?

_____ years old

96. Have you stopped having monthly periods?
( ) Yes
( ) No

If so, for what reason?
( ) Natural menopause
( ) Surgery

At what age did you stop having periods?

_____ years old

97. Have you ever used birth control pills?
( ) Yes
( ) No

If yes, how many years did you use them?

_____ years

98. Have you ever used female hormones (estrogens)?
( ) Yes
( ) No

If yes, how many years did or have you used them?

_____ years

99. When your mother was pregnant with you, did she use the female hormone diethylstilbestrol (DES)?
( ) Yes
( ) No
( ) Unknown

100. Below are two lists of problems.

Have you had any of these problems in the last six months?

Female organs

Itching on the outside of your vagina ( ) Yes ( ) No

Bleeding or spotting between your menstrual periods ( ) Yes ( ) No

Unusual vaginal discharge ( ) Yes ( ) No

Bleeding or spotting after sex or after douching ( ) Yes ( ) No

Breasts

Lump or thickening in breast or armpit ( ) Yes ( ) No

Pain or tenderness (other than before periods) ( ) Yes ( ) No

Discharge from nipple(s) ( ) Yes ( ) No

Change in the skin of your breast, such as dimpling or puckering ( ) Yes ( ) No

Changes in nipple appearance ( ) Yes ( ) No

Women, please skip to question 102.

Men only

101. Below is a list of problems. Have you had any of these in the past six months?

Lump or thickening in either testicle ( ) Yes ( ) No

Pain or swelling of either testicle ( ) Yes ( ) No

Undescended testicle at any time during your life ( ) Yes ( ) No

Enlarged prostate gland ( ) Yes ( ) No

Sore or irritation on the penis that is not healing ( ) Yes ( ) No

EXPOSURES

102. Have you ever been involved in any of the following occupations or avocations or been exposed to any of the chemicals for at least six months' duration? (Check all that apply.)

   a. Artist
   ( ) Yes ( ) No ____ years
   b. Asbestos
   ( ) Yes ( ) No ____ years
   c. Benzene
   ( ) Yes ( ) No ____ years
   d. Cable-making industry
   ( ) Yes ( ) No ____ years
   e. Carpentry
   ( ) Yes ( ) No ____ years
   f. Chemical industry
   ( ) Yes ( ) No ____ years
   g. Chemotherapy drugs
   ( ) Yes ( ) No ____ years
   h. Chimney sweep
   ( ) Yes ( ) No ____ years
   i. Lifeguard
   ( ) Yes ( ) No ____ years
   j. Lumber industry/heavy wood dust
   ( ) Yes ( ) No ____ years
   k. Mining
   ( ) Yes ( ) No ____ years
   l. Nickel smelting
   ( ) Yes ( ) No ____ years
   m. Outdoor occupation
   ( ) Yes ( ) No ____ years
   n. Painting
   ( ) Yes ( ) No ____ years
   o. Pesticide spraying or manufacturing
   ( ) Yes ( ) No ____ years
   p. Petroleum industry
   ( ) Yes ( ) No ____ years
   q. Plastic industry
   ( ) Yes ( ) No ____ years
   r. Plumber
   ( ) Yes ( ) No ____ years
   s. Printing
   ( ) Yes ( ) No ____ years
   t. Radiation or x-rays
   ( ) Yes ( ) No ____ years
   u. Roofing or road repair
   ( ) Yes ( ) No ____ years
   v. Rubber industry
   ( ) Yes ( ) No ____ years
   w. Shipbuilding
   ( ) Yes ( ) No ____ years
   x. Shoemaking or leather work
   ( ) Yes ( ) No ____ years
   y. Tanning or taxidermy
   ( ) Yes ( ) No ____ years
   z. Textile weaving
   ( ) Yes ( ) No ____ years
   aa. Welding
   ( ) Yes ( ) No ____ years

Cancer Prevention/Early Detection Materials Specifically for African Americans

AMERICAN CANCER SOCIETY, INC.

Can They Stop Smoking? Can You? This publication is about three African American women of different ages who tell their story in the context that anyone can quit if they really want to. Tips on how to quit are on the back page. Order code 2662.

Don't Miss Out On Your Sunset Years . . . Together is a pamphlet for the older African American audience that describes what men and women can do to protect themselves against colorectal cancer. The message is positive and details the steps to take for early diagnosis. Order code 2666 for pamphlets and 2124 for posters.

Got a Few Minutes? This is a pamphlet on breast self-examination (BSE) directed towards African American women. It clearly explains and illustrates the basic steps of BSE. BSE's two-fold purpose of early detection and increased awareness of the body is stressed. This pamphlet is intended to accompany BSE programs. Order code 2078.

It's My Life . . . My Choices is intended to encourage African American women to get a regular Pap test. Furthermore, older women are encouraged to see a doctor at the first sign of abnormal bleeding because of the risk of endometrial cancer. Order code 2079.

Listen to Your Body lists the seven warning signals and indicates the type of cancer that could be causing them. The approach that is taken is very positive and reassuring; emphasis is placed on the high cure rates for early cancer and on the benign diseases that cause the same symptoms as cancer. Order code 2067 (should be valuable at all programs for adults).

Quit Cigarettes—Live Longer is easy-to-read, informative, and frank in exposing the dangers of cigarette smoking while emphasizing the benefits of quitting. Order code 2041 (the folder can be used effectively wherever special population groups congregate . . . health centers, schools, exhibits, churches, and companies).

Smoking and Genocide is a companion pamphlet to the powerful "Genocide" poster for the African American male audience. Written by an African American man, this pamphlet deals with the special meaning of the word for the African American family and community with hard-hitting facts about smoking and lung cancer. Order code 2664 for pamphlets and for posters 2132.

When a Woman Smokes communicates in a sympathetic manner the ACS's health concerns for women who smoke. Increased risks for lung cancer and heart disease and harm to unborn babies are discussed, along with the alarming rise in smoking among teen-age girls. For those who want to stop smoking, this pamphlet provides suggestions on quitting. Order code 2093.

Your Health is Your Business These two folders provide cancer facts for (1) low-income men, and (2) women from disadvantaged areas. The message is "life is tough enough . . . don't kill yourself by neglecting your health." Calls for more information on cancer are referred to the local ACS unit. Order codes for women 2034, for men 2035.

Alive! Pap Test This is a poster designed to emphasize the importance of the Pap test to African American women that features a powerful close-up of an attractive African American woman using strong, contemporary colors. Order code 2103 (can be displayed wherever women congregate, including churches, hospitals, schools, or community health centers).

Like Mother, Like Daughter This poster for African American women shows the power of role models in smoking. It depicts a child who copies the smoking mother by using a crayon and contains the caption, "Why don't you quit before she starts?" Order code 2120.

It Only Hurts You If You Don't Have it PAP TEST is an upbeat message for African American women to encourage them to have the test and find out how frequently they should repeat it. Order code 2134 Poster.

Life . . . The One Race You Lose By Finishing First . . . Don't Smoke This poster for African American youth makes a telling point by contrasting the high speed photo of a young man crossing the finish line with fresh-approach copy by an African American writer on the realities of smoking. Order code 2122.

There's Lots of Loving and Living Ahead . . . Why Cut It Short This poster features a young African American couple in an outdoor setting, to carry the message that life is beautiful without cigarettes. Order code 2152.05.

Five Minutes For Self-Examination Narrated by a health guide, this film is meant to encourage low-income women to practice BSE. The film focuses on a young housewife who discovers a lump in her breast. After her physician examines her and finds nothing abnormal, she is shown how to perform BSE. Order code 2377 for 16mm, 2377.08 for 8mm, 2377.88 for Super 8mm, and 2377.98 for Super 8mm, technicolor.

The Cancer No One Talks About Narrated by Dr. LaSalle D. Leffall of Howard University, this film openly discusses many previously unspoken aspects of colorectal cancer in order to motivate people over 40 to have regular procto exams and to use the do-it-yourself quaiac slide kit. Order codes 2351 for 16mm, 2351.08 for 8mm, 2351.88 for Super 8mm, and 2351.98 for Super 8mm, technicolor.

No Time For Privacy This film contains graphics of the human body and a patient-physician discussion to explain how three tests aid in the early detection of colorectal cancer; narrated by Harry Belafonte. Order code 2343.00.

Take The Time This film on cervical and endometrial cancer, narrated by Phylicia Rashad, takes place in a gynecological clinic with a variety of women from various backgrounds. Order code 2367.00.

Check It Out is a "Rap" style film for youth on the effects of smokeless tobacco. Order code 2398.00

Be a Hero Lyrics slide set or videotape. Audiences can sing along with Cissy Houston; on the videotape, the lyrics "light up" as each line is sung. Order code 2516.07 for the slide set; 2516.14 for the tape.

Cancer? Who Me? This pamphlet on the Minority Cancer Education Program was prepared by the Department of Cancer Control and Epidemiology, Roswell Park Memorial Institute and Special Population Subcommittee, American Cancer Society, Buffalo, NY.

Get In Touch With Your Body Stunning art emphasizes the important message about monthly breast self-examination in this poster for African American women. Order code 2133.

What Black Americans Should Know About Cancer—This publication answers many questions individuals have about cancer and what they can do to guard against it. The approach is positive and reassuring. A glossary of terms is provided along with telephone numbers for the Cancer Information Service. Order DHEW (NIH) 78-1635.

Community Resources

Mass Communication—Television (public and private) and radio. Experts have found that television is most people's primary source of cancer information. African American radio stations that address the listening needs of various age groups can also be used to disseminate information on cancer. The messages must be non-threatening and culturally sensitive. When at all possible the use of a public figure who the African American community knows and respects should be used. Many cable companies have a health information station and may provide their services free of charge.

Magazines and Newspapers—Magazines that target the African American audience, such as *Ebony*, *Jet*, and *Essence*, can be found in many homes and are an excellent source for cancer information. Local African American newspapers and magazines should also be used. School newspapers/letters, union newsletters, and church bulletins are another resource. Listings can be found in local telephone directories.

Minority Cancer Control, The SHARE Harlem Health Project Coalition, New York, NY—This program, conducted by the Memorial Hospital for Cancer and Allied Diseases, aims to reduce cancer risks by promoting health among African Americans and Hispanics in Harlem.

Public Education Programs—These programs are designed to inform the public about cancer and what they can do to protect themselves, as well as to demonstrate related health habits and lifestyles. Emphasis is currently on the following six sites: colon and rectum, lung, breast, uterus, oral cavity and skin. The program focuses on prevention, early detection, and risk reduction.

Youth Programs—These are designed to target youth of various ages and school levels. The programs provide scientific, comprehensive cancer education with emphasis on cancer risks. Educational strategies are designed to teach good health habits, help youth to make health-enhancing lifestyle decisions, and help them understand health behavior as it relates to cancer risk reduction. The programs are usually conducted in the schools and often include activities to be used in the home and community.

Road to Recovery—Under this program, volunteer drivers assist patients in getting to and from medical appointments.

Ostomy Rehabilitation Program—In cooperation with the United Ostomy Association and enterostomal therapists, trained volunteers who have had similar surgery offer help to other ostomy patients on a one-to-one basis, assisting them in their physical and psychological adjustment.

Laryngectomy Rehabilitation Program—Former laryngectomy patients provide support and education programs to other patients pre- and/or post-operatively. A program to inform employees about re-employability of laryngectomies is also available.

Reach To Recovery—(Approval of attending physician required.) This program provides rehabilitation support to women who had mastectomies. Volunteers will visit in the hospital or home to demonstrate rehabilitation exercises and provide a temporary prosthesis. Literature to help husbands, children, and friends of breast cancer patients is also available.

Can Surmount—This is a short-term visitor program for patients, and the families of patients, with many types of cancer. Hospital and home visits are made with the approval of the physician. The one-to-one visit by a person who has experienced the same type of cancer offers functional, emotional, and social support.

I Can Cope—This American Cancer Society program provides information on cancer therapy, treatment, side effects, nutrition, availability of resources, and other topics of interest to cancer patients and their families.

Cancer Care, Inc. of the National Cancer Foundation—This group provides counseling and planning services to patients and their families, as well as financial assistance, nursing care, homemakers, home health aides, and a housekeeper.

Mastectomy Counseling for Men—Counseling through this program is on a one-to-one basis or in a group of men whose wife, mother, sister, or significant other is having a mastectomy. Clients are referred from the ACS Reach To Recovery program.

YM/YWCA—Many of these organizations offer exercises and swim programs for the rehabilitation of cancer patients. Check the local chapter for services provided.

American Lung Association—The ALA provides smoking cessation programs and educational materials, and works with various organizations to achieve a common goal of cleaning up the air.

Community Organizations—Civic organizations within the community provide numerous services. The local chamber of commerce and some local health agencies can provide a listing of such services. Some known to provide various health-related services for African Americans are: the National Council of Negro Women, Inc., National African American Coalition Party, and the National Black Nurses Association.

Religious Organizations—Many consider the church to be a seminal influence on the African American community. It is one institution from which an enormous amount of support, health information, and services can be distributed.

Make Today Count—This is a nonprofit organization that provides counseling and peer support services to terminally ill patients, their families, and health care professionals.

Comprehensive Cancer Centers—These offer a broad range of services for cancer prevention, diagnoses, treatment, and rehabilitation; they also conduct scientific research.

Community-Based Cancer Control Programs—The creation of these programs, which are funded by the National Cancer Institute, was based on the concept that cancer patients can be most effectively and efficiently cared for if local resources are combined in a cooperative effort. Maximum use is made of community physicians, clinics, hospitals, and other local resources. These health professionals help to prevent, detect, and diagnose cancer; they also provide continuing care and rehabilitation for cancer patients.

Cancer Control programs are listed in local telephone directories.

State and Local Departments of Health and Social Services—These agencies provide information and a variety of services for patients with cancer and their families. A listing can be found in local telephone directories.

Cancer Prevention and Screening Among Hispanic Populations

This chapter provides an overview of Hispanic culture, its beliefs, values, customs and more, as they relate to health and illness beliefs. This is knowledge that can be useful to oncology nurses, to nurses in general, as well as to other health practitioners who care for Hispanic patients. It is important to understand Hispanic health-seeking behaviors as well as cultural responses to health and illness. Only when we understand, are sensitive to, and respectful of the patients' cultural values and beliefs, can we provide effective health care.

Cancer in the Hispanic community is increasing. It is imperative that prevention and early detection be of primary concern to health providers, especially those involved in the health care of Hispanics. As a Hispanic who has been very involved with cancer and with the Latin American countries, I remember when cancer of the breast among Hispanic women was rare, while there was somewhat more cancer of the cervix. There were theories then, that because Latin American women breast-fed their babies this was a deterrent to breast cancer. The fact that women had rather large numbers of children beginning rather early, this could predispose or even bring about cancer of the cervix. All that is changing. The authors state that although cancer of the breast has a low incidence among Hispanic women, the mortality rate is very high. This of course is related to the lack of early detection of the cancer, and to getting help too late to make any difference. Unfortunately, this was the case in my cousin's wife. The need for information, education, and prevention of cancer among Hispanics for early detection of cancer is a paramount necessity for the Hispanic community. Hispanic men are equally at risk for prostate and stomach cancer and other sites. Lately, in my own experience, I have known three Hispanic men with cancer of the breast. The authors emphasize the need for education for the Hispanic population, and a knowledge base of the culture on the part of the health care professionals, to help Hispanics prevent the incidence and high mortality rate of cancer among them.

It is a well known fact, and it has been documented, that Hispanics do not seek medical help for cancer problems until it is too late to do them any good. Therefore prevention and early detection cannot be emphasized too much. This has to be the first line of defense against cancer among Hispanics. Teachers and supervisors working with students and young nurses should find this article a great help in classroom teaching and in the clinical area supervision. It has much good material about Hispanic cultural beliefs and behavioral modes that influence their health and illness behaviors.

The authors have made it clear that there is diversity among the Hispanic group that needs to be taken into consideration when working with them. As a Representative of Central and South American Countries and the Caribbean, on the Board of Directors of the International Society of Nurses in Cancer Care, I have first-hand knowledge of the cancer problems and difficulties in the Latin American area of the world. Being so closely related to the Hispanic problems and their difficulties in trying to resolve them, I am convinced that information, education, prevention, and early detection is the key to decrease the incidence and mortality of cancer among Hispanic people. To this end the article gives nurses, and other health professionals, a good overview of Hispanic culture, values, and beliefs to help them be sensitive and effective in their nursing and health care to Hispanics.

I would like to again emphasize the need of nurses in general, and oncological nurses in particular, to become knowledgeable about Hispanic culture and Hispanics health-seeking behaviors. Their beliefs about health and illness influence how they react and behave when faced with the incidence of cancer. We need more literature like this in relation to minorities, which is a neglected area in our profession.

Ildaura Murillo-Rohde, Ph.D., CS, FAAN

Dean and Professor Emeritus,
State University of New York, Brooklyn;
International Society of Nurses in Cancer Care,
Board of Directors, Latin America Representatives

Cancer Prevention and Screening Among Hispanic Populations

REBECCA J. COHEN
JACQUELINE A. ROHALY

"HISPANIC": A GENERIC TERM—A DIVERSE CULTURE

The United States population is a heterogeneous melting pot of cultures and ethnicities. The Hispanic population is one of the fastest growing minority groups in the country. "Hispanic," a generic term created by the U.S. Bureau of the Census for the 1970 census, refers to the numerous cultures in the Western Hemisphere of Spanish descent including Mexican, Puerto Rican, Cuban, and Central and South American. The unique aspects of each Hispanic culture challenge health care professionals to provide holistic care.

DEMOGRAPHICS
Population Statistics

According to the U.S. Bureau of the Census (1989) and the National Coalition of Hispanic Health and Human Services Organizations (COSSMHO, 1988), "Hispanic" is an umbrella term for several subgroups in the U.S. Persons of Mexican origin, the largest of these sub-

groups, represent nearly 63% of the Hispanic population; Puerto Ricans comprise 12%; and Cubans make up 5%. All the "other" subgroups comprise 20% of the total Hispanic population.

The Hispanic population has been growing five times as fast as the rest of the country for the past decade, and in 1989 totaled 20 million in the 50 states and the District of Columbia (Puerto Rico and other associated areas are not included). This group increased 39% from the 1980 census to the 1990 census, with half the growth attributable to immigration and the rest to births (Table 5-1). By the year 2000, this population is expected to reach 31 million, making it the largest U.S. minority group (Rich, 1989).

There are two major reasons for the rapid growth of the Hispanic population. *First*, some Hispanic countries (i.e. Mexico, Cuba) lie in close proximity to the U.S. borders. Nearly a half million persons of all ethnic origins immigrate legally to the U.S. each year, and an estimated half million more enter the coun-

TABLE 5-1 Hispanic Origin for the United States: 1980 vs. 1990 Census Findings

Race	1990 Census Number	1990 Census Percent of pop.	1980 Census Number	1980 Census Percent of pop.	Number Change	Percent Change
All persons	248,709,873	100.0	226,545,805	100.0	22,164,068	9.8
White	199,686,070	80.3	188,371,622	83.1	11,314,448	6.0
African American	29,986,060	12.1	26,495,02	11.7	3,491,035	13.2
Native American	1,878,285	0.8	1,364,033	0.6	514,252	37.7
HISPANIC ORIGIN						
Hispanic origin*	22,354,059	9.0	14,608,673	6.4	7,745,386	53.0
Mexican	13,495,938	5.4	8,740,439	3.9	4,755,499	54.4
Puerto Rican	2,727,754	1.1	2,013,945	0.9	713,809	35.4
Cuban	1,043,932	0.4	803,226	0.4	240,706	30.0
Other Hispanic	5,086,435	2.0	3,051,063	1.3	2,035,372	66.7
Not of Hispanic origin	226,355,814	91.0	211,937,132	93.6	14,418,682	6.8

*Persons of Hispanic origin may be of any race.
From U.S. Department of Commerce, Bureau of the Census: *Census and You* 26(9):3, September 1991.

try illegally. A *second* reason for the rapid growth is this population's high birth rate. According to the Bureau of the Census (1988), immigration represents only 50% of the population increase; the other 50% is due to new births. A significant percentage of Hispanic women are in their childbearing years and they begin having children at an early age, contributing to the rapid growth of this population.

Geographical Distributions

The Hispanic population is concentrated in nine states. Nearly 63% of Hispanics live in the southwestern states of California, Texas, Arizona, New Mexico, and Colorado. Another 25% of the population is located in New York, New Jersey, Illinois, and Florida, and the remaining 12% is scattered throughout the country.

Education, Employment, and Income

In 1970, only 32% of the Hispanic population had completed four years of high school, and only 5% had completed four years of college. However, by 1990, 51% had completed high school and 9% had completed college (U.S. Bureau of the Census, 1991) (Table 5-2 presents a breakdown by subgroup).

In March 1990, Hispanics age 16 years and older had a higher unemployment rate than non-Hispanics in the same age group (8.2% and 5.3%, respectively). However, the 1990 rate of 8.2% for Hispanics was much lower than it was for this group in March of 1983, which was 16.5% (U.S. Bureau of the Census, 1991).

Among Hispanic males, the unemployment rate in March 1990 was also higher than that for non-Hispanic males (8% versus 5.7%), but also lower than the

TABLE 5-2   Educational Level in 1988 of Hispanic U.S. Residents, Age 25 and Over, by Ethnic Group

Ethnic Group	Percent Completed Less Than 5 Years	Percent Completed 4 Years of High School	Percent Completed 4 Years of College
Mexican American	16	43	6
Puerto Rican	10	54	10
Cuban American	4	63	20
Non-Hispanic	2	79	22

From U.S. Bureau of the Census: The Hispanic Population in the United States, *Current Population Reports*, Washington, DC, 1989, U.S. Government Printing Office.

March 1983 rate of 16.5%. A similar pattern is evident among females: about 8.5% of Hispanic females were unemployed in March of 1990, compared to 4.9% of non-Hispanic females (U.S. Bureau of the Census, 1991).

There is no statistically significant difference in the unemployment rate for males of different Hispanic subgroups. Among Hispanic females, however, Mexican females had a higher unemployment rate (9.8%) than did Cuban, Central and South American, or other Hispanic females (U.S. Bureau of the Census, 1991).

The average Hispanic earns 10%-60% less than other U.S. workers (Table 5-3). According to the U.S. Bureau of the Census (1989), 25% of Mexican Americans, 22% of Puerto Ricans, and 54% of Cuban Americans—or a total of 1.2 million Hispanics—live below the poverty level; this is estimated to be 2.5 times the number of non-Hispanic families in poverty (9%) (COSSMHO, 1988).

Family Composition

The traditional Hispanic family is large, nuclear, and patriarchal (U.S. Bureau of the Census, 1991); however, this is changing. In March, 1990, there were 66 million families in the U.S.; 7% of these families were Hispanic and 93% were of other ethnic groups. About 7 of 10 Hispanic families were married-couple families, compared to about 8 of 10 non-Hispanic families. Twenty-three percent of all Hispanic families were maintained by a female householder with no husband present, compared to 16% of non-Hispanic families. Approximately 7% of Hispanic and approximately 4% of non-Hispanic families were maintained by a male with no wife present (U.S. Bureau of the Census, 1991).

Among the Hispanic subgroups, families of Puerto Rican origin were the least likely to be maintained by a married couple (57%) and the most likely to be maintained by a woman with no husband present (39%) (U.S. Bureau of the Census, 1991).

Hispanic families on the average were larger than non-Hispanic families—3.82 persons and 3.12 persons, respectively. About 28% of Hispanic families had five or more members, compared to about 13% of non-Hispanic families. Among the subgroups, Mexican families had the

TABLE 5-3   Family Income of U.S. Residents in 1988 (Percent)

Ethnic Group	Less Than $10,000	$10,000–$24,000	$25,000–$49,000	$50,000 and Above	Median
Mexican American	20	38	33	10	$21,025
Puerto Rican	29	33	27	11	18,932
Cuban American	17	30	28	24	26,858
Non-Hispanic	10	26	37	27	33,142

From U.S. Bureau of the Census: The Hispanic Population in the United States, *Current Population Reports*, Washington, DC, 1989, U.S. Government Printing Office.

highest proportion of families with five or more members (33%); about one of every six Mexican families had six or more members (U.S. Bureau of the Census, 1991).

Health Status

Although Hispanics live about as long as Caucasian non-Hispanics, they tend to die of different causes. Among both groups, heart disease and cancer rank first and second, respectively, as causes of death, but these diseases cause 60% of Caucasian non-Hispanic deaths and 40% of Hispanic deaths. Accidents kill nearly 10% of Hispanics, but only 4% of Caucasian non-Hispanics. And although homicide strikes Hispanics more than non-Hispanic whites, Hispanics do not commit suicide as often. Acquired Immunodeficiency Syndrome is the sixth leading cause of death among Hispanics of all ages, but is not even among the top 10 causes of death for Caucasian non-Hispanics (*The Washington Post*, 1991) (see Figure 5-1).

In general, Hispanics are less likely to have medical insurance than any other group. In 1988, the latest year for which statistics are available, 13% of the U.S. population lacked health insurance over-

all: 10.2% of Caucasians; 20% of African Americans and 32% of Hispanics. Uninsured Hispanics tend to be less educated, poorer, and sicker than the uninsured of other cultures. Experts once believed that Hispanics did not go to doctors because they choose instead to go to a **curandero** (folk healer) or an **herbalista,** both of which are **folk medicine practitioners** in Hispanic culture. However, the Hispanic Health and Nutrition Examination Survey found that only 4.2% of Mexican Americans had seen a folk healer in the previous year (Estrada, Trevino, and Ray, 1990; Higginbotham, Trevino, and Ray, 1990).

EPIDEMIOLOGY OF CANCER

Tracing cancer incidence among Hispanics is difficult for several reasons. First, the term "Hispanic" was only introduced in 1970; before that the Hispanic population was not identified as a distinct minority group. For this reason, data on cancer incidence among Hispanics were not aggressively recorded nor did this data differentiate between the five ethnic subgroups—Mexican-American, Puerto Rican, Cuban, Central/South American, and other.

Generally, the incidence of cancer is

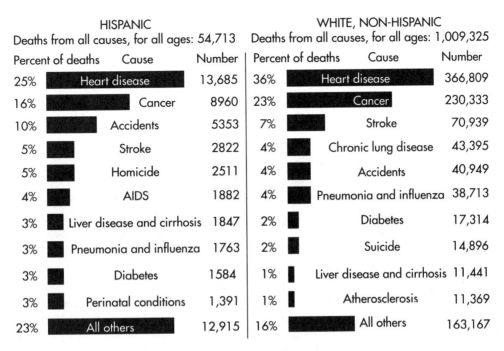

HISPANIC
Deaths from all causes, for all ages: 54,713

Percent of deaths	Cause	Number
25%	Heart disease	13,685
16%	Cancer	8960
10%	Accidents	5353
5%	Stroke	2822
5%	Homicide	2511
4%	AIDS	1882
3%	Liver disease and cirrhosis	1847
3%	Pneumonia and influenza	1763
3%	Diabetes	1584
3%	Perinatal conditions	1,391
23%	All others	12,915

WHITE, NON-HISPANIC
Deaths from all causes, for all ages: 1,009,325

Percent of deaths	Cause	Number
36%	Heart disease	366,809
23%	Cancer	230,333
7%	Stroke	70,939
4%	Chronic lung disease	43,395
4%	Accidents	40,949
4%	Pneumonia and influenza	38,713
2%	Diabetes	17,314
2%	Suicide	14,896
1%	Liver disease and cirrhosis	11,441
1%	Atherosclerosis	11,369
16%	All others	163,167

Figure 5-1   Top ten causes of death in 1988: Hispanics and Caucasian non-Hispanics. From *Top ten causes of death in 1988: Hispanics and White non-Hispanics*, January 15, 1991, Washington Post.

low among Hispanics compared to the Caucasian and African American populations. According to Markides and Coriel (1986), the Hispanic population has a *lower* incidence of cancer than the Caucasian and African American populations, but *higher* incidence than that for Native Americans. This trend is notable because the Native American and Hispanic groups share a common genetic heritage. However, among Hispanic women cancer mortality rates for all disease sites are slightly *higher* than those for Caucasian and African American females.

According to Martin and Suarez (1987), most Hispanics delay seeking treatment for symptoms and continue to use folk remedies as their first choice in health care. Samet, Key, Hunt, and Goodwin (1987) concluded that a Hispanic patient's decision to seek early diagnosis or delay diagnosis may depend, in part, on their ethnic (subgroup) origin.

The largest concentrated population of Hispanics in the U.S. resides in Los Angeles County, California. Hispanics from this county are primarily of Mexican and Central American origin. A study of cancer incidence trends and risk ratios for this group identified cancers of high, intermediate, and low incidence in the population. The group faced a high risk of gallbladder, liver, cervical, and stomach cancers; an intermediate risk of pancreatic and prostate cancers; and a low risk of melanoma and colorectal, lung, and reproductive cancers (Mack, Walker, Mack, and Berstein, 1985).

Gallbladder Cancer

Hispanic men and women are both at high risk for gallbladder cancer (Mack et al., 1985). Devor and Buechley (1980) found a genetic predisposition for gallbladder cancer in this group after observing the incidence trends for the disease among Hispanic New Mexicans. They reviewed state mortality rates and found 521 cases of gallbladder cancer in New Mexican residents from 1957-1977. Nearly 46.3% of the cases involved Hispanic individuals, an incidence rate higher than that found in the Native American and Caucasian population. Further investigation revealed that northern New Mexico accounted for the largest percentage of gallbladder cancer cases. Hispanics of this region were found to be Native American in ancestry. The isolation of this population and the resulting inbreeding accounted for a pattern of gallbladder cancer that demonstrated familial tendencies. As a result, the researchers proposed that gallbladder cancer had a genetic basis in this population.

Findings of another study that examined the incidence of biliary tract cancer in the Los Angeles County area (Menck and Mack, 1982) were similar to those of Mack et al. (1985). Menck and Mack (1982) identified epidemiologic characteristics, such as gender and ethnic background that indicated that Hispanics were at high risk for biliary tract cancer. They found females to be at higher risk for biliary cancer than males. Also, risk for this cancer began to rise at an earlier age in Hispanic females than other ethnic groups, and place of birth appeared to have a strong effect on incidence rates.

Liver Cancer

Hispanics face a high risk for liver cancer. The Hispanic population, regardless of gender, has an incidence rate for liver cancer that is three times the rate of the Caucasian population. Liver cancer occurs primarily in Mexican males of lower socioeconomic status who immigrated late to the U.S. (Mack et al., 1985). Suarez and Martin (1987) concluded that liver cancer incidence rates in Mexican males through age 50 were similar to those found in the U.S. Caucasian population; however, after age 50, the incidence rate for the Mexican male increases dramatically. It has been estimated that the incidence of liver cancer in Mexican males is 2.2 times higher than that for Caucasians, while the incidence rate among Mexican females is 2.8 times higher (Suarez and Martin, 1987).

Cervical Cancer

Another type of cancer that occurs frequently in the Hispanic population is cervical cancer. According to Mack et al. (1985), Hispanic females face a higher risk of cervical cancer than both Caucasian and Native American females. One 1986 study found that cervical cancer was the third leading cancer diagnosed in U.S. Latina women, and that these women, specifically those from Central and South America, exhibited a cervical cancer incidence rate that was 7.3 times greater than that for Caucasian women (Peters, Thomas, Hagan, Mack, and Henderson, 1986). The researchers also noted that in comparison to Caucasian women, Hispanic women with the disease were younger, less educated, and had fewer sexual partners, but were younger when they first had sex, and had more children. The Hispanic women also had fewer visits to physicians and fewer Pap tests. The researchers concluded that these findings accounted for advanced disease at diagnosis and the increased cervical cancer mortality recorded.

Savitz (1986), who focused on a different Hispanic subgroup, noted that Hispanic females in Colorado also had a higher rate of cervical cancer than the Caucasian population. It is noteworthy that during the 1970s the incidence rate of cervical cancer among Hispanics rose from 1.7 to 2.0; the corresponding rate for Caucasians declined dramatically.

Stomach Cancer

Stomach cancer is a serious threat to all subgroups of the Hispanic population, and the incidence of it does not appear to differ between foreign- or native-born residents of the U.S. (Mack et al., 1985). Savitz (1986) found that during the 1970s, the stomach cancer incidence rates for Hispanic men declined from 31.6% to 18.3%, but the incidence rate for Hispanic females increased during this same period. Because this disease appeared to affect all Hispanic subgroups, Savitz proposed that the risk was associated with cultural factors such as diet.

Pancreatic and Prostate Cancers

Cancer of the pancreas is common only among certain subgroups of the U.S. Hispanic population, primarily Mexican Americans. According to Mack et al. (1985), pancreatic cancer occurs predominantly among the lower socioeconomic class/segment of this population, along with those who immigrated later in their adult life.

The U.S. Hispanic population also faces an intermediate risk of prostate cancer (Mack et al., 1985), which affects men as they age. The incidence rate for prostate cancer correlates more strongly to place of residence than to ethnicity.

Other Types of Cancer

The Hispanic population faces a low risk of colorectal cancer. A study comparing colorectal cancer incidence among Puerto Rican natives to that among Puerto Ricans living in New York showed that the incidence rate was higher among those living in New York than among the Puerto Rican natives, but both rates were less than that for the Caucasian population (Warshauer, Silverman, Schottenfield, and Pollack, 1986).

Mexican Americans also exhibit a lower incidence rate for colorectal cancer than Caucasians. Martin and Suarez (1987) found that among Mexican Americans living in Texas, the death rate for colon cancer was 50% lower than that for the Caucasian population.

Another cancer that occurs infrequently among Hispanics is lung cancer, although this has not always been the case. During the 1950s, both Hispanic males and females who smoked exhibited a very high rate of lung cancer. In fact, the incidence rate was estimated to be three times as high as that for the Caucasian population (Holck, Warren, Rochat, and Smith, 1982). More recently, a dramatic change in lung cancer incidence rates has been noted in Mexican American women. According to Marcus and Crane (1985), Mexican American women born before 1900 demonstrated unusually high rates of cigarette smoking, early adoption of the habit, and use of substitutes for tobacco when necessary. However, as this subgroup immigrated to the U.S., smoking patterns changed for Hispanic women. Hispanic women today have the lowest smoking rate of women in any U.S. ethnic group, and therefore the lowest incidence of lung cancer (Marcus and Crane, 1985).

Breast cancer presents unique problems to the Hispanic population. Although the incidence rate of the disease is low in this population, the mortality rate is high. According to Newell and Mills (1987), Hispanics have a lower breast cancer rate than either Caucasians or African Americans. Several hypotheses have been proposed to explain this low incidence rate: early age at menarche, early age of first pregnancy, and high fertility rate (Newell and Mills, 1987). These factors may protect the Hispanic woman against the development of breast cancer.

Access to health care services may explain the high breast cancer mortality rate among Hispanic women. In a sample of 600 Hispanic women 55 years of age and older 50% had not had a breast exam during the previous year (Richardson, et al., 1987). Nearly 74% had not had a mammogram, and only 47% indicated they performed monthly self-examinations. Richardson and his colleagues (1987) found that older Hispanic women

presented with larger tumors and metastases at time of diagnosis. The researchers suggested that age, education, and acculturation influenced mortality rates in this group.

Daly, Clark, and McGuire (1985) also examined breast cancer incidence and mortality among Hispanic women. They, too, found that Hispanic women over the age of 50 presented with larger, more advanced tumors. They suspected that cultural factors and delays in seeking medical care were responsible for the elevated mortality rates.

Malignant melanoma is another disease that occurs infrequently in the Hispanic population. Among Hispanics, the incidence rate for malignant melanoma is one sixth that of the Caucasian population (Pathak, Samet, Howard, and Key, 1982). Between the years 1969-1977, 495 cases of melanoma were reported in New Mexico; only 42 of them were diagnosed in Hispanic persons. More recently, Black, Goldhahn, and Wiggins (1987) confirmed that the incidence rate for this disease among Hispanics was still one sixth that of the Caucasian population. Data suggest Hispanics who were diagnosed with melanoma tend to have advanced disease and poor prognosis.

CULTURAL HEALTH BELIEFS

Generalizations about any ethnic group can be misleading, as diverse family patterns and coping behaviors are common. Within the Hispanic population, there are many poor families and some that are wealthy. Some families speak strictly Spanish, some only English, and others incorporate both into their lives. Differences in ancestry also exist. Some Hispanics have a purely Spanish background, while others have Native Central or South American ancestors. In addition, although many Hispanics no longer believe in or practice the folk medicine of their ancestors, a large percentage still hold fast to these traditional beliefs. Regional, historical, political, and socioeconomic factors, as well as the degree to which the individual adheres to traditional, ethno-medical beliefs and practices, will all influence beliefs about illness (Gonzales-Swafford and Gutierrez, 1983).

The Role of Family and the Community in Treating Illness

Women have always been and continue to be the primary caregivers in Hispanic society. When a family member's illness is too great for the woman to handle alone, she may ask the extended family to help care for the sick individual. Historically, Hispanics have used home remedies as the first line of treatment. When this did not work, they often sent for a traditional folk medicine healer (the **curandero** or the **herbalista**); and, if these avenues failed, they sought Western physicians. More recently, studies have suggested that cultural assimilation has resulted in the tendency to select Western medical interventions before using more traditional healers (Marsh Hentges, 1988; Gomez and Gomez, 1985; Hautman, 1979).

Beliefs About the Causes of Illness

Many Mexican-Americans believe illness is dependent upon lifestyle (Gonzales-Swafford and Gutierrez, 1983). Homeostasis, or the balance of elements within the individual, promotes health; disruption in the system produces illness. The concept that a disease is the will of God is also a widely accepted principal.

Hautman (1979), has identified several categories by which this ethnic group classifies diseases: hot and cold imbalances, dislocation of internal organs, magical origin, emotional origin, folk disease, and scientific illnesses.

The concept of **hot and cold imbalances** resembles the concept of Yin and Yang in the Chinese culture. In the healthy body, an equilibrium exists between hot and cold elements; when this is disrupted, illness occurs. Internal factors, such as a change in body temperature, and external factors, such as foods eaten, can both affect the hot/cold balance. For example, a stomach ulcer is a "hot illness," which many Hispanics believe is caused by eating too much hot foods. A "cold disease," on the other hand, may be caused by the night air touching the flesh (Gonzales-Swafford and Gutierrez, 1983; Hautman, 1979).

Dislocation of organs is a very common health disorder in the Hispanic culture. **Empacho,** or a blocked intestine, occurs when undigested food sticks to the walls of the intestine; this, in turn, is caused by eating improperly cooked foods or by eating foods at the wrong times. The symptoms of this disease are bloating of the stomach, nausea, and diarrhea (Marsh and Hentges, 1988). The treatment consists of massaging the stomach and giving the person mint tea.

Caida de mollera, or fallen fontanelle, occurs when a baby pulls away from the breast or nipple too quickly, or when the baby is held improperly. The signs of this disease are inability to suck, restlessness, and irritability (Marsh and Hentges, 1988). This is treated by manually pushing up the palate in the baby's mouth. **Aire de oido,** or air in the ear, is caused by air entering the ear canal. The symptoms include popping of the ears and earaches. The treatment includes blowing smoke into the ear (Marsh and Hentges, 1988).

The third category of diseases consists of those caused by **magical interventions.** An example of this is **mal de ojo** or evil eye. This occurs when someone with a strong glance looks improperly at a child; it is believed to be a manifestation of witchcraft. The child is then affected by evil spirits. The symptoms are fever, vomiting, and listlessness. The treatment consists of the ceremonial ritual of passing an egg over the affected person's body while reciting prayers (Marsh and Hentges, 1988).

A second illness of this nature is **susto** or sudden fright. This occurs when a person feels an unexpected fright that dislodges the person's spirit. The symptoms are depression, anxiety, and irritability (Foreman, 1985). Susto is treated in several stages. The first stage of treatment includes bed rest and a cleansing of the soul through confession of what caused the fright. The second phase of treatment includes rituals and prayers that help drain the evil spirit and return the person's soul. Finally, the person is slowly reintroduced into society (Foreman, 1985).

Emotional illnesses are divided into two specific subgroups: mental and moral. According to Gonzales-Swafford and Gutierrez (1983), mental illnesses are inevitable, and the affected person is viewed as a victim of consequence. The disease is explained as the disruption of a person's equilibrium by some supernatural force. Such illnesses need traditional medical attention. Moral illnesses, on the other hand, are caused by the person himself, and thus the treatment is the responsibility of the family members. An example of this type of disease is alcoholism (Gonzales-Swafford and Gutierrez, 1983).

Finally, the **scientific diseases** are those that cannot be treated by the traditional medical practices of the culture; they must be diagnosed by the Western health care system. However, even though the disease has been diagnosed by the medical system, Hispanics may still believe that the disease is the result of some indiscretion against God. This is especially true of terminal illnesses. The Hispanic population, in general, views illness very fatalistically; it is the will of God and therefore it goes against principle to aggressively treat the disease (O'Brien, 1982; Gonzales-Swafford and Gutierrez, 1983; Sugarek, Deyo, and Holmes, 1988).

Table 5-4 illustrates the correlation between individual health beliefs and health practices. The table reflects content analysis of a 28-page document that resulted from a 5-hour focus group of 10 Hispanic nurses who attended cancer courses for nurses working with minority groups (Frank-Stromborg and Olsen, 1988).

TABLE 5-4 Health Beliefs and Practices of Hispanic People

Health Belief	Health Practice
DISEASE	
1. The causes of problems are external, i.e., bad luck, God's will, and/or the supernatural forces. Approach to health and illness is fatalistic, i.e., "what will be, will be." Faith and prayer make the disease go away. Destiny and fate determine what happens to a person. God will provide and care for each person. Disease may be a punishment for past sins. Illness can be caused by the "evil eye" **mal de ojo,** e.g., skin cancer; or by fright **(espanto),** e.g., loss of appetite, lethargy, depression. A soul can be jarred out of the body by terror **(susto** = fright or soul loss). An illness may be due to someone placing a hex on another person. Curses (evil spells) can cause serious or incurable disease, such as mental illness. Miracles exist and will help heal illness.	a. Talismans, religious articles, and/or pictures are used to protect against illness. b. Religious rituals (blessings) are used to ensure good results with medicines. c. Prayer and calling upon God and the saints are used to supplement healing. d. **Limpías** (sweeping) used to reduce a fever: a raw egg is passed over the body in a cross-like movement and prayers are recited.
2. Health is a reward for good behavior. Healthy is being well enough to work. When you get old, you get sick. "Illness won't happen to me." Illness is a sign of weakness.	a. Will stay home only when too sick to see a doctor. b. Treatments are often avoided in order to avoid pain and discomfort; it is felt that the treatment is worse than the disease. c. Avoid psychological care because it means the person is "crazy." d. Tend to ignore signs and symptoms of illness.
3. A real illness must produce pain or fever. If you feel ok, nothing is wrong. Illness is a state of discomfort. If a person has a fever and nothing relieves it, it's the "evil eye" creating the fever. It is good to sweat or perspire when experiencing a fever.	a. Fevers will be sweated out by rubbing the entire body with lard and then wrapping the person in blankets overnight. b. May not follow through with medical therapies. c. Take medicine only until they feel better. d. Cold is avoided to avoid illness. e. Will not sleep with their hair wet because lesions may develop. f. Will not step on cold water barefooted for fear of developing a fever.
4. The only thing that matters is today. When I get sick, I will take care of it. Today I feel fine.	a. Often do not carry health insurance and do not practice prevention. Tend to be crisis-oriented. b. Exercise is usually not viewed as necessary.
5. Massage of an area of pain or injury is helpful in promoting healing.	a. Vick's Vaporub is warmed and rubbed into a painful area to relieve pain.

Continued.

TABLE 5-4 Health Beliefs and Practices of Hispanic People—cont'd

Health Belief	Health Practice
DISEASE—cont'd	
6. Medicines should cure illness rapidly and effectively. Infections are better than oral medicines. Doubt the efficacy of medicines. Penicillin can cure everything.	a. Save old medicines to cut down on future expense. b. Mexican Americans use medicine bought in Mexican pharmacies because it is cheaper there than in the United States. c. Will use someone else's medicine—if it worked for them, it should work for me. d. Use plants instead of medicines if they are thought to be more helpful. e. Will use Anglo medicine along with Hispanic health practices and beliefs. f. Will start themselves on antibiotics at the first sign of fever. g. Do not take prescription drugs correctly.
7. Disease affects the core and extended family. Illness makes a sick individual a burden to the family and brings shame to the family, so family should not be told when a member is sick. Illness should not be spoken of outside of the family.	a. Denial plays a significant role in Hispanic culture. It is better not to know; if you go to the doctor, you might find out something is wrong. b. Extended family will be involved in making health care decisions, often before going to a doctor; the family's recommendations may be taken over the doctor's.
8. Physical touch will promote healing. People can have a spiritual healing influence, i.e., can have healing hands. Healers can diagnose an illness by "laying on of the hands." God heals through healers.	If medical providers do not touch during their visit, then Hispanic patients may feel that they did not derive any benefit from that visit.
9. We all have to die of something, sometime; life after 50 is a gift. Planning for death is abandoning hope and may result in death. Autopsies should not be done—the body should not be desecrated for any reason.	a. Have less fear of dying than the general public, and so feel the need for fewer treatments. b. Suspicious of organ donations—are less willing to donate their organs or those of family members.
CANCER	
1. Family members, especially elders, should not be informed of their "real" diagnosis (i.e., cancer); it will only make them sicker. Cancer is a death sentence. Cancer is deadly and engenders great fear. There is a stigma surrounding cancer. Cancer is God's punishment for sins; "I deserve to suffer, I was bad."	a. Some Cuban and Puerto Rican physicians will write orders not to tell the patient about their cancer diagnosis. b. The family will often forbid health care workers to mention the diagnosis in front of the client. c. The family encourages the patient's denial and often will not discuss the illness at all to protect the patient. d. Penance and prayers are offered to heal cancer.

TABLE 5-4   Health Beliefs and Practices of Hispanic People—cont'd

Health Belief	Health Practice
2. Cancer may be contagious. Cancer is caused by many things and is, therefore, hard to prevent. Going to see the doctor early serves no purpose in dealing with cancer. Sex at an early age and infections may predispose a person to cancer. Cancer is not hereditary. Chemotherapy does not work. Radiation therapy causes cancer. Cancer will remain even after surgery is performed to remove it. Certain cancer treatments may have side effects that can be passed to family members, e.g., having radiation treatment may make the family members radioactive from being around the patient. Opening surgical wounds exposes a person to cancer. Cancer care is too costly.	a. Because of misconceptions about what causes cancer, may become fearful when having minor symptoms related to other diseases. b. Younger women may not seek mammography because they believe breast cancer only happens to older women. c. Cigarette smoking is common among males because it is viewed as cool; they start at young age and feel very "macho" (manly). d. Cigars are smoked because it is believed that they are not harmful.
DIET 1. Food eaten has an influence on healing. Home remedies are common and are often used to treat illness before seeking a medical assessment. Illness is caused when there is a "hot" and "cold" imbalance in the body. This is most common in pediatric and Ob/Gyn. illness. To treat illness, the proper hot or cold food and medicine must be used. Herbs or spices are useful to treat illness; they are often used before, or in conjunction with, traditional medicine. Eating the wrong things can cause **empacho** (stomach ache). The Mexican diet can cure anything.	a. Drink "cabellos de elote" (hair from an ear of corn" or boiled corn-silk) for bladder infections. b. Cactus ointment or juices are used for healing (especially for diabetes). c. Herbal teas are considered good for specific ailments, especially by Mexican Americans (e.g., **Gordolobo** for coughs; **manzanilla** for colic; **yerbabuena** for stomach pains; **estafiate** for stomach cramps and diarrhea; anise tea, boiled and then cooled to help with a delivery; **unis** for cramps; **estafiate** teas for diarrhea; mint for sores in the mouth; onion tea to lower a diabetic's sugar level. d. Garlic is good for insect bites and controlling hypertension. e. Hot potatoes on the side of the head are good for treating the flu and fever. f. Hot tomatoes, mashed on the neck are curative. g. Cool ashes and an egg in a glass on the stomach drain the heat out of the body (for fevers).

Continued.

TABLE 5-4   Health Beliefs and Practices of Hispanic People—cont'd

Health Belief	Health Practice
DIET—cont'd	h. Honey and lemon in warm drinks will soothe a cough and bring up phlegm.
	i. Use a malta mix drink (corn meal with condensed milk) for terminal patients.
	j. Oil will help stomach aches.
	k. For chicken pox, grind flour, place it in a bag, and dust the pox.
	l. Boiled sour cane (**ganya aya**) is used for fever blisters and loose teeth.
	m. Olive oil and herb rubs help insomnia.
	n. Rice water or oatmeal water will cure a baby's vomiting and diarrhea.
	o. Raw eggs rubbed on the body will lower a fever.
	p. Old cold coffee dropped in an eye will relieve "pink eye."
	q. Toothpaste rubbed on a burn will reduce pain and enhance healing.
2. Fat is healthy. Obesity means health and wealth, especially in older individuals. The quantity of food is more important than the quality. Weight loss is not a sign of cancer. Fasting is a good way to handle illness.	a. Chicken fat is used on burns. b. Diet has higher than recommended fat content; e.g., high use of quick fixed foods; high intake of cheeses but low intake of other dairy products. c. Poorly balanced diet due to low income. d. Preference for beer over mixed drinks.
3. The spice chile is unhealthy but can cure some illnesses. Eating certain spicy foods predisposes a person to cancer.	a. Hot spicy foods are often eaten in large quantities, even though there is a belief that chile is unhealthy. b. Chile used to cure colds and stomach ailments. Hot sauce (picante sauce) is used to treat colds.
4. Vitamins and local healers can help when traditional measures aren't successful and when funds are low.	Vitamins are used to cure abnormal vaginal bleeding.
5. Enemas should be performed regularly. Don't get close to the stove when cooking, especially after taking a shower, or you will get sick. "Knots" in the back of the legs come from food sticking to the lining of the stomach.	

TABLE 5-4   Health Beliefs and Practices of Hispanic People—cont'd

Health Belief	Health Practice
SEX, SEXUAL/REPRODUCTIVE ORGANS, AND EXAMINATIONS OF "PRIVATE PARTS"	

1. Touching one's own body is taboo.
  Pelvic exams are a sexual act.
  No one except a husband or lover should touch a woman's breasts.
  A gynecological exam should not be done before marriage.
	a. Rectal exams for men are insulting and embarrassing, so men may avoid them.
	b. Women may be very reluctant to have physical examinations.
	c. Some husbands don't want their wives examined by a male doctor.
	d. Patients may be very embarrassed about or fearful of looking at or touching bodies.
	e. Women may be very uncomfortable having doctors examine them during gynecological and breast exams.
	f. Mammography and routine annual gynecological exams are used infrequently.
	g. Women may not believe in, or may be unaware of, Pap smears.

2. A hysterectomy will make a woman "less of a woman."
  Sexual activity can drain a male of his "power or health" during healing and sickness.
  Women should remain virgins until marriage.
  Birth control is against God's law.
  Sex should not be discussed.
  Having many children is a sign of virility.
	a. Women may need to obtain permission from their husbands to have a treatment that will affect their sexuality.
	b. Withdrawal is used as a form of birth control.
	c. Women are often blamed for STDs and genitourinary cancers even if their male partner was the contact.
	d. Birth control practices, when used, are approved or disapproved by the male partner.
	e. In some families, girls can't get wet, wash their hands or feet, or take a bath when they are menstruating.

3. Pregnant women who experience "morning sickness" will have a baby with lots of hair. It is not necessary to get prenatal care.	a. Men do not participate in labor and delivery because it is not necessary. b. Women use midwives for home delivery—receive poor or no prenatal care. c. Apply warm compresses and oil to an infertile woman's abdomen to help her conceive. d. Pin a holy medal on the pregnant woman's underwear.
CHILDREN	
1. An infant that cries too much might have **empacho** (a stomach ache).	a. Massage the lumps in the back of the leg to cure stomach aches.

Continued.

TABLE 5-4 Health Beliefs and Practices of Hispanic People—cont'd

Health Belief	Health Practice
2. The fallen **mollera** or fontanelle will fall down to the roof of the mouth. A fallen fontanelle will cause physical obstruction, i.e., vomiting, diarrhea, dehydration (belief most common among Puerto Ricans). A fallen fontanelle is known as **caida de mollera** and occurs only in infants before the fontanelles close.	a. For a sunken soft spot, apply salt to the area and then have a healer suck the soft spot up. Cigarette paper is placed over the area and left in place for one week.
3. Children should not be tickled (especially infants) or they will become stutterers. Cutting a child's fingernails causes nearsightedness. Letting a male child's hair grow will protect him from harm. Breastfeeding is the only way to feed infants. If the baby makes a dry sucking sound when eating, it must be turned upside down and shaken three times. A red cloth on the forehead will cure colic and hiccoughs. Cover a baby's head to avoid cool air when going outdoors—cool air will make a baby sick.	
HOSPITALS, DOCTORS, AND HEALTH CARE	
1. There is no need to be seen by a physician unless you are very ill. If you feel good, you don't need a doctor.	a. Preventive health care is often not practiced or sought. b. Seek medical attention only after illness or symptoms develop and/or when individual can no longer care for the signs and symptoms alone (i.e., when the person is nonfunctional). c. Do not seek health care for health promotion information or early detection, but, rather, for treatment of illness/injury. Frequent use of emergency rooms.
2. Only receive as much health care as can be afforded. Health care is available only to those with money or insurance. Doctors are too expensive; they are only for very sick people. Do not believe in taking charity, i.e., free treatment.	a. Concern about financial security during illness and fear of dependency on society. If there is no money to pay the doctor, care will not be sought. b. Care-seeking behavior is a low priority for some; other needs are more urgent. c. May not have health insurance due to the cost.

TABLE 5-4   Health Beliefs and Practices of Hispanic People—cont'd

Health Belief	Health Practice
3. Hospitals and health care providers will act in a retaliatory manner if criticized. It is not appropriate to question those giving care about the condition. Family members should spend a lot of time in attendance when a relative is hospitalized. God plays an important role in the health/illness continuum and is more important than the health team.	a. Do not get second opinions or ask the doctor questions. b. Physician's word is never questioned. c. Mexican American patients usually have family members accompany them when they seek medical care; the extended family provides protection, assistance, care, and support. d. Mexican American patients tend to let a family member speak for them when consulting their family physician. e. Passive and dependent upon health care provider.
4. People go to the hospitals to die. Hospitals are a last resort for treatment. The American health system is destructive.	a. Like to have candles in the patient's room. b. Place trust in clinics in Mexico.
5. Mom knows best, often better than nurses or doctors.	a. The Mexican American wife or mother usually makes the decision to seek medical care for the children or other family members; the men make all other decisions for the family.
6. The family should take care of its own. One should seek out a doctor who understands the problem and to whom one can relate. Doubt the accuracy of instructions, tests, etc., due to the language barrier.	a. Elderly parents are rarely placed in nursing homes. b. Tend to seek out doctors from their own culture. c. Don't always let English-speaking health care professionals know they do not comprehend what is being said or done. d. Go to certain health facilities or practitioners when recommended by a friend or relative, rather than by need; will "shop" for a doctor. e. Language barrier limits use of medical services. f. Some mistrust Anglo Americans and traditional American medicine, especially when the health care provider does not speak Spanish.

Table 5-4 reflects content analysis of 28 pages of typed transcription from a 5 hour focus group of 10 Hispanic nurses chosen to attend the *Cancer Courses For Nurses Working With Minority Groups* (Frank-Stromborg, M. and Olsen, S. Cancer courses for nurses working with minority groups. National Cancer Institute, National Institutes of Health, 1988-1991, CA 09554-03S1). The focus group was devoted to identifying the unique health beliefs and practices of Hispanics and how these influenced prevention/early detection of cancer. Nurses provided 308 comments related to health practices and 352 comments on health beliefs that have been divided into similar content groups, correlating beliefs with practices.

CULTURAL HEALTH PRACTICES

In her study of health and illness among different ethnic groups, Spector (1977) noted that, "Each of us interprets health illness according to our own cultural background." Traditional Hispanic people look for answers to illness within their own culture and traditions. This population often turns to traditional medical practices to treat sick family members. Only certain trained or gifted individuals in the community practice traditional medicine. Although each ethnic subgroup within the Hispanic culture suffers from the same illnesses and every healer performs essentially the same rituals, each subgroup has a different name for the "medicine man" or woman.

TRADITIONAL MEDICAL PRACTICES

According to Marsh and Hentges (1988), for nearly 50% of the Hispanic population folk healing methods are the first treatment choice. The Hispanic healing system, called **curanderismo,** is based on eight philosophical premises about wellness and illness (Manduro, 1983). Among these premises are the beliefs that disease is caused by evil forces beyond one's control and that disruption in peace of the soul causes sickness. These premises guide the Hispanics' preference for family involvement in health care and indicate the need for open communication between the healer and the sick individual (Manduro, 1983).

Some Mexican-Americans subscribe to the care of a **curandero,** who receives his or her skills through an apprenticeship or as a gift from God. A curandero is knowledgeable in the use of herbs, diet, massage, prayer, and rituals (Gomez and Gomez, 1985). This person can treat all traditional folk illnesses but often refuses to treat illnesses caused by magical influences. Curanderos are admired and respected members of the community and will not risk losing balance and good grace with God (Gomez and Gomez, 1985).

The Puerto Rican population seeks medical treatment through **espiritismo** (Gomez and Gomez, 1985), a folk healer with the gift of contacting the spirit world and healing through the powers of spirits. According to Hautman (1979), the espiritista also has a special gift that enables him or her to analyze dreams and foretell the future. These healers also use medals, prayers, and amulets.

The Cuban population seeks medical help from a **santero,** a medicine man who works with the spirits of good within a system to promote wellness (Gomez and Gomez, 1985). The santero uses animal sacrifices, rituals, chanting, and prayers to aid in healing. The santero bases his or her practice on a body of practices called **santaria,** a mixture of Catholic rituals and tribal African beliefs (Gomez and Gomez, 1985).

Other healers who are common to all subgroups of the Hispanic culture but have less influence than the curandero, espiritista, or santero are the **yerbero** and the **sobador.** The former is a herbalist who cures and heals through the natural powers within herbs (Hautman, 1979); the latter is similar to a chiropractor; he treats by using massage and manipulation of bones (Hautman, 1979).

High-Risk Behaviors in the Hispanic Population

Much of the literature on Hispanics characterizes this population as a homogeneous group (COSSMHO, 1988). In fact, the lifestyles, beliefs, and values of members of this group vary according to country of origin. Few researchers have investigated the differences between the major subcultures within this population. When applying the risk behavior information provided here to their Hispanic clients, health care workers should keep in mind that differences do exist between ethnic subgroups.

Diet. The traditional Hispanic diet is high in fiber and carbohydrates from such staples as rice, beans, and corn; however, this diet contains few leafy green vegetables. Beans provide a substantial source of protein; dairy intake tends to be limited. The use of lard and the common practice of frying foods both contribute to the high fat content in the Hispanic diet.

Obesity is a common problem among Hispanics in the United States. Roberts and Lee (1980) suggest this is due both to the nature of the diet and to a lack of physical activity in this group. Although a large percentage of Hispanic males are manual laborers, there is little emphasis in this culture on performing additional physical activity. Overall, this group accepts obesity as part of the natural aging process and feels little motivation to lose weight (COSSMHO, 1988).

As noted earlier, as many as one in four Hispanic families lives in poverty, an economic condition that has been associated with alcohol abuse (COSSMHO,

1988). Alcohol contributes to cancers of the esophagus and pancreas. It is not culturally acceptable for Hispanic women to drink (COSSMHO, 1988); however, Hispanic men tend to drink at younger ages than Caucasians and tend to consume larger amounts of alcohol more often.

Cigarette smoking. Although Hispanic men and women do not currently face a high risk of lung cancer, cigarette smoking is increasing in this group. Adult Hispanics generally smoke less than either Caucasians or African Americans (see Table 5-5); however, smoking is on the rise among Hispanic adolescents (COSSMHO, 1988; Haynes, Harvey, Montes, Nickens, and Cohen, 1990).

Sexual practices. Hispanic women face a high risk for cervical cancer. Factors associated with the development of this neoplasm include early onset of sexual activity with multiple partners; and infections with human papilloma virus, her-

TABLE 5-5 Prevalence of Cigarette Smoking Among Racial/Ethnic Groups by Sex, 1987

	Both Sexes	Male	Females
All Races	28.8	31.2	26.5
Caucasians (Non-Hispanic)	29.0	30.6	27.5
African Americans (Non-Hispanic)	33.5	38.9	28.2
Hispanics (Total)	24.0	30.0	18.0
Mexican American	23.7	30.5	16.8
Puerto Rican	29.3	35.4	23.2
Cuban	20.1	21.9	18.2
Other	22.8	29.0	16.5

From Inter-university Consortium for Political and Social Research: *Health interview survey*, Hyattsville, Md, 1987, National Center for Health Statistics.

pes simplex II, and other sexually transmitted diseases. Other important but indirect risk factors include low socioeconomic status and low levels of education. Studies have documented infrequent Pap smears, infrequent use of barrier contraceptives, and the lack of reporting of genital warts in this population; one researcher has suggested that because many young Hispanic women receive little education, they lack the knowledge to follow these precautions (Peters, et al., 1986). The box on pp. 223-224 outlines the lifestyle characteristics of many members of the Hispanic population and the implications for cancer prevention and early detection.

Barriers to Health Care

Numerous factors inhibit Hispanic patients from entering the Western health care delivery system.

Acculturation and language. Acculturation refers to the process by which one culture adopts the characteristics of another as a result of continuous contact between the two groups. Although this definition does not specify the type, degree, or direction of change that occurs, some researchers presume that Hispanics who adopt the behavioral practices and values of the dominant society are more likely to utilize health services.

Deyo, Diehl, Hazuda, and Stern (1985) report that use of or preference for the dominant language typically comprises one dimension of acculturation, and that this element is the most important behavioral indicator of acculturation. In addition, Solis, Marks, Garcia, and Shelton (1990) have reported that preference for speaking English (which they identify as one variable of acculturation) was associated with greater recency in utilization of preventive health services by Hispanic individuals. However, utilization of health services varies depending upon the subgroup studied. Among Cuban American men, the ability to speak English did correlate with the degree to which they used health services; however, this was not the case for Cuban American women or Puerto Ricans. Language, but not ethnic identification, was the important predictor of the use of medical services by Mexican Americans (Solis et al., 1990). Among all three Hispanic subgroups, language skills clearly influenced the decision to participate in screening programs; that is, participation increased as acculturation increased (Solis et al., 1990).

Socioeconomic status. One in four American Hispanics live at or below the poverty level. The cost of being sick includes not only the amount of money needed for care, but also loss of money due to time missed from work and ancillary costs such as transportation to a health care facility (Rodriguez, 1983). Many members of the Hispanic population fear that because of their economic status and ethnicity, they may receive inferior care in the U.S. medical system (Mardiros, 1984).

Modesty. Perhaps the most important reason why Hispanics do not enter the U.S. medical system is personal modesty. They generally do not like being touched by others or having to touch themselves, are not comfortable being examined by a health care professional of

LIFESTYLE CHARACTERISTICS AND THEIR IMPLICATIONS FOR CANCER PREVENTION AND EARLY DETECTION

LIFESTYLES

1. Diet unbalanced: large amount of pork products; frequent meals of red meats; low use of vegetables and fruits; high use of cheeses in cooking; spicy foods enjoyed; low fiber; high salt content.
2. Infrequent participation in exercise activities.
3. High, and increasing, incidence of substance abuse, especially among the young: alcohol, smoking (i.e., smokeless tobacco, cigarettes, cigars), drug abuse.
4. Over-exposure to sun (outside work; living in sunny, warm climate).
5. Frequent exposure, due to occupation and poor living conditions, to chemical carcinogens (paint, oils, asbestos, lead pipes, pesticides, herbicides, etc.).
6. Families frequently in lower socioeconomic levels due to lack of education, low-paying jobs as unskilled laborers, migratory status, many dependents to support, language barriers, and unemployment.
7. Family frequently does not have health insurance, because employers often do not offer health insurance; the family may not be able to afford it; the family may not know how to get insurance, why it is needed, or when it should be acquired; or family is proud and does not like to use social welfare programs.
8. Unable to read English, and only limited ability to read Spanish.
9. Strong belief in God's influence on health, home remedies, and "healers"/faith healing. Result is often prolonged delay in seeking medical care and lack of attention to symptoms of illness. Prevention is not practiced. Crisis orientation and thinking only of "today" are common.
10. Frequent sense of fatalism and, as a consequence, low use of medical facilities/services such as mammography screening, breast self-examination, annual gynecological exams, and Pap tests.
11. Belief that the health care professional is all-powerful and knowing; doctor's word is never questioned.
12. High level of modesty and embarrassment about the body. Because of prevalence of "macho" image, males tend not to do testicular self-examination or to have annual physicals, and are reluctant to touch their own bodies. Many Hispanic women do not like to be examined by a male practitioner; men do not like to be examined by a female practitioner.
13. Immigrant, migratory status often creates a great deal of stress, isolation, and depression; medical records are unavailable or incomplete.
14. Hispanic society is paternalistic: family and community acts as a strong support network. The mother is the primary source of health information and makes most of the health decisions, with collaboration from other family members.
15. Often lack transportation due to financial condition, making it difficult to get to the clinics and/or hospital.
16. Double standard in relation to sex: women should wait until they are married to have sex and are often chaperoned while dating; men often have early sexual activity and frequent sexual partners, even while married. Talking about sex is taboo.
17. Early pregnancy and multiple pregnancies are common for Hispanic women.
18. Men do not like to wear a condom.
19. High respect for elders in the community.

Continued.

LIFESTYLE CHARACTERISTICS AND THEIR IMPLICATIONS FOR CANCER PREVENTION AND EARLY DETECTION—cont'd

IMPLICATIONS FOR CANCER PREVENTION AND EARLY DETECTION

1. Risk for **breast, colon/rectal, uterine, ovarian, and stomach cancer** due to diet. Provide information about: proper nutrition; importance of a balanced diet; need to reduce intake of fat; benefits of increasing intake of fruits, vegetables and fiber; and how to have a healthy, balanced diet on a low income.
2. High risk of **gallbladder cancer** possibly due to diet and hereditary factors.
3. High risk of **liver cancer** due to alcohol abuse. Provide information about dangers of alcohol and drug abuse and importance of counseling for withdrawal.
4. Risk of **lung cancer** due to use of tobacco (cigarettes and cigars); **oral cancer** due to use of smokeless tobacco. Discuss importance of participating in smoking cessation programs.
5. Intermediate risk of **pancreatic and prostatic cancer.**
6. **Skin cancer** can occur due to increased sun exposure. Teach clients about the use of sun blocks; the effect the sun can have on the skin and signs and symptoms of skin cancer; and how to perform a self-assessment of skin.
7. Spicy foods predispose Hispanic people to **oral cancer.**
8. Sexual promiscuity and infrequent use of condoms by males predispose both males and females to sexually transmitted diseases (STDs), including AIDS. Infections and early onset of sexual activity among females place Hispanic women at high risk for **cervical cancer.** Provide education about the importance of using condoms to prevent (STDs), especially AIDS. Include information about signs and symptoms of STDs and reproductive cancer and possible complications of STDs (e.g., sterility, frequent pelvic inflammatory diseases, problems in getting pregnant, fetal abnormalities and death, etc.).
9. Decreased rate of early detection results in delay in treatment and poor prognosis, especially for cancers of the **breast, testicles, scrotum, colon/rectum, uterus, cervix, and skin.** Educate clients about signs and symptoms of cancer, why they should have routine examinations, how to perform a self-assessment, and the importance of engaging in preventive activities.
10. Provide information about health insurance, and how to apply for public assistance for health care; discuss issues related to possible reluctance to use government support programs.
11. Provide information about possible risks, diseases, and injuries that can occur in dangerous residences and at work, and how to lower incidence of illness and injury.

The above information reflects content analysis of 14 pages of typed transcription from a 5 hour focus group of 10 Hispanic nurses chosen to attend the Cancer Courses for Nurses Working with Minority Groups (Frank-Stromborg, M. and Olsen, S. Cancer courses for nurses working with minority groups. National Cancer Institute, National Institutes of Health, 1988-1991, CA 09554-03S1). Study questions and work assignments previously sent to the participants enabled them to come prepared to share information about life-styles of Hispanic people. Nurses provided 273 comments related to life-styles.

the opposite sex, and are often embarrassed by invasive procedures or the exposure of body parts during an examination (see Tables 5-6, 5-7, and 5-8).

PHYSICAL ASSESSMENT

The Hispanic population presents unique challenges to U.S. health care professionals. Despite the size and diversity of this minority, many of its members still maintain a strong affinity for traditional cultural beliefs. Medical treatment must therefore balance modern medical therapies with valued folk remedies; traditional beliefs and practices must be respected during examinations and/or procedures.

Martaus (1986) proposes six steps for introducing Hispanic clients to the U.S. health care delivery system. First, health care workers must communicate their acceptance of the patient's value system; this will help establish trust. Second, care providers should incorporate a culturally relevant interview into the admission process; this defines the patient's perceptions of illness and allows the health care professional to establish a workable treatment plan. Third, the treatment plan must have a family focus; in the Hispanic culture, illness intensifies the need for family involvement. Fourth, many Hispanics are very religious and so may view treatment without prayer as ineffective. Fifth, the health care worker must take responsibility for finding a common ground that incorporates traditional beliefs and modern health care. Finally, it is important for health care workers to realize that many Hispanics have a great fear

TABLE 5-6 Cancer Screening—Digital Rectal Exams of Males Age 40 and Older by Race, 1987

	Never Had Test		Had Procedure for:			
				Screening Purpose		
	Never Heard of	Heard of but Never Had	Health Problem	<1 yr	1-3 yrs	>3 yrs
All Races	22.8	19.1	10.9	17.1	10.4	19.6
Caucasians (Non-Hispanic)	20.2	19.0	11.0	18.1	11.3	10.4
African Americans (Non-Hispanic)	38.2	16.4	10.8	15.7	5.9	13.0
Hispanics	29.3	28.5	10.5	8.4	7.2	16.1
Mexican American	38.5	29.8	8.8	4.7	6.1	12.1
Puerto Rican	23.8	23.8	14.7	9.5	7.1	21.1
Cuban	7.6	42.5	6.5	10.0	7.3	26.1
Other	30.8	22.7	12.2	12.0	8.8	13.6

From Inter-university Consortium for Political and Social Research: *Health interview survey*, Hyattsville, Md, 1987, National Center for Health Statistics.

TABLE 5-7   Cancer Screening—Mammography for Women Age 40 and Older by Race, 1987

| | Never Had Test | | Had Procedure for: | | | |
| | Never Heard of | Heard of But Never Had | Health Problem | Screening Purpose | | |
				<1 yr	1-3 yrs	>3 yrs
All Races	15.6	47.5	6.6	16.6	6.4	7.3
Caucasians (Non-Hispanic)	12.2	48.9	7.0	17.4	6.9	7.6
African Americans (Non-Hispanic)	29.4	40.9	5.6	14.2	3.9	5.9
Hispanics:	31.6	42.2	3.1	12.9	3.1	7.1
Mexican American	38.3	40.0	2.7	10.8	2.1	6.1
Puerto Rican	52.2	23.3	2.4	11.4	5.6	5.0
Cuban	19.3	61.0	1.1	10.1	3.5	5.0
Other	20.9	44.8	4.6	16.9	3.0	9.9

From Inter-university Consortium for Political and Social Research: *Health interview survey*, Hyattsville, Md, 1987, National Center for Health Statistics.

TABLE 5-8   Cancer Screening—Pap Smears for Females Age 18 or Older by Race, 1987

| | Never Had Test | | Had Procedure for: | | | |
| | Never Heard of | Heard of But Never Had | Health Problem | Screening Purpose | | |
				<1 yr	1-3 yrs	>3 yrs
All Races	4.0	7.3	7.8	48.0	17.0	15.8
Caucasians (Non-Hispanic)	2.1	6.9	7.6	47.9	17.8	17.7
African Americans (Non-Hispanic)	4.1	7.8	10.6	52.8	15.4	9.2
Hispanics:	15.1	9.6	7.4	44.8	12.9	10.3
Mexican American	16.4	9.8	8.6	46.1	11.5	7.6
Puerto Rican	15.0	7.1	6.7	49.9	9.9	11.5
Cuban	8.7	23.2	6.1	31.1	14.4	16.5
Other	15.5	5.4	6.1	45.0	16.4	11.7

From Inter-university Consortium for Political and Social Research: *Health interview survey*, Hyattsville, Md, 1987, National Center for Health Statistics.

of authority. They may believe that disease occurs because it is God's will, and also place great emphasis on treating doctors with respect.

When performing a physical examination on a person of Hispanic origin, caregivers should also make an effort to promote and maintain dignity of the patient and provide a non-judgmental, private environment. Because of the differences in the subgroups within the Hispanic population, it is important to recognize the terminology used by each individual patient. In addition, caregivers should supply written materials to augment any verbal instruction they provide.

Skin Assessment

The health care professional should assess all areas of the skin, including the scalp, soles of feet, and ears. These areas are often overlooked but are a necessary part of the examination. Examination of the skin should not be a separate assessment, but rather performed throughout the entire procedure. Educate the patient and/or family member on how to do a self-assessment of skin. The health care worker should explain the results of the assessment as soon as they are known (Frank-Stromborg and Olsen, 1988).

Oral Assessment

The health care professional must be very cautious of proximity; closeness may be embarrassing for the patient. If the patient is elderly, dentures must be removed. Several high-risk behaviors of the Hispanic population may compromise the health of the oral cavity. Dental

caries are very common in younger Hispanics. It is important for the caregiver to recognize these problems and to educate patients about appropriate techniques for performing an oral assessment and care of the oral cavity. A mirror is an important part of this procedure (Frank-Stromborg and Olsen, 1988).

Lung Assessment

Because the lungs are located within the chest, it is very important that the health care professional recognize this culture's "hot/cold" theory of disease causation and help the patient avoid drafts. Females must cover their breasts. Warm the instruments to be used during the examination. The examination should begin and end with explanation of procedure and results found. Finally, the health care professional should not express his/her opinion about smoking and offend the client. Rather, discuss the topic in a matter-of-fact, non-judgmental manner; present the signs and symptoms of tobacco-related problems; discuss the dangers of smoking; and explain the value of smoking cessation programs (Frank-Stromborg and Olsen, 1988).

Breast Examination

For women. Before this examination, the health care professional should take time to establish a rapport with the patient and stress the importance of this procedure. The room should be private with no drafts, and only the breast that is being examined should be exposed. Use professional terminology when referring to the breasts. Educate the patient on the importance of breast self-examination and demonstrate it to her. If the physician is male, a female assistant should be in the room before the patient exposes herself (Frank-Stromborg and Olsen, 1988).

For men. The health care professional needs to explain the importance of the procedure and perform it as accurately and as quickly as possible. The breast examination may embarrass the male patient (Frank-Stromborg and Olsen, 1988).

Colorectal Examination

The examiner should begin by explaining the procedure for the examination, and taking dietary and defecation histories. The diet history should include education about proper dietary requirements. The caregiver should proceed slowly with this procedure and only expose the area needed for the examination. Education about the home hemoculture test is also a priority, although this test may make the patient uneasy (Frank-Stromborg and Olsen, 1988).

Prostate and Testicular Examination

If possible, only male health care professionals should perform this examination on Hispanic clients. The procedure should not be rushed and only performed after rapport and a safe, secure environment have been established. Education and explanation of each step of the procedure are also recommended. It is important not to expose other areas of the body during this examination. The patient needs to be reassured that the procedure is being performed using sterile techniques (Frank-Stromborg and Olsen, 1988).

Gynecological Examination

If possible, only female health care professionals should perform this examination. The examiner should first establish a rapport with the patient and explain the procedure by drawing pictures to describe the technique. This procedure cannot be rushed; sensitivity to the patient's modesty is vital. It is also important to give the patient the results of the examination as soon as they are available (Frank-Stromborg and Olsen, 1988).

The box on pp. 229-233 summarizes the special needs of Hispanic people before a physical assessment. The information reflects content analysis of a 22-page transcript from a focus group consisting of 10 Hispanic nurses in a special seminar funded by the National Cancer Institute (NCI) (Frank-Stromborg and Olsen, 1988). Before the courses, the participants received study questions and work assignments and were asked to describe pre-physical assessment needs that they thought were particularly important for Hispanics. The nurses provided 339 comments; these were then analyzed for content, divided into categories related to body systems, and put into table format for easy reference.

STRATEGIES AND RESOURCES FOR CANCER PREVENTION AND DETECTION

Health education strategies and materials can play a significant role in fulfilling the health needs of minority groups.

PRE-ASSESSMENT AND ASSESSMENT GUIDELINES FOR USE WITH HISPANIC PATIENTS

1. Hispanic patients tend to consider exams invasive. Before performing any assessment, the patient should have the procedure and its importance explained. All questions should be answered in terms they comprehend.
2. Hispanic clients tend to be very modest. They need exams in a room by themselves and should be provided with a gown or sheet.
3. Ask clients about their perceptions of the assessment, the illness, and/or any abnormal findings.
4. If a child is being examined, be sure that at least one parent is there, preferably the father.
5. Explain what is going to be done and why before conducting the procedure.
6. Include a significant other in all decision making and consultations regarding care.
7. Expose only the body area being examined—keep the rest of the body covered as much as possible.
8. If the health care professional does not speak Spanish, make sure that an interpreter is available. However, bilingual staff are important.
9. Whenever possible, try to have a female health care professional examine female Hispanic patients.
10. Many Hispanic clients approach the clinic with underlying beliefs and cultural expectations; they may think that the health provider is socially "higher" and so will act very respectful. They may not offer additional information unless asked, or communicate their own disbelief of or disagreement with what the professional says. Some will believe a professional can just look at the patient and know what is wrong, so they may withhold valuable historical and symptomatic information.
11. Respect cultural amenities. Greet the patient formally and discuss socially appropriate issues first, e.g., the family and the weather. It is considered rude and impolite to barge in and start on the chief complaint without these amenities.
12. Be nonjudgmental and use terms with which the patient will be comfortable.
13. Maintain space between the examiner and patient—try not to invade the patient's "personal space" unless necessary.

LUNG ASSESSMENT

1. Be aware of the feelings of the patient concerning the hot/cold theory: i.e., do not expose the patient to cold air and drafts.
2. Women should have their breasts covered.
3. Have the patient listen to how their lung and heart sound.
4. Undress the male chest or remove his shirt only for the examination.
5. Do not moralize regarding cigarette smoking but do support smoking cessation programs and activities. Be sure to get a smoking and work history.
6. When taking the medical history, a Hispanic patient may hide a personal or family history of TB. TB is treated as a disease to be hidden.
7. Explain to the patient the importance of listening to all areas of their chest.
8. If significant others are present in the exam room, explain all procedures to them, also.
9. Allow the patient to bring a family member with them to the exam if they so desire. Female patients may want to bring another female with them.
10. Prior to initiating the assessment, ask the client for permission to perform the examination.
11. Give facts on prevention or early signs and symptoms during the examination.
12. Demonstrate to the patient proper breathing technique for the exam: i.e., how to breathe in and out.

Continued.

BREAST ASSESSMENT

1. Expose only the breast being examined. Provide for privacy and help maintain dignity of patient. When exposing the patient, avoid prolonged periods of exposure. Work quickly and smoothly.
2. Allow the patient to bring another female with her to the exam.
3. Many Hispanic females prefer having a female practitioner conduct breast examinations.
4. Use models for demonstration. Explain that the purpose of breast self-examination is to be aware of the normal state of their breasts, that the exam will allow them to find problems early and that the model will help them learn what lumps are normal.
5. Try to do as much of the breast examination with the gown on and the examiner placing her hands under the gown to perform the exam.
6. Give a demonstration of the breast assessment which will be done on the model before doing the procedure on the patient.
7. Teach breast self-examination while you are doing the breast assessment.
8. Be understanding of the patient's reluctance to touch herself. Hispanic women may not know what the body part looks like or how it functions. May feel more comfortable if the exam can be explained in detail before the assessment.
9. Tell the patient the results of the assessment, i.e., whether they do or do not have any lumps present.
10. If a male physician must do the exam, make sure that a female is present.
11. Have the patient provide a return demonstration on the model and show you lumps which they may have found.
12. Reassure the patient that embarrassment about the exam is all right and that you will do everything you can to maintain their privacy.
13. Prior to initiating the breast examination, gain permission from the patient to touch her breasts. Then proceed gently. Apologize for invading the patient's privacy.
14. Talk to the woman about the issue of avoidance of touching one's breasts. Explain the importance of breast self-examination. It may help to touch one's own breast to show that it is normal and okay. Include comments about the fact that sometimes it's embarrassing when a patient first touches herself but it's also interesting to learn how really different parts of the breast feel. Show how to do breast self-examination on yourself and the model.
15. Use professional terms when speaking to the patient, i.e., breasts should be referred to as "senos," "pechas," "busto." Do not use derogatory terms.
16. When doing a breast examination on males, palpate firmly, quickly and make sure that you explain the purpose of the examination.

COLORECTAL ASSESSMENT

1. Explain the procedure thoroughly. Use enough lubricant and avoid as much exposure as possible. Explain the reason for the procedure.
2. Have the same-sex practitioner do the exam.
3. Male clients usually prefer that female nurses are not present during the exam. Provide for a male assistant to be present when doing a male exam, if possible.
4. Provide for the privacy of the patient. Expose only the area to be examined.
5. Demonstrate the procedure on a model prior to performing it on the patient.

PRE-ASSESSMENT AND ASSESSMENT GUIDELINES FOR USE WITH HISPANIC PATIENTS—cont'd

6. Inform patient what you plan to do. Make sure patient understands preparation required prior to procedure (may need to empty bowels; special diet) what will be done during exam, physical sensations the patient may have during exam, and post exam feelings.
7. Request permission to touch the body; drape the patient carefully. Apologize for invading the patient's privacy.
8. For hemoculture tests, patient may have an aversion to sampling his/her own stool. Make sure the patient will carry out the test properly; make sure clear, concise instructions are provided.
9. Explain to the patient what will help procedure go smoothly, i.e., deep breathing will help, push against examiner's finger, relax.
10. Encourage a diet with fiber, e.g., corn tortillas, high amount of raw fruits, vegetables, lower amount of fats and oils.
11. Explain signs and symptoms which would indicate problems such as bleeding or change in bowel habits.
12. Explain signs and symptoms of problems such as hemorrhoids. If the patient has such, explain proper care, importance of diet and cleanliness, when to see a doctor.
13. Discuss causes of colorectal cancer.
14. When explaining this exam, one must be careful of the terminology used to describe the procedure and be aware of your facial expressions.
15. If a male practitioner conducts a rectal exam on a female patient, make sure that a female assistant or family member is present.

PROSTATE ASSESSMENT

1. Give a demonstration on a model prior to completing the exam on the patient.
2. This exam should be done by a male only.
3. Protect the privacy of the patient. Expose only the area to be examined.
4. Be gentle, tactful, develop good rapport with the patient.
5. Allow the patient to empty his bladder prior to the rectal exam. Explain the procedure before performing it on the patient.
6. Explain the importance of screening procedures, what information the exam will provide, and how often it should be done.
7. Use proper terminology.
8. Do all explanations before doing the examination, not during it.
9. Give the patient the results of the exam as soon as it is completed.

TESTICULAR ASSESSMENT

1. This exam should be done by a male only.
2. Provide for the patient's privacy. Uncover only the parts of the body to be examined.
3. Before asking questions about the testicular assessment, discuss the high percentage of testicular cancers occurring, and the high cure rate if found quickly.
4. Teach the patient how to do a self-testicular examination. Use a model for demonstration.
5. Ask the patient for permission to perform the examination before touching the patient. Apologize for invading the client's privacy.
6. Some males may be too macho to have the examiner touch them.
7. Always use proper terminology, not derogatory terms, for body parts.
8. Explain why and how the procedure should be done. Explain findings immediately.

Continued.

PRE-ASSESSMENT AND ASSESSMENT GUIDELINES FOR USE WITH HISPANIC PATIENTS—cont'd

GYNECOLOGICAL ASSESSMENT

1. This assessment should be done by a female. If it is not possible, a female should be assisting and/or present.
2. Protect the patient's privacy. Uncover only the body part to be examined. Provide for proper draping.
3. Make sure that all specula are warm before using.
4. Give a demonstration of the procedure on a model before proceeding on the patient. Explain the procedure and tell the patient why it is important.
5. Allow client to empty her bladder prior to the examination.
6. Hispanic women tend to be very modest about their bodies. It will help if the procedure is explained in detail, a model is used to show the procedure, questions are answered, and possibly pictures of the body parts are shown to the patient before doing the assessment.
7. Assess the patient for risk factors.
8. Apologize for invading the patient's privacy.
9. Use proper terminology for body parts. Do not use derogatory terms.
10. Provide patient education while carrying out the assessment. Discuss the importance of going to a doctor if there is any unusual vaginal discharge and explain what signs and symptoms the patient should observe for. As each part of the exam is done, discuss signs and symptoms which could indicate problems and which the patient should report.
11. Discuss the importance of having Pap smears done, how often, and why.
12. Make sure the patient knows that many women are embarrassed about having a gynecological exam. Try to help her feel proud that she came in for her examination. Tell her how she is helping herself, and that you will complete the assessment as quickly as possible.
13. Give the client the results of the assessment as soon as possible.

GENITOURINARY ASSESSMENT

1. Protect the patient's privacy. Only uncover the body part to be examined. Provide for proper draping.
2. Females should have a female examiner. Males should have a male examiner. If not possible, make sure that someone of the same sex is in the room.
3. Ask permission from patients to touch them.
4. Give a demonstration of the procedure on a model prior to assessing the patient. Use pictures where helpful. Answer the patient's questions. Explain the procedure in detail: what will be done and why.
5. Use proper terminology for body parts.
6. Apologize for invading the patient's privacy.
7. Provide patient education regarding signs and symptoms to report to the doctor, e.g., blood in urine, discharge, rash, pain on urination, etc.
8. Be careful about offending the male patient's sexuality. Both male and female Hispanic patients may be very embarrassed to have a GU assessment performed. Be gentle, professional, respectful, very matter-of-fact, and get the procedure done as quickly as possible with little talk during the procedure.

PRE-ASSESSMENT AND ASSESSMENT GUIDELINES FOR USE WITH HISPANIC PATIENTS—cont'd

ORAL ASSESSMENT

1. It may be embarrassing for the patient to have a health care professional so close to their face.
2. Oral care may be poor due to smoking, drinking, and use of smokeless tobacco.
3. Teach the patient how to examine themselves. Use a mirror and point out what they are looking for and why, e.g., lesions, discoloration, etc.
4. Oral care is often not a priority in Hispanic people.
5. If the patient has dentures, it maybe very embarrassing for them to have to remove them.
6. Tell the patient the results of the assessment as soon as possible, i.e., the status of their teeth, gums, oral cavity.
7. Explain what will be done and why. Discuss signs and symptoms of problems which should be reported to the doctor.
8. Allow the patient to rinse their mouth before the assessment. Use gloves to do the assessment.
9. Explain to the patient the importance of good oral hygiene and discuss what "good oral hygiene" includes.
10. Many Hispanic patients are embarrassed to open their mouths widely. Demonstrate on yourself and explain that if the patient says "ah," the examiner can see better. Wet the tongue blade to lower discomfort. Try not to induce the gag reflex.
11. Ask the patient about risk factors. Don't be judgmental or condemning.

SKIN ASSESSMENT

1. Include scalp, soles of feet, and ears.
2. Teach the patient how to do a self-examination and explain what they are looking for and why.
3. Give the results of the assessment as soon as possible.
4. Cover the body appropriately. Protect the patient's privacy. Avoid unnecessary exposure. Do not leave body parts exposed.
5. Explain what will be done and why before proceeding with the exam. Use proper terminology for body parts.
6. Ask the patient about risk factors. Inquire as to whether the patient knows of any lumps, changes in moles, rashes, etc. that are present.
7. Apologize for invading the patient's privacy.
8. Be sure not to expose the patient to cold drafts.
9. Before the examination, demonstrate on a model, or on yourself, how you will look at the skin. Show how everyone has spots and marks on the body.

The above information reflects content analysis of 22 pages of typed transcription from a 5 hour focus group of 10 Hispanic nurses chosen to attend the Cancer Courses for Nurses Working with Minority Groups (Frank-Stromborg, M. and Olsen, S. Cancer courses for nurses working with minority groups. National Cancer Institutes, National Cancer Institutes of Health, 1988-1991, CA 09554-03S1). Study questions and work assignments previously sent to the participants enabled them to come prepared to share information about special pre-physical assessment needs of Hispanic people. Nurses provided 339 comments related to these needs that then were analyzed for content and divided into categories related to systems.

However, health professionals often use strategies that are not appropriate for the particular population, or educational materials that are not culturally sensitive. In particular, the strategies and health materials that have been developed for use with Hispanic people often fail to meet their needs or reflect their cultural beliefs. Although many organizations translate their publications into Spanish, literal translations are frequently insensitive to cultural, linguistic, and other factors that may influence attitudes about and behaviors regarding health.

The box on pp. 234-235 suggests strategies for providing cancer prevention and health promotion information to Hispanic patients. These strategies were also suggested by nurses at the cancer courses presented by NCI (Frank-Stromborg and Olsen, 1988). Strategies that may be inadequate or inappropriate are also noted.

The nurses attending the cancer courses funded by NCI also identified printed materials that they felt were relevant for the ethnic sub-group with which they worked. Hispanic nurses identified several topics related to cancer prevention and detection that are summarized in the box on p. 236 on cancer-related topics.

The Office of Minority Health Resource Center publishes a list of agencies that produce or distribute health promotion materials in Spanish. This publication, *Sources of Spanish Language Health Materials* (U.S. Department of Health and Human Services, 1989), contains a range of materials, including pamphlets, brochures, booklets, fact sheets, videos, and other items provided by public agencies and private organizations. It is not an exhaustive list, but rather, identifies those resources utilized by the Center. Appendix 1 includes a summary of that publication along with resources identified by nurses at the cancer courses for nurses working with Hispanic people (Frank-Stromborg and Olsen, 1988).

COMMUNITY-BASED STRATEGIES FOR PROVIDING PREVENTION AND HEALTH PROMOTION INFORMATION TO HISPANICS

1. Present cancer prevention or health promotion street theaters, or **teatras.**
2. Serve healthy food at community presentations and events, especially when held at churches.
3. Try disseminating information at health fairs in the community, even though prevention is not a widely accepted concept in the Hispanic culture, and attendance at screening programs tends to be low.

4. Use Spanish-language radio and TV public service announcements to disseminate information; radio is the best approach, as it is most popular. "Novelas" (dramas or soap operas) can be a vehicle to provide cancer prevention/health promotion information.
5. Identify influential people within the community and include them in community programs and presentations.

COMMUNITY-BASED STRATEGIES FOR PROVIDING PREVENTION AND HEALTH PROMOTION INFORMATION TO HISPANICS—cont'd

6. Make sure that screening programs include health professionals who have in-depth knowledge of the Hispanic culture and language.
7. Provide cancer prevention information at schools, community business organization meetings, and newsletters, and nursing programs.
8. Contact the American Cancer Society for information on cancer prevention and detection for Hispanics; information can be provided in pamphlets, handouts, and presentations.
9. Present information on cancer prevention and detection to the Catholic Youth Organization and involve its members in the development of community programs.
10. Use visual materials, including pictures of people, to present information.
11. Present information to children at children's theaters using muppets/puppets to gain attention and promote retention of information; distribute materials at school for students to take home to parents and siblings.
12. Make sure that health care facilities for Hispanics have bilingual staff available.
13. Consider establishing small, informal family interaction meetings to provide health promotion messages; meetings may be held at health care facilities, churches, or private homes.
14. Develop small novellas (books, pamphlets) that contain information on cancer prevention and health promotion for distribution throughout the community. Use a "soap opera" format involving characters and a story line.
15. Make sure that waiting rooms and patient rooms in health care facilities have cancer prevention and health promotion pamphlets, handouts, posters, pictures, etc.
16. Provide health promotion programs, such as "staying healthy after 50," to senior citizen groups.
17. Develop and distribute tables and charts explaining good vs. poor nutrition to women. Focus on health care facilities, school meetings, church functions, and youth activities.
18. Health information can be displayed on billboards in Spanish neighborhoods.
19. Post health information, including posters, brochures, and pamphlets, in Hispanic stores.
20. Use Spanish newspapers, magazines, and newsletters to disseminate cancer prevention information.

1. The above information reflects content analysis of 23 pages of typed transcription from a 5 hour focus group of 10 Hispanic nurses chosen to attend the Cancer Courses for Nurses Working with Minority Groups (Frank-Stromborg, M. and Olsen, S. Cancer courses for nurses working with minority groups. National Cancer Institute, National Institutes of Health, 1988-1991, CA 09554-03S1). Studying questions and work assignments previously sent to the participants enabled them to come prepared to share information about resources and strategies specifically designed for Hispanic people. Nurses provided 310 comments related to resources and strategies which then underwent content analysis.
2. 2-hour interview with Guadalupe Palos for Frank-Stromborg, M. and Olsen, S. Cancer courses for nurses working with minority groups, National Cancer Institute, National Institutes for Health, 1988-1991, CA 09554-03S1.

TOPICS RELATED TO CANCER PREVENTION AND DETECTION IDENTIFIED AS IMPORTANT FOR HISPANIC PEOPLE

1. Breast self-examination: including the importance of the exam and how to do it.
2. Breast cancer: signs, symptoms, treatment, and screening procedures (mammography).
3. Testicular examination: why it is conducted and how.
4. Testicular cancer: signs, symptoms, treatment, and screening procedures.
5. Seven warning signs of cancer.
6. Smoking and cancer: smoking cessation programs.
7. Pap smear exams: why, how, when they should be done.
8. Gynecological cancers: signs, symptoms, treatment, and screening procedures.
9. Sigmoidoscopy/colorectal exams and cancer.
10. Chemotherapy: types, side effects, benefits, and statistics related to effectiveness.
11. Cancer: what to know, and what to do about it, including risk factors, prevention, what to do if you have a sign/symptom, resources for care, importance of screening programs, and early detection.
12. Lung cancer: signs and symptoms, relation to smoking, treatment, prevention.
13. Prostatic cancer.
14. Protecting yourself against cancer: dietary intake, avoiding alcohol, sun exposure, smoking.

From Frank-Stromborg M, Olsen S: Cancer courses for nurses working with minority groups, National Cancer Institute, 1988-1991. National Institutes of Health.

REFERENCES

1. Black WC, Goldhahn RT, Wiggins C: Melanoma within a southwestern Hispanic population. *Arch Dermatol* 123:1331-1334, 1987.
2. Cox C: Physician utilization by three groups of ethnic elderly, *Med Care* 24(8):667-676, 1986.
3. Daly MB, Clark GM, McGuire WL: Breast cancer prognosis in a mixed Caucasian-Hispanic population, *J Natl Cancer Inst* 74(4):753-757, 1985.
4. Devor EJ, Buechley RW: Gallbladder cancer in Hispanic New Mexicans: I. General population, 1957-1977, *Cancer* 45:1705-1712, 1980.
5. Deyo R, Diehl A, Hazuda H, Stern M: A simple language-based acculturation scale for Mexican Americans: Validation and application to health care research, *Am J Public Health* 75(1):51-55, 1985.
6. Estrada A, Trevino F, Ray L: Health care utilization barriers among Mexican Americans: Evidence from HHANES 1982-1984. *Am J Public Health* 80 (suppl):27-31, 1990.
7. Foreman JT: Susto and the health needs of the Cuban refugee population, *Top Clin Nurs* 7(3):40-47, 1985.
8. Frank-Stromborg M, Olsen S: Cancer courses for nurses working with minority groups. Final Report to funding agency, 1988-1991, National Cancer Institute, National Institutes of Health, CA 09554-03S1.
9. Gomez GE, Gomez EA: Folk healing among Hispanic Americans, *Public Health Nurs* 2(4):245-249, 1985.
10. Gonzales-Swafford MJ, Gutierrez MG: Ethnomedical beliefs and practices of Mexican-Americans, *Nurse Pract* 8(10):29-30, 32, 34, Nov-Dec, 1983.
11. Palos G: Cancer prevention and detection, M.D. Anderson Hospital, Houston, Tex, 2 hour interview for Frank-Stromborg M, Olsen S. Cancer courses for nurses working with minority groups, National Cancer Institute, National Institutes of Health, 1991.
12. Hautman MA: Folk health and illness beliefs, *Nurse Pract* (4):23, 26-27, 31, 34, July/Aug, 1979.
13. Haynes S, Harvey C, Montes H, Nickens H, Cohen B: Patterns of cigarette smoking among His-

panics in the United States: Results from HHANES 1982-1984, *Am J Public Health* 80 (suppl):47-53, 1990.

14. Higginbotham J, Trevino F, Ray L: Utilization of curanderos by Mexican Americans: Prevalence and predictors findings from HHANES 1982-1984, *Am J Public Health* 80 (suppl):32-35, 1990.

15. Holck SE, Warren CW, Rochat RW, Smith JC: Lung cancer mortality and smoking habits: Mexican-American women, *Am J Public Health* 72(1):38-42, 1982.

16. Inter-university Consortium for Political and Social Research: *Health Interview Survey*, Hyattsville, Md, 1984, National Center for Health Statistics.

17. Johnston M: Folk beliefs and ethnocultural behavior in pediatrics: Medicine or magic, *Nurs Clin North Am* 12(1):77-84, 1977.

18. Mack TM, Walker A, Mack W, Berstein L: Cancer in Hispanics in Los Angeles County, *Natl Cancer Inst Monograph* 69:99-104, 1985.

19. Manduro R: Curanderismo and Latino views of disease and curing, *The West J Med* 139(6):868-874, 1983.

20. Marcus AC, Crane LA: Smoking behavior among U.S. Latinos: An emerging challenge for public health, *Am J Public Health* 75(2):169-172, 1985.

21. Mardiros M: A view toward hospitalization: The Mexican-American experience, *J Adv Nurs* 9:469-478, 1984.

22. Markides KS, Coriel J: The health of Hispanics in the southwestern United States: An epidemiologic paradox, *Public Health Rep* 101(3):253-265, 1986.

23. Marsh WW, Hentges K: Mexican folk remedies and conventional medical care, *Am Fam Pract* 37(3):257-262, 1988.

24. Martaus TM: The health-seeking process of Mexican-American migrant farm workers, *Home Healthcare Nurse* 4(5):32-36, 1986.

25. Martin J, Suarez L: Cancer mortality among Mexican Americans and other Whites in Texas, 1969-80, *Am J Public Health* 77(7):851-853, 1987.

26. Menck HR, Mack TM: Incidence of biliary tract cancer in Los Angeles, *Natl Cancer Inst Monograph* 62:95-99, 1982.

27. National Coalition of Hispanic Health and Human Services Organizations: *Delivering preventive health care to Hispanics: A manual for providers*, Washington, D.C., 1988, The Coalition.

28. Newell GR, Mills PK: *Low cancer rates in Hispanic women related to social and economic factors*, pp 23-25, 1987, Haworth Press.

29. O'Brien ME: Pragmatic survivalism: Behavior patterns affecting low-level wellness among minority group members, *Adv Nurs Sci* 13-26, April 1982.

30. Pathak DR, Samet JM, Howard CA, Key CR: Malignant melanoma of the skin in New Mexico, 1969-1977, *Cancer* 50(7):1440-1446, 1982.

31. Peters RK, Thomas D, Hagan DG, Mack TM, Henderson BE: Risk factors in invasive cervical cancer among Latinas and non-Latinas in Los Angeles County, *J Natl Cancer Inst* 77:1063-1077, 1986.

32. Richardson JL, Marks G, Solis JM, Collins LM, Birba L, Hisserich JC: Frequency and adequacy of breast cancer screening among elderly Hispanic women, *Prev Med* 16:761-774, 1987.

33. Roberts RE, Lee ES: Health practices among Mexican Americans: Further evidence from the laboratory studies. *Prev Med* 9:675-688, 1980.

34. Rodriguez J: Mexican Americans: Factors influencing health practices, *J Sch Health*, pp 130-139, 1983.

35. Samet JM, Key CR, Hunt WC, Goodwin JS: Survival of American Indian and Hispanic cancer patients in New Mexico and Arizona, 1969-82, *J Natl Cancer Inst* 79(3):457-463, 1987.

36. Savitz D: Changes in Spanish surname cancer rates relative to other Whites, Denver area, 1969-71 to 1979-81. *Am J Public Health* 76:1210-1215, 1986.

37. Solis J, Marks G, Garcia M, Shelton D: Acculturation, access to care, and use of preventive services by Hispanics: Findings from HHANES 1982-1984, *Am J Public Health* 80 (suppl):11-19, 1990.

38. Spector RE: Health and illness among ethnic people of color, *Nurs Educ* 10-13, 1977.

39. Suarez L, Martin J: Primary liver cancer mortality and incidence in Texas Mexican Americans, 1969-80, *Am J Public Health* 77(5):631-633, 1987.

40. Sugarek NJ, Deyo RA, Holmes BC: Locus of control and beliefs about cancer in a multi-ethnic clinic population, *Oncol Nurs Forum* 15(4):481-486, 1988.

41. Top Ten Causes of Death in 1988; Hispanics and White, Non-Hispanics." January 15, 1991, *Washington Post*.

42. US Bureau of the Census: Current population reports, *The Hispanic population in the United States*, Series p 20, No 449, Washington, DC, March 1991. US Government Printing Office.

43. US Bureau of the Census: Current population reports, *The Hispanic population in the United States*, Washington, DC, March 1989, US Government Printing Office.

44. US Department of Commerce Bureau of the Census: *Census and you* 26(9), Washington, DC, September 1991.

45. US Department of Commerce Bureau of the Census: *The Hispanic population in the United States: March 1988 (advanced report)* Series P-20, No 431,

Washington DC, August 1988. US Government Printing Office.

46. US Department of Health and Human Services: *Sources of Spanish language health materials*, Washington, DC, 1989, The Department.

47. Warshauer ME, Silverman DT, Schottenfield D, Pollack ES: Stomach and colorectal cancers in Puerto Rican born residents of New York City, *J Natl Cancer Inst* 76(4):591-595, 1986.

Community Resources for Printed and Multimedia Health Information Materials for Hispanic People

GENERAL INFORMATION BEFORE SELECTING PRINTED AND MULTIMEDIA RESOURCES

1. Make sure that reading material is geared to the 5th-6th grade level of reading ability (use FOG or SMOG Indices).
2. To enhance identification, try to utilize materials that are not geared toward Caucasians. Hispanic individuals should be included and clearly visible.
3. Printed material should have good illustrations explaining important aspects of information.
4. Materials should be culturally sensitive.
5. Make sure that information is not presented using medical terminology. Even though it is in Spanish, clients still may not understand the material if the language used is too technical.

MULTIMEDIA RESOURCES

1. American Association of Retired Persons
   1909 K Street, NW
   Washington, DC 20049
   (202) 872-4700
   Makes available *Su Hogar, Su Ellecion: Manual Para Personas de Edad y Sus Familias (Your home, your choice: A workbook for older people and their families.*

2. American College of Radiology
   1891 Preston White Drive
   Reston, VA 22091
   (800) 227-7762
   (703) 648-8900
   Distributes the pamphlet, *Mamografia: Guia para Pacientes ante el Examen Radiologico de la Mama (Mammography).*

3. American Cancer Society
   3340 Peachtree Road, NE
   Atlanta, GA 30026
   (800) 227-2345
   Offers a wide variety of materials on cancer, cancer prevention and treatment, the Pap test, and smoking; also educational materials on breast, colorectal, mouth, skin, and uterine cancers and on breast self-examination (in Spanish and English).

4. American Diabetes Association
   Diabetes Information Center
   1660 Duke Street
   Alexandria, VA 22314
   (800) 232-3472
   Provides a number of materials in Spanish concerning proper nutrition, meal planning, and all aspects of diabetes and diabetic care. Also, contact local association affiliate.

5. American Dietetic Association (ADA)
   216 W. Jackson Boulevard, Suite 800

Chicago, IL 60606-6995

(312) 899-0040

Makes available several publications related to proper nutrition and meal planning.

6. American Heart Association
7320 Greenville Avenue
Dallas, TX 75231-4599
(214) 706-1220
Makes available materials on exercise, heart disease, high blood pressure, nutrition, stroke, weight reduction.

7. American Lung Association
DC Chapter
475 H Street, NW
Washington, DC 20001
(202) 682-LUNG
Publications available on tuberculosis, tuberculin test, smoking and pregnancy, and smoking cessation.

8. American Red Cross
National Headquarters
17th and D Streets, NW
Washington, DC 20006
(202) 737-8300
Distributes pamphlets in Spanish about AIDS, what you should know before donating blood, first aid, and other topics.

9. Amigas Latinas en Accion Pro-Salud (ALAS)
47 Nichols Avenue
Watertown, MA 02172
(617) 926-6046
Develops health education materials in Spanish and bilingual formats. Topics include: AIDS, family planning, use of condoms and vaginitis. ALAS and local community activists also produce videos on topics including AIDS, nutrition, women's health, and patient's rights.

10. Asociacion Nacional Pro-Personas Mayores
2727 West Sixth Street, Suite 270
Los Angeles, CA 90057
(213) 487-1922
Publishes a series of health fact sheets on a wide range of topics including accident prevention, alcohol abuse, cancer facts, dental care, dietary supplements, drug interaction protection, eye diseases, medical safety, nutrition, sexuality, skin care, prostate problems, and others.

11. Channing L. Bete Company, Inc.
200 State Road
South Deerfield, MA 01373
(800) 628-7733
Distributes scriptographic booklets and coloring books on numerous topics. Spanish language materials are available on alcohol and drug abuse, contraception, pregnancy and childbirth, infant and child health, child abuse and neglect, nutrition, sexually transmitted diseases, smoking and smoking cessation, women's health, mammography, and other topics.

12. Colorado Department of Health
Alcohol and Drug Abuse Division
4210 East 11th Avenue
Denver, CO 80220
(303) 331-8238
Provides a listing of Spanish-language materials on numerous topics.

13. Eli Lilly and Company
Lilly Corporate Center
Indianapolis, IN 46285
(317) 261-2663

Has Spanish language booklets and pamphlets on diabetes, meal planning, and nutrition.

14. Environmental Protection Agency
    401 M Street, SW
    Washington, DC 20460
    (202) 382-3080
    Makes available materials on air pollution, lead, noise, pesticides, solid waste disposal, toxic substances, and water pollution.

15. ETR Associates Network Publications
    PO Box 1830
    Santa Cruz, CA 95061-1830
    (408) 438-4060
    Provides educational materials on family life and sexuality to school district programs, health organizations, and agencies serving youths that focus on AIDS, STDs, contraception, family planning, menstruation, sex education, and sexuality. "The Latino Family Life Education Curriculum Series," which strongly affirms Latino culture and family values, is also available.

16. Krames Communications
    312 90th Street
    Daly City, CA 94015-1898
    (800) 433-0490
    Offers publications on several topics including: AIDS, breast lumps, contraception, gallbladder, hysterectomy, mammography, Pap test, radiology procedures, pelvic sonogram, pregnancy, STDs, and other topics.

17. Leukemia Society of America
    733 Third Avenue
    New York, NY 10017
    (212) 573-8484
    Offers a pamphlet on what everyone should know about leukemia and the patient aid program.

18. National Cancer Institute
    Office of Cancer Communications
    Building 31, Room 10A-21
    9000 Rockville Pike
    Bethesda, MD 20892-3100
    (301) 496-5583
    Provides informative materials on all types and aspects of cancer and cancer treatment.

19. National Coalition of Hispanic Mental Health and Human Services Organizations (COSSMHO)
    1030 15th Street, NW, Suite 1053
    Washington, DC 20005
    (202) 371-2100
    Makes available the publication: *Bibliography: Selected Health Materials in Spanish.*

20. Lange Productions
    7661 Curson Terr.
    Hollywood, CA 90046
    Provides a pamphlet on breast health.

21. National Dairy Council
    6300 Northriver Road
    Rosemont, IL 60018-4289
    (708) 696-1020
    Offers materials on calcium, child nutrition, proper nutrition, and other topics.

22. National Heart, Lung and Blood Institute
    Education Programs and Information Center
    4733 Bethesda Avenue, Suite 530
    Bethesda, MD 20814
    (301) 951-3260
    Provides [resources for] Spanish-lan-

guage materials on high blood pressure, cholesterol, smoking, and multiple risk factors.

23. National Institute on Aging (NIA)
    Federal Building, 6th Floor
    9000 Rockville Pike
    Bethesda, MD 20892
    (301) 496-1752
    Spanish-language consumer materials on accident prevention, skin care, foot care, and various other topics including cancer and breast examination.

24. International Cancer Information Center
    National Cancer Institute, National Institutes of Health, U.S. Department of Health and Human Services, Information Specialist
    Bloch Building, Room 102
    Bethesda, MD 20892
    (301) 496-7403
    Disseminates results of cancer research; produces a monthly current awareness bulletin with abstracts on cancer research.

25. Health Risk Appraisal Activity
    Centers for Disease Control
    U.S. Department of Health and Human Services
    Building 3, Room B43
    1600 Clifton Road, NE
    Atlanta, GA 30333
    Has developed computerized health risk appraisals that can be used with multiple ethnic and special targeted populations. Assesses risk of death from cancer, heart disease, and other medical conditions.

26. Office of Minority Health Resource Center

Information Specialist
PO Box 37337
Washington, DC 20013-7337
(800) 444-6472
Available to answer questions concerning minority health resources at the state, federal, and local levels. Bilingual staff (Spanish/English) available.

27. Rural Health Office
    University of Arizona
    3131 East Second Street
    Tucson, AZ 85716
    Provides a directory of patient education resources in Spanish and English.

OTHER RESOURCES

28. M.D. Anderson Hospital, Austin, Texas
29. Local Hospice Organizations
30. National Migrant Referral Project, Inc.
    Migrant Clinicians Network
    2512 South 1H-25 Suite 220
    Austin, TX 78704
31. Texas Department of Health
32. Community medical centers and clinics.
33. Local "I Can Cope" programs offered through hospitals and health centers.
34. Educational departments of local hospitals: Ask for pamphlets, brochures, posters and/or videos on cancer, either in English or Spanish. Also ask if they know of other resources that provide bilingual materials.
35. American Cancer Society support groups, such as "Reach for Recovery" for mastectomy patients. These

groups may be listed in phone books, or call the local chapter of the ACS or a hospital for referral to the closest support group.

36. Specialty health care organizations such as the Dental Society for oral cancer or Medical Society for specific information about other cancers. Start with the local organization; if they do not have materials, ask for the national association address.

37. Local church groups might have access to cancer information/resources. In heavily Spanish congregations, bulletins might be good resources.

38. Brochures available in doctors' offices, especially in Spanish areas.

39. State and local public health departments.

40. Drug companies, such as Searle, which publishes "Auto Examen Del Seno."

Office of Minority Health Resource Center, *Sources of Spanish Language Health Materials.* August, 1989. U.S. Department of Health and Human Services, Office of Minority Health, P.O. Box 37337, Washington, D.C. 20013-7337. Appendix I also reflects content analysis of 21 pages of typed transcription from a 5 hour focus group of 10 Hispanic nurses chosen to attend the Cancer Courses for Nurses Working with Minority Groups (Frank-Stromborg M, Olsen S: *Cancer courses for nurses working with minority groups,* National Cancer Institute, National Institutes of Health, 1988-1991, CA 09554-03S1). Study questions and work assignments previously sent to the participants enabled them to come prepared to share information about patient education materials and resources specifically designed for Hispanic people. Nurses provided 188 comments related to resources, 151 comments related to printed materials and 106 comments related to indicating resources and types of multimedia available. Content analysis of these comments has been done to provide a comprehensive list of resources.

CHAPTER 1   Resources

American Cancer Society
South Dakota Chapter
Rapid City, South Dakota

This chapter of the ACS had BSE booklets printed in Lakota Sioux, but these have not been reprinted. The organization also has a slide presentation on TSE with a Native American pictured on the slide.

For TSE slide tape contact: Tom Colhoff, Director, Black Hill Training Center, c/o Sioux San, 3200 Canyon Lake Dr., Rapid City, SD 57701.

American Indian Health Care Association
245 E. 6th St., Suite 499
St. Paul, Minnesota 55101
(612) 348-1900

This nonprofit organization, which was established in 1975, works in cooperation with CDC, ANA, IHS, NCI to develop materials on cancer prevention and screening for Native Americans. With funding from the CDC, the group has developed brochures, posters, comic books, and magnets on AIDS (contact Joan Myric), and participates in programs to promote the Year 2000 Health Objectives (contact Sherri Scott). The IHS has provided funding for the implementation of the Health Risk Appraisal in urban populations and to study the health status of elderly Native Americans.

With a 5-year grant from the National Cancer Institute, the group is developing urban cervical screening for Native American women in urban areas (1990-1995). With a 3-year grant from the National Heart, Lung and Blood Institute (1989-1990) the organization is conducting a study entitled "Strategies for Smoking Cessation in Native Americans." The target audiences will be pregnant females, the elderly, teenagers, and urban adult Indian smokers. The organization will be developing brochures and videos.

The association also publishes several quarterly newsletters *(News briefs; AIDS briefs; Prac-tice Management Forum)*. These newsletters are an excellent resource for learning about new publications, programs, and statistics relating to Native Americans.

Association on American Indian Affairs, Inc.
P.O. Box 284
Norwood, New Jersey 07648-9967

The purpose of this nonprofit corporation is advocacy for Native Americans. It publishes a quarterly newsletter and is involved in the following activities: technical assistance, small grants, legal assistance, *amicus curiae* briefs to U.S. Supreme Court, public education, national studies, legislation drafting, advice to agencies working with tribes, cooperation with Indian organizations, scholarship programs, and Congressional testimony.

Indian Health Service Chart Series Book, April, 1987.
Indian Health Service, U.S. Department of Health and Human Services
Washington, DC.

This publication provides basic statistics and information on the Indian Health Service (IHS) and its work with the Native American and Alaska Native people. The tables in the book provide detailed data, and the charts show significant relationships. A table and its corresponding chart appear next to each other. However, some charts that are self-explanatory do not have a corresponding table. The book includes information on IHS structure, the demographics of Native American and Alaska Native populations, patient care, and community health care. Historical trends are depicted, and comparisons to other population groups are made when appropriate.

The tables and charts are grouped into six major categories: IHS Structure; Population Statistics; Natality and Infant/Maternal Mortality Statistics; General Mortality Statistics; Patient Care Statistics; and Community Health Statistics.

Single copies of this publication are available at no cost from the Indian Health Service, Division of Program Statistics, 5600 Fishers Lane, Rm 6A-30, Rockville, MD 20857; (301) 443-1180.

The Native American Research and Training Center (NARTC)
1642 East Helen Street
Tucson, Arizona 85719
(602) 621-5075

The center conducts research and training programs in health and rehabilitation for disabled and chronically ill Native Americans. It also publishes a monograph series, produces training videotapes, and cosponsors annual conferences and workshops on a variety of rehabilitation issues. For more information and order forms contact NARTC.

Native American Rights Fund
1506 Broadway
Boulder, Colorado 80302
(303) 447-8760

This nonprofit agency is the national legal defense fund working directly with Native American tribes, villages, groups, and individuals in cases of major significance to a great many Native people. Their five priorities are: (1) the protection of tribal existence; (2) the protection of tribal resources; (3) the protection of Native American human rights and basic freedoms, including religious freedom; (4) the accountability of the federal government to live up to its responsibilities to native people; and (5) the development of Native American law.

Nutrition Education for Native Americans: A Guide for Nutrition Educators
Health Resources and Services Administration: U.S. Department of Health and Human Services,
Washington, DC, 1984, U.S. Government Printing Office,
p 67.

The purpose of this guide is to help professionals involved in nutrition education in food assistance programs. The guide contains three major sections. Section I provides background information on Native Americans, including cultural characteristics, basic health and diet-related illnesses, and traditional and contemporary dietary practices. The section also contains some information on lifestyles and food behavior, adaptation of materials for Native American cultures, and current nutrition education activities in various programs or delivery systems that may be of help to nutrition educators. Section II describes several counseling strategies offered by individuals who work with Native Americans in different geographic locations. This section was developed specifically for educators who have never worked with Native Americans. References pertaining to counseling are provided at the end of the section. Section III lists a variety of both government and private sector resources for nutrition educators. Each section has a reference list at the end.

This publication is available through interlibrary loan from the Food and Nutrition Information Service, National Agricultural Library, Rm. 304, 10301 Baltimore Blvd., Beltsville, MD 20205; (301) 344-3719.

Nutrition Education Resource Guide for American Indians and Alaska Natives: A Selected Annotated Bibliography for the Food Distribution Program on Indian Reservations.
Nutrition Science and Education Branch, U.S. Department of Agriculture
Washington, DC, 1988, U.S. Government Printing Office, p 75.

This bibliography describes culturally relevant nutrition education materials written for and/or by Native Americans and Alaska Natives. The print and audiovisual materials listed in this guide are divided into two categories: one for consumers, and one for nutrition educators. The material for consumers is subdivided into seven separate sections including ones on infant feeding and child feeding; weight control and obesity; general nutrition, diet, and health; and foods and food preparation. All of the materials for educators are grouped together in a separate section. The appendices contain an alphabetized title index and a handy checklist for use by persons writing new materials or revising or adapting materials from this guide for use with a specific tribe or reservation.

Copies of this publication are available through interlibrary loan from the Food and Nutrition Information Service, National Agricultural Library, Rm. 304, 10301 Baltimore Boulevard, Beltsville, MD 20205; (301) 344-3719.

U.S. Department of Health and Human Services
Public Health Service
Indian Health Service (IHS)
5600 Fishers Lane
Rockville, MD 20857

The IHS is the federal health agency responsible for administering the health program for more than one million Native Americans. Its mission is to provide a comprehensive health services delivery system for American Indians and Alaska Natives, while increasing opportunities for tribes to develop and manage programs to meet their own health needs.

CHAPTER 2   Resources

AIDS International Information Distribution Service
PO Box 2008
Saratoga, CA 95070
(408) 866-6303

Distributes AIDS-related publications prepared by other sources, including, *Don't Gamble with AIDS. . .It's a Stacked Deck* (Chinese, Filipino, Japanese, Korean, Tagalog, and Vietnamese).

Adult Health System
Hypertension Control Program
714 P Street, Room 616
Sacramento, CA 95814
(916) 322-6851

Materials related to hypertension and ethnic foods high in potassium are available in English and Chinese.

Al-Anon Family Group Headquarters, Inc.
P.O. Box 862, Midtown Station
New York, NY 10018-0862
(212) 302-7240

This organization offers alcoholism-related materials approved by the Al-Anon/Alateen Conference (Chinese, Portuguese, Korean, and Japanese).

American Association of Retired Persons
Minority Resource Directory
NCBA
P.O. Box 64846
Chicago, IL 64846
        or
Minority Resource Directory
AARP—Area V Office
2720 Des Plaines Ave.
Des Plaines, IL 60016

A directory of minority agencies and organizations in the greater Chicago area is available for free and includes information of importance to Asian-Americans.

American Cancer Society—California Division
PO Box 2061
Oakland, CA 94604
(415) 893-7900

American Cancer Society—San Francisco Unit
973 Market Street
San Francisco, CA 94103
(415) 974-1592

Distributes materials on basic facts about cancer (Chinese, Japanese, Tagalog, and Vietnamese.) Materials on quitting smoking, colorectal cancer, breast cancer, prostate cancer, and nasopharyngeal cancer (Chinese). Breast health materials (Chinese and Vietnamese).

American Cancer Society—San Gabriel/Poma Valleys Unit
50 North Hill Avenue
Pasadena, CA 91106

An informative guide book has been designed for health care professionals to provide to Japanese and Chinese individuals with cancer. Four areas of cancer are covered: chemotherapy, nutrition, pain control, and ostomy. The materials have been translated, are easily duplicated, and stored in 2 three-hole binder.

Asian American Health Forum
835 Jackson Street
San Francisco, CA 94133
(415) 391-8494

Provides Asian language materials on tuberculosis, thalassemia, and hepatitis B.

Asian Health Project
T.H.E. Clinic
3860 W. Martin Luther King Boulevard
Los Angeles, CA 90008
(213) 295-6571

Makes available general brochures about AIDS (Japanese, Thai, and Vietnamese). Provides materials on birth control methods, natural family planning, sterilization, sexually transmitted diseases, cancer prevention in women, sexual hygiene, and mental hygiene (Cambodian, Japanese, Lao, Thai, and Vietnamese). Also provides the booklet, *A Guide to Translated Publications: A Directory of Health-Related Materials in Asian/Pacific Languages.*

Asian Health Services, Inc.
310 8th Street, Suite 200
Oakland, CA 94607
(415) 465-3271

Distributes pamphlets on common health problems, perinatal topics, and family planning (Chinese, Korean, and Vietnamese). Specific topics include controlling high blood pressure, diabetes, weight control, nutrition during pregnancy, and birth control methods. Also has a brochure on AIDS (Korean).

Association of Asian/Pacific Community Health
Organizations 310 8th Street, Suite 200
Oakland, CA 94607
(415) 272-9536

Provides copies of *Health Education Materials in Asian Languages-Maternal and Child Health Topics: Catalog of Evaluated Materials*, which describes audiovisual and written materials on accident prevention and safety, family planning, newborn care, immunization, nutrition, and prenatal care. Also distributes pamphlets on substance abuse (Chinese, Korean, Tagalog, Vietnamese). Currently developing a materials list on thalassemia.

Bureau of Refugee Services
Iowa Department of Human Services
1200 University, Suite D
Des Moines, IA 50314
(515) 371-3117

Distributes materials on a variety of health topics, including: birth control, nutrition, and diabetes (Hmong, Khmer, Lao, Thai, and Vietnamese). Offers a guide to other sources.

Children's Hospital of San Francisco
Bessie Woo, RN
San Francisco, CA 94118

Ms. Woo developed a 20-minute videotape for Chinese patients and their families about chemotherapy. The videotape discusses the goals, methods, and potential side effects of chemotherapeutic regimens. It is available in either Cantonese or Mandarin narration; both have English subtitles.

Chinatown Health Clinic
Health Education Department
89 Baxter Street
New York, NY 10013
(212) 732-9547

Distributes pamphlets on AIDS, the health hazards of smoking, angina, cholesterol, heart attack, sodium, stress and hypertension, hypertension medications, diabetes, and gestational diabetes (Chinese).

Chinese Hospital
845 Jackson Street
San Francisco, CA 94133

The hospital is bilingual in all its departments, and all health care communications are available in both English and Chinese. The hospital sponsors national conferences on health care issues related to Chinese medicine and Chinese-Americans.

Cooperative Extension University of California
2615 South Grand Avenue, Suite 400
Los Angeles, CA 90007
(415) 670-5200

Provides materials on nutrition and diet (Chinese).

Division of Outpatient and Community Services
San Francisco General Hospital
San Francisco, CA

Distributes a 29-page pamphlet, *Sodium Values of Common Asian/Pacific Islander Foods* compiled by Janice Louie, RD, MA, Rozane Gee, and the Division of Outpatient and Community Services. Includes the food and a description of the food, measurements sodium content is based on, sodium content, and ethnic names in Chinese, Japanese, Filipino, Vietnamese, Cambodian, and Laotian.

Ethnic Minority Health Committee, Utah Department of Health
Box 16660
288 North 1460 West
Salt Lake City, UT 84116
(801) 538-6305

Distributes a listing of Asian language health materials available from various sources.

Health Center #4
San Francisco Department of Public Health
1490 Mason Street
San Francisco, CA 94133
(415) 558-2308

Publishes a booklet on proper nutrition for good health (Chinese, Cambodian, Lao, Vietnamese, and English).

International District Community Health Center
416 Maynard Avenue South
Seattle, Washington 98104
(206) 461-3617

A brochure *Asians and Aids* is available that provides multilingual, culturally sensitive health care information for Asian/Pacific Islander populations. Clients served include Japanese, Samoan, Korean, Khmer, Lao, Vietnamese, Chinese, Filipino.

International Refugee Center of Oregon
1336 East Burnside
Portland, OR 97214
(503) 234-1541

Provides consumer health pamphlets on topics including breast self-examination, birth control, child health, sexually transmitted diseases, immunization, infectious hepatitis, and tuberculosis. Makes available a series on after-care for emergency room patients that includes individual titles on eye injuries, sprains and fractures, and wounds (Cambodian, Lao, Vietnamese).

Merck Sharp & Dohme
Pharmaceutical Company

Brochures for Asian-Americans related to the prevention of hepatitis B are produced in cooperation with the American Liver Foundation. These booklets are translated into different languages. Health care professionals can contact the local drug company representative for information on ordering the material.

Multicultural Health Coalition
1017 Wilson Boulevard, Suite 407
Downsview, Ontario, Canada M3K 1Z1
416-630-8835

This group developed a series of fact sheets topics including alcohol, cancer, diabetes, nutrition, second-hand smoke, and stress (Chinese and Vietnamese).

National Institute on Aging
Federal Building, 6th Floor
9000 Rockville Pike
Bethesda, MD 20892
(301) 496-1752

Provides titles from the "Age Page" series on cancer, high blood pressure, and diabetes (Chinese).

Pacific Basin Maternal and Child Health Resource Center.
671-734-4717
PO Box 5143, UCOG Station Mangilao, Guam 96923.

The Pacific Basin Maternal and Child Health Resource Center, established in 1984 on the University of Guam campus in Mangilao village, is a regional resource center that focuses primarily on maternal and child health. The center serves the following Pacific Basin jurisdictions: American Samoa; Commonwealth of the Northern Mariana Islands (CNMI); Federated Republic of Belau; and Republic of the Marshall Islands. The center is responsible for developing and providing educational services, information, and technical assistance to health professionals in the Pacific Basin jurisdictions. The center maintains a collection of materials on maternal and child health, including books; pamphlets; brochures; vertical files; slides; videos; 16-mm films; flipcharts; posters; and professional journals and newsletters from regional, national, and international organizations concerned with maternal and child health. The center also conducts computerized searches through DIALOG. Another important mandate of the center is to develop culturally relevant health education materials on selected maternal and child health topics for use by the jurisdictions. Although most of its information is designed for health professionals in various settings, the center also provides information to other consumers on request and allows them to use its resource materials.

PUBLICATIONS: The center's newsletter, *MCH NEWSPAC,* is published twice a year and provides an overview of maternal and child health activities in the Pacific jurisdictions. The center also produces the *Resource Directory of Maternal and Child Health Programs.* Other publications include brochures, posters, and charts on topics such as breast-feeding, cancer, and smoking. These materials are available in the following languages: English, Samoan, Yapese, Marshallese, Kosraen, Trukese, Pohnapean, Palauan, Chamorro, and Carolinian.

The Queen's Cancer Institute
1301 Punchbowl Street
Honolulu, HI 96813

This health care institution produces publications related to cancer and Asian-Americans, such as the brochure and poster, *Enjoy Food for Life.*

Rainy Day Press
P.O. Box 574
Pohnpei, Federated States of Micronesia 96941

This company publishes books related to the Pacific Islanders including: *Micronesian Customs and Beliefs,* an explanation of 99 customs involving childbirth, land and food, marriage, skills, legends, and funerals on Micronesian islands, written by Micronesians ($9.95); *Pohnpei—An Island Argosy,* on the history, natural features, flora and fauna, government and education, culture, customs and languages, places of interest, and a list of selected readings ($9.95).

Refugee Health Issues Center
American Refugee Committee
2344 Nicollet Avenue, South, Suite 350
Minneapolis, MN 55404
612-872-7060

Publishes a brochure on sudden infant death syndrome (SIDS) (English, Khmer, Hmong, and Vietnamese), brochures on domestic violence and sexual assault (Cambodian, Hmong, Lao, and Vietnamese), and educational materials on sexual assault prevention (English, Chinese, Khmer, Lao, and Vietnamese).

Refugee Immigrant Health Program
Hawaii Department of Health
1250 Punchbowl Street
Honolulu, HI 96813
(808) 548-2074

Materials on nutrition, hepatitis, and health concerns of newly arrived immigrants are available (Chinese, Lao, and Vietnamese).

South Cove Community Health Center.
617-482-7555
885 Washington St., Boston, MA 02111

Founded in 1972, SCCHS is dedicated to providing comprehensive and preventive health care services to the residents of Boston's Asian and South Cove communities. The center is also committed to advocating for patients at local hospitals and health care and social service agencies. The center's services include pediatrics, adolescent medicine, school health, obstetrics/gynecology, internal medicine, and eye care. Mental health services are available for adults and children as well as the mentally retarded. The center also offers nutrition and health education, community outreach, and a variety of social services. The SCCHS is a member of the Association of Asian/Pacific Community Health Organizations.

PUBLICATIONS: The SCCHS has developed a English/Chinese brochure for patients that includes information on center services, cholesterol, cancer, and smoking.

Washington State Commission on Asian American Affairs
110 Prefontaine Pl. S. #202
Seattle, Washington 98104
(206) 464-5820
    or
1515 S. Cherry Street
Olympia, Washington 98504
(206) 753-7053

This organization produces informational brochures on a number of topics including: Chinese Americans, Filipino-Americans, Japanese Americans, Korean Americans, South Asian Americans, Southeast Asian Americans, South Pacific Americans.

Your Guide to Good Nutrition During and After Cancer Treatment. A bilingual nutritional handbook.
Susana Chan, RN, MS, and Holley Wysong, RD
California Pacific Medical Center
P.O. Box 7999
San Francisco, Calif. 94120
Phone 415-750-6036

The authors, working in an oncology department with a large Chinese population, have

compiled culturally specific instructional material that can be used by all health care professionals. Includes:

- Parallel English-Chinese format for use by non-Chinese speaking health care workers.
- Sample menu and recipes.
- List of ethnic Chinese foods high in protein and calories.
- Chinese health beliefs.
- Suggestions for coping with poor appetite, weight loss, dry mouth, etc.

CHAPTER 3   Resources

Alu Like, Inc.
1024 Māpunapuna Street
Honolulu, HI 96819
808-836-8940

This is a private service and training agency for Native Hawaiians. Among its various programs, Alu Like currently has a program on Substance Abuse Prevention and an Elderly Services Program for Native Hawaiians.

E Ola Mau, Inc.
1374 Nu'uanu Avenue, Suite 201
Honolulu, HI 96817
808-533-1628

This is a private, nonprofit consortium of Native Hawaiian health providers whose mission is to ensure that Native Hawaiians achieve lōkahi (healthful harmony of self, with others and all of nature) and function effectively as citizens and leaders in their aina (homeland).

Hawaii State Department of Health
Community Cancer Program of Hawaii
(American Cancer Society, Hawaii Division)
3627 Kilauea Avenue, Suite 304
Honolulu, HI 96816
(808) 735-5303

Publishes brochures on cancer prevention/detection (Chinese, Japanese, Korean, Hawaiian, Lao, Vietnamese, Samoan, Tongan). Two booklets are also available to assist the health professional in communications with Asian-Americans: *Chinese Phrases for Nurses—Patient Conversation,* and *A Quickie Guide to Commonly Used Phrases, Mandarin.*

Kamehameha Schools/Bernice Pauahi Bishop Estate
Kapālama Heights
Honolulu, HI 96817
808-842-8211

This is a private 12-year school for Native Hawaiian children established under the estate of Princess Pauahi. The school offers classes in Hawaiian language, culture, and history. It has a Hawaiian Studies Institute that produces materials and research on Hawaiian culture. The school also has a large Hawaiian collection of publications and other resource materials.

Native Hawaiian Culture and Arts Program
650 Iwilei Road
Honolulu, HI 96817
808-532-5630

This is a federally funded program developed to assist in the research and perpetuation of Native Hawaiian culture. It has offered several grants to individuals and groups on a wide range of culturally related topics.

Office of Hawaiian Affairs
711 Kapi'olani Blvd., Suite 500
Honolulu, HI 96813
808-586-3777

This is a semi-autonomous state agency dedicated to the betterment of the Hawaiian people. It is governed by an elected board of trustees and has several administrative priority programs including health and human services. It publishes a monthly newspaper, *Ka Wai Ola O OHA,* which contains monthly articles concerning Native Hawaiian health issues.

Office of Hawaiian Health
Hawai'i State Department of Health
50 Kukui Plaza, 208-B
Honolulu, HI 96817
808-586-4800

This is a government office located within the Department of Health to ensure that the health care system for the state is responsive to the health needs of Native Hawaiians. Its programs are developed to assist the improvement of services within the department to Native Hawaiians. This office publishes articles and other informational materials periodically on various subjects concerning Native Hawaiian health care.

Papa Ola Lōkahi
Kawaiaha'o Plaza
567 South King Street
Honolulu, HI 96813
808-536-9453

This is a federally funded office under the Native Hawaiian Health Care Act. It is governed by a consortium board of public and private agencies concerned with Native Hawaiian Health care and assists in the planning and development of Native Hawaiian health care systems statewide utilizing federal funding.

State of Hawai'i Library System
478 South King Street
Honolulu, HI 96813
808-586-3500

This is a statewide public library system with a central library located in Honolulu. A reserve-reference collection on Hawaiian and Pacific Island materials is deposited at the central library with other lending materials.

University of Hawai'i at Mānoa
Center for Hawaiian Studies
1890 East-West Road
Moore Hall 428
Honolulu, HI 96822
808-956-6825

This is a multidisciplinary program offering a B.A. degree and emphasizing the study of both traditional and modern Hawaiian society, language, and culture.

University of Hawai'i at Mānoa
Hamilton Library
2550 The Mall
Honolulu, HI 96822
808-956-7203

This library has an extensive Hawaiian and Pacific Island collection that includes rare books, prints, and other materials not usually found at other repositories in the state.

CHAPTER 4   Resources

Public Education Programs—designed to inform the public about cancer, what they can do to protect themselves and demonstrate related health habits and lifestyles. Emphasis is currently on the following six sites; colon and rec-

tum, lung, breast, uterus, oral cavity, and skin. Prevention, early detection, and risk reduction is the program's focus.

Adult Programs—reached through the workplace, clubs and organizations, at home and in neighborhoods, and through programs with other health agencies. Programs can be provided to a small group or on a one-to-one basis involving two-way communication and interaction. Whenever possible, volunteers are selected on the basis of skills that can be readily adapted to society work such as ex-smokers with group experience who can help in smoking cessation programs, and nurses who can teach breast self-examination to groups of women.

A variety of films, slides, pamphlets, and posters that are site specific and directed to African Americans are available.

Cancer Among Blacks and Other Minorities: Statistical Profiles.
National Cancer Institute, National Institutes of Health, U.S. Department of Health and Human Services
Washington, DC, 1986, U.S. Government Printing Office
p. 273.

This report presents data collected on the cancer experiences of different racial/ethnic groups. The statistics presented are descriptive and intended to document discrepancies in the cancer experiences of different populations, including blacks, Hispanics, Native Americans, and Asian and Pacific Islanders. The data presented in this report fall into three categories: incidence data collected by the Surveillance, Epidemiology and End Results Program (SEER); mortality data collected by the National Center for Health Statistics; and survival data on how long patients live after the diagnosis of cancer. The data collected cover both cross-sectional comparisons of cancer rates and time trends for the eight ethnic groups covered by the SEER program.

Single copies are available at no cost from the Office of Cancer Communications, National

Cancer Institute, Bldg. 31, Rm 10A-18, 9000 Rockville Pike, Bethesda, MD 20892 (301) 496-5583. Single copies are also available for no cost from the Office of Minority Health Resource Center, P.O. Box, 37337, Washington, DC 20013-7337; (1-800) 444-6472.

Delta Sigma Theta Sorority, Inc.
202-483-5460
1707 New Hampshire Avenue, NW,
Washington, DC 20009

The Delta Sigma Theta Sorority, founded in 1913 at Howard University, is a private, non-profit organization that provides services and programs that promote human welfare. The sorority, whose membership consists of more than 125,000 predominantly black college-trained women, currently has 725 chapters in the United States and chapters in West Germany, the Virgin Islands, the Bahamas, and West Africa. The organization focuses on educational development, economic development, physical and mental health, political awareness and involvement, and international awareness and involvement. The sorority has also established the Delta Research and Educational Foundation, which focuses on programs for family welfare, research and service projects in educational development, and research and study programs to increase international awareness—particularly of African and Caribbean countries. Several local chapters have established Life Development Centers, which provide counseling services for families, programs on preventing teenage pregnancy, health screening, health education, and career counseling and referral services. Some chapters hold health fairs and comprehensive screening programs in their local communities. The sorority has also conducted a series of projects to address the problems of high cancer incidence and mortality rates among blacks. Delta Sigma Theta is working closely with the National Cancer Institute on a project to make people aware of ways to prevent cancer.

National Black Women's Health Project (NBWHP)
404-753-0916
1237 Gordon St., NW, Atlanta, GA 30310

The NBWHP was established in 1981 as a health advocacy organization committed to improving the health status of Black women. The NBWHP has developed wellness programs designed to address the related effects of being black, female, poor, and unhealthy. These programs have been developed from a black woman's perspective and designed on a self-help framework. The organization works to gather and disseminate useful information to health care providers and educators, help define workable prevention programs, and motivate black women to assume responsibility for their own health care. The organization, which now operates 52 local chapters, has also developed programs and disseminated materials on issues, such as prevention of adolescent pregnancy, cervical cancer, safe sex, HIV infection, and others. The NBWHP also convenes national and regional conferences.

PUBLICATIONS: The NBWHP disseminates brochures on various health-related subjects and publishes *Vital Signs,* a quarterly newsletter highlighting health issues affecting Black women.

CHAPTER 5   Resources

National Cancer Institute
Office of Cancer Communications
Building 31, Room 10A-21
9000 Rockville Pike
Bethesda, MD 20892-3100
(301) 496-5583

Provides informative materials on all types and aspects of cancer and cancer treatment.
Cancer prevention materials include:
1. *A Time of Change/De Nina A Mujer (88-2466),* 1988. A bilingual fotonovela was

developed specifically for young women. It discusses various health promotion issues such as nutrition, smoking, exercise, and pelvic, Pap, and breast examinations.

2. *Guia Para Dejar De Fumar (88-3001)*. A full-color, self-help smoking cessation booklet prepared specifically for Spanish-speaking Americans. it was developed by the University of California, San Francisco, under an NCI grant. 36 pages.

3. *La Prueba Pap (90-2694)*, 1988. This booklet, in Spanish, answers questions about the Pap test, including how often it should be done, and what are significant results. 16 pages.

4. *Lo Que Usted Debe Saber Sobre El Cancer (What You Should Know About Cancer) (83-1828)*. This bilingual booklet, directed toward people of Hispanic origin, answers questions on cancer causes, prevention, and treatment. Includes glossary. 33 pages.

National Coalition of Hispanic Mental Health and Human Services Organizations (COSSMHO)
1030 15th Street, NW, Suite 1053
Washington, DC 20005
(202) 371-371-2100

Makes available the publication: *Bibliography: Selected Health Materials in Spanish.*

Lange Productions
7661 Curson Terr
Hollywood, CA 90046

Provides a pamphlet on breast health.

National Dairy Council
6300 Northriver Road
Rosemont, IL 60018-4289
(708) 696-1020

Offers materials on calcium, child nutrition, proper nutrition, and other topics.

Compendium of Resources

This compendium describes additional government and nongovernment organizations that may be of assistance to health professionals working with minority populations.

American Association of Retired Persons
Minority Affairs Initiative
1909 K. Street N.W.
Washington, D.C. 20049
(202) 728-4808

American College of Obstetricians and Gynecologists (ACOG)
Resource Center. 202-863-2518. 202-863-2519
409 12th St. SW, Washington, DC 20024

The ACOG Resource Center is a clearinghouse for information on women's health care that maintains a large collection of books, serials, reference files, ACOG archives, and other special collections. The center provides national data on such topics as consumer health, statistics on obstetrics and gynecology, Caesarean section rates, perinatal mortality, natality, and ob/gyn manpower. The center also provides information on ACOG publications, audiovisual materials for health care workers and consumers, physician referral, continuing medical education opportunities, and automation information to fellows, ACOG staff, professional groups, and the general public. Staff at the center can respond to specific requests by subject, title, or format, and can provide general source lists.

PUBLICATIONS: The ACOG Resource Center has produced several video tapes on the history of obstetrics and gynecology in America. It also distributes *ACOG Patient Education Pamphlets*, which inform patients on several topics related to obstetrics, gynecology, and women's health, including smoking and cancer. Spanish-language materials are available on several topics. The ACOG home video and audio programs deal with exercise for pregnant and postpartum women, balanced fitness, and childbirth education. Each program is offered in video cassette, audio cassette, or record album, with accompanying instruction booklet. All other professional and technical books and journals published by ACOG are also available at the center.

SERVICE LIMITATIONS: There is a fee for all publications and audiovisual materials.

Cancer Care, Inc.
Program Coordinator, 212-302-2400
1180 Avenue of the Americas, New York, NY 10036

Cancer Care, Inc. is a social service agency founded in 1944 to help cancer patients and their families and friends cope with the impact of cancer. Program staff offer professional counseling and guidance to patients and their families. Eligible families can also receive financial assistance to help with certain home care, transportation, and medical treatment costs. The agency also conducts programs of professional consultation and education, community education and awareness, social research, and public affairs on a local and national basis. The Hispanic Outreach Program, for example, is a bilingual, bicultural program providing education, counseling, and financial assistance to help Hispanic patients better cope with the diagnosis and treatment of cancer. Other programs are the Community Education Program, Adolescent Outreach Program, and the Breast Cancer Outreach Program. Cancer Care, Inc. is entirely supported by gifts, grants, and contributions from the public; government funds are not accepted. Cancer Care has offices in New York City, New Jersey, and Long Island.

PUBLICATIONS: Cancer Care, Inc. publishes a quarterly newsletter and distributes brochures and informational literature on cancer to organizations and individuals.

SERVICE LIMITATIONS: Fees are determined based on the service provided and ability to pay.

Cancer Facts and Figures 1986 for Minority Americans
American Cancer Society
New York, NY: 1986, 25 p.

This publication contains information about cancer in the Black, Hispanic, Asian/Pacific Islander, and Native American populations. The first section of the book provides basic information on the general populations such as etiology, treatment, incidence, survival trends, and prevention measures. The second section provides statistical information on minority populations, including incidence, mortality, and survival rates; race, ethnic, and gender variations; Black and Hispanic populations' perceptions and knowledge about cancer; and trends in survival by site of cancer. A variety of charts and tables included in this section provide a better understanding of the information offered. The last section in this book deals with cancer and the environment. The publication also contains a list of comprehensive cancer centers and chartered divisions of the American Society.

Free copies of this publication are available from the American Cancer Society, 3340 Peachtree Rd, NE, Atlanta, GA 30026; (1-800) 227-2345; (404) 320-3333.

Cancer in the Socioeconomically Disadvantaged Initiative, American Cancer Society.
Director, Special Group Relations, 404-320-3333; 1-800-ACS-2345
1599 Clifton Road, NE Atlanta, GA, 30329

The American Cancer Society (ACS), founded in 1913, is dedicated to the control and eradication of cancer. The ACS has conducted activities aimed specifically at minority populations, including national conferences on cancer in Black Americans, Alaska Natives, Native Americans, Asians, Hispanics, and Pacific Islanders. Other ACS activities have included: a national survey of the attitudes of Blacks toward cancer; a national workshop on cancer in Hispanics; and the enlistment of thousands of Blacks and Hispanics in Cancer Prevention Study II which assessed lifestyle and environmental influences on cancer.

PUBLICATIONS: The ACS has published *Cancer Facts and Figures for Minority Americans 1986,* which provides incidence, mortality, and survival statistics for specific minority populations. The organization has also published reports on cancer in the economically disadvantaged. The ACS has developed public education materials including pamphlets, posters, handbooks, and audiovisuals. The ACS has also developed specific materials for African-Americans on quitting smoking and breast self-examination and Spanish-language materials on topics such as smoking, prostate cancer, breast self-examination, and skin cancer.

SERVICE LIMITATIONS: Requests for materials should be made through local ACS chapters. There are 57 ACS state offices and over 3,400 local offices. Bulk quantities of publications are available for a fee.

Cancer in the Economically Disadvantaged: A Special Report.
Subcommittee on Cancer in the Economically Disadvantaged, American Cancer Society
New York, NY: 1986, 31 p.

This report presents detailed data relating racial and socioeconomic factors to cancer incidence and survival. One major question that this report addresses is the extent to which economic status accounts for the differences in survival and mortality between racial groups. A set of recommendations formulated by the ACS subcommittee is presented in this report. Appendix A of this publication contains the executive summary of the report, and appendix B outlines differences in cancer mortality rates by income in Baltimore from 1949-51 to 1979-81.

Free copies of this publication are available from the American Cancer Society, 3340 Peachtree Rd, NE, Atlanta, GA 30026; (1-800) 277-2345; (404) 320-3333.

Cancer Information Service (CIS)
1-800-4-CANCER; 1-800-638-6070 in Alaska; 1-800-524-1234 in Hawaii; 301-496-8664 (Administrative Office)
9000 Rockville Pike, Executive Plaza North, Rm. 239D
Bethesda, MD 20892-4200.

The CIS is a national toll-free telephone inquiry service supplying information about cancer to cancer patients and their families, the general public, and health professionals. In addition to information on specific types of cancer, diagnosis, treatment, and prevention, each CIS office can provide information on cancer-related resources in its region. Health professionals and trained volunteers respond to inquiries. CIS staff are also trained to help callers quit smoking. Staff fluent in both Spanish and English are available to callers from California, Florida, Georgia, Illinois, and Texas. Some of the CIS' 25 regional offices also conduct information and education activities on cancer, some of which target minorities.

PUBLICATIONS: A flyer and a questions-and-answers fact sheet about the CIS are available. The CIS also distributes consumer and professionals materials produced by the Office of Cancer Communications, National Cancer Institute.

Disease Prevention/Health Promotion: The Facts.
Office of Disease Prevention and Health Promotion, U.S. Department of Health and Human Services.
Palo Alto, CA: Bull Publishing Co., 1988, 331 p.

The health data presented in this report illustrate that prevention is a much more efficacious approach to managing disease than treatment. The report contains sections on health promotion, health protection, prevention services, age groups, minority populations, diseases, and health care settings. Included are chapters on specific diseases including cancer and AIDS. Each discussion of specific disease contain information on incidence and prevalence, risk factor prevalence, and interventions. The report also includes chapters on specific populations, such as Asian Americans, Black Americans, Hispanic Americans, and Native Americans. These chapters contain demographic data, socioeconomic data, mortality data, morbidity data, risk factor data, and significant trends. References are listed at the conclusion of each chapter.

Copies of this publication may be ordered for $24.95 plus $2.75 shipping and handling from Bull Publishing Company, P.O. Box 208, Palo Alto, CA 94302-0208; (415) 322-2855.

Food and Nutrition Information Center (FNIC) U.S. Department of Agriculture.
Nutritionist, 301-344-3719
National Agricultural Library Building, Rm. 304
Beltsville, MD 20705

The FNIC was established in 1971 to serve as a source of information about human nutrition, food service management, and food technology. The center acquires and lends books, journal articles, and audiovisual materials. The collection ranges from children's books to materials for professionals. Users may also photocopy materials at the center for a fee. The FNIC maintains a 24-hour answering service to monitor requests during non-business hours. The center also has a demonstration center where individuals can examine food, nutrition, and human ecology microcomputer programs by appointment.

PUBLICATIONS: The FNIC produces resource guides for consumers on various aspects of nutrition, fad diets, cancer, alcohol, dietary fat, children's nutrition, and other topics. Professional materials include resource guides on the same topics and a guide to education and training programs. A bibliographic series, *Pathfinder*, guides consumers and professionals through the initial stages of searching for information or resources on a particular topic. Topics in the "Pathfinder" series include: diet and cancer; nutrition and cancer; nutrition and alcohol; and nutrition for infants and toddlers. The FNIC has also prepared other special bibliographies, such as *Nutrition Education Resource Guide:*

An Annotated Bibliography of Educational Materials for the WIC and CSF Programs, Nutrition and the Elderly: A Selected Annotated Bibliography for Nutrition and Health Educators, and *Promoting Nutrition Through Education: A Resource Guide to the Nutrition and Education Program.*

SERVICE LIMITATIONS: Bibliographies prepared by the FNIC must be purchased through the U.S. Government Printing Office. Users must return borrowed materials in their original container and pay the postage.

Health Risk Appraisal Activity Program, Centers for Disease Control (CDC), U.S. Department of Health and Human Services.
Program Analyst, 404-639-3452
Building 3, Room B43, 1600 Clifton Road
NE Atlanta, GA 30333

Staff of the Health Risk Appraisal Activity Program develop software for computerized health risk appraisals (HRAs) programs to predict the individual's risk of death from several medical conditions, including cancer based on personal risk factors. The staff also instruct health professionals in various locations on the use of HRAs, provide technical assistance in their use through state and regional contacts, and disseminate general information on HRAs. Current activities include: supporting the development of a state-of-the-art, public domain HRA at the Carter Center of Emory University; integrating occupational risk appraisal with lifestyle risk appraisal; and evaluating the effect of HRA use on communities. This office also supports the development of HRA programs for Native Americans and Alaska Natives, Black women, Hispanics, Native Hawaiians, teenagers, children, and industrial workers. The CDC also operates a computer bulletin board/conference for researchers and other professionals interested in the study, development, and use of HRAs. The CDC also offers an HRA software package for individuals interested in working with HRAs. Individuals desiring to use the CDC's HRA can obtain a list of state and regional contacts from the CDC.

PUBLICATIONS: The Carter Center of Emory University publishes *Healthier People,* a HRA available for a fee. The proceedings from the HRA Users Conference (March 1983) at the CDC, the Health Risk Appraisal Community Evaluation Study (May 1986) at the University of Illinois at Urbana-Champaign, and other studies or conference proceedings are also available free to professionals from the CDC.

SERVICE LIMITATIONS: The HRA is not a substitute for a physical examination by a medical doctor. Publications and some HRAs are for research and professional use only.

ICI Pharma
A business unit of ICI Americas Inc.
Wilmington, Delaware 19897 USA

A booklet for patients titled *Prostate Cancer: What it is and how it is treated.* Booklet is 17 pages long and includes information on what is prostate cancer, how treatments are chosen, coping with prostate cancer, cancer support services and simple definitions of medical terms. Booklet is available in English and Spanish.

International Cancer Information Center (ICIC), National Cancer Institute (NCI), National Institutes of Health, U.S. Department of Health and Human Services.
Information Specialist, 301-496-7403
Bloch Building, Room 102, Bethesda, MD 20892

The ICIC was established in 1984 to disseminate cancer research information useful in the prevention, diagnosis, and treatment of cancer to research scientists and clinicians throughout the world. The center collects information on the results of cancer research conducted in any country in its International Cancer Research Data Bank, and disseminates it to cancer researchers, cancer centers, or appropriate organizations worldwide.

PUBLICATIONS: The ICIC produces a number of serial publications, including: *Cancergrams,* a monthly bulletin with abstracts on can-

cer research; *Oncology Overviews,* specialized annotated bibliographies of recent publications on cancer topics; and *Recent Reviews,* a fully indexed and categorized annual compilation of abstracts selected from *Cancergrams. NCI Monographs* contains supplementary reports on conferences and meetings or on closely related research fields, or presents a related group of papers on specific subjects. *Cancer Treatment Reports* and the *Journal of the National Cancer Institute* have been combined into a new journal, simply entitled *The Journal,* which presents original, unsolicited, and previously unpublished basic and clinical cancer research. Back issues of *Cancer Treatment Reports* are also available.

SERVICE LIMITATIONS: Subscriptions to serial publications published by the ICIC must be purchased through the U.S. Government Printing Office.

Minority Outreach Initiative, American Lung Association.
212-315-8700; 202-393-1260
1740 Broadway New York, NY 10019-4374
1029 Vermont Ave., NW, Ste. 710
Washington, DC 20005-3517

The Minority Outreach Initiative of the American Lung Association (ALA) works to reduce lung disease in minority populations through public advocacy and on-going programs. The ALA is the oldest national voluntary health agency in the United States dedicated to the prevention, cure, and control of all lung diseases and their related causes, including smoking, air pollution, and occupational lung hazards. The association provides selected programs, publications, and materials that address issues of minority health, including materials on air pollution, school health education, lung disease, and smoking. The Minority Outreach Initiative, in particular, is a national effort based on the premise that many respiratory diseases can be prevented and controlled, and that survival rates can be improved through individual and institutional change. The initiative publishes and disseminates audience-specific multilingual educational materials to increase knowledge about lung disease and its serious impact on the health and longevity of minority Americans. It also provides educational materials and training programs on environmental health hazards; tobacco and marijuana smoking; and early detection, prevention, and control of respiratory diseases such as lung cancer and AIDS-related disorders. The Minority Outreach Initiative also works to: increase the representation of minority populations in the ALA and its network of local associations; ensure the inclusion of minority professionals in the conduct of research funded by the ALA; and advocate for increased funding of federal programs to improve the health status of minority populations.

PUBLICATIONS: The ALA provides a variety of education programs and public information materials under the umbrella of the Minority Outreach Initiative. Education materials include brochures, flyers, posters, and video presentations on topics such as air pollution, marijuana, and lung cancer. The ALA also promotes a number of smoking cessation and prevention programs.

National Clearinghouse for Primary Care Information (NCPCI).
Information Specialist, 703-821-8955
8201 Greensboro Drive, Ste. 600, McLean, VA 22102

Established in 1983, the NCPCI supports the planning, development, and delivery of high quality ambulatory care in areas underserved by the health care system. The NCPCI works with administrators of two federally funded programs—the Community Health Center Program and the Migrant Health Program. The Community Health Center Program provides preventive, therapeutic, and rehabilitative primary care services to families living in rural and urban areas where health resources are scarce or nonexistent. The Migrant Health Program provides a comprehensive range of primary care services to migrant and seasonal farm workers

and their families in rural areas. The clearinghouse informs administrators of recent developments in federal primary care policies; identifies resources to support health services and offers information on clinical, administrative, and financial management systems.

PUBLICATIONS: The NCPCI distributes several BHCDA project administrative documents. The clearinghouse also distributes an annual directory of community health centers funded by the Community Health Center Program. Professional program planning materials are available on many health topics. The clearinghouse also distributes medical phrase books for practitioners in English/Spanish and English/Haitian Creole, as well as Spanish-language materials on pesticide safety, migrant health, childhood injury prevention, and AIDS. Consumer materials are distributed on nutrition, cancer, and AIDS. The clearinghouse also publishes a quarterly newsletter, *Primary Care Perspectives*, and an annotated publications list.

SERVICE LIMITATIONS: Although the clearinghouse will respond to requests from others, activities are directed toward BHCDA project grantees.

National Institute on Aging (NIA), National Institutes of Health (NIH), U.S. Department of Health and Human Services.
Information Officer, 301-496-1752
Federal Bldg., 6th Fl., 9000 Rockville Pike
Bethesda, MD 20892.

The NIA was established to fulfill the mandates of the Research on Aging Act of 1974. The institute was created to conduct and support biomedical, social, and behavioral research and training programs on the aging process and the special problems and needs of the aged. Scientists at the institute's Gerontology Research Center (GRC) conduct research on biomedical, psychological, social, and economic and educational aspects of aging. The intramural program also supports postdoctoral scientists seeking experience in basic or clinical research on aging at the GRC. In addition, the NIA's extramural program funds clinical and basic research projects and training programs at universities, hospitals, medical centers, and other organizations through grants and contracts.

PUBLICATIONS: Consumer materials are available free of charge; some have been translated into Spanish and Chinese (Mandarin). Topics include: nutrition, cancer, menopause, osteoporosis, *Minorities and How They Grow Old,* and other conditions related to aging. Professional materials on Alzheimer's disease and on self-help groups are also available. A publications list is available upon request.

NHLBI Smoking Education Program: Strategy Development Workshop for Minorities. Summary Report.
National Heart, Lung, and Blood Institute, National Institutes of Health, U.S. Department of Health and Human Services
Washington, DC: U.S. Government Printing Office, 1988, 59 p.

This report contains the proceedings of a workshop held in March of 1987 at the National Institutes of Health, Bethesda, MD. Participants at the Workshop learned how to develop minority-specific educational programs on cigarette smoking cessation for minorities. The participants divided into working groups on each minority category: Black, Hispanic, Asian/Pacific Islanders, and Native American/Alaska Native; the body of the report is organized according to the same four categories. The suggestions and comments made by each minority working group are incorporated into the following subsections:

Patient/Professional Education, Worksite and Community-Based Programs, and Schools. Recommendations for each minority working group are condensed at the end of each section. A summary section reviews the cross-cutting themes and issues that emerged during the workshop. In addition, appendix C contains the notes from each minority working group's small group discussion.

Single copies of this publication are available

free of charge from the National Heart, Lung, and Blood Education Program Information Center, 4733 Bethesda Ave., Ste. 530, Bethesda, MD 20814; (301) 951-3260.

National Resource Center on Women and AIDS
Center for Women Policy Studies, (202) 872-1770
2000 P St., NW, Ste. 508, Washington, DC 20036

The National Resource Center on Women and AIDS, created by the Center for Women's Policy Studies is the first national organization to focus exclusively on AIDS and women. The Resource Center develops materials and activities to serve local activists who work with minority and low income women as they confront the AIDS crisis; it also seeks to influence the development and implementation of policies concerning minority women. Local and state projects on women and AIDS can receive assistance from the center. The center also presents workshops on women and AIDS at the national conferences of organizations representing minority groups, social service and health care providers, educators, and policy makers. The center also conducts a series of Washington policy seminars that bring together concerned legislators, service providers, and activists; a speakers bureau and speakers assistance service; and Washington internship programs.

PUBLICATIONS: The National Resource Center on Women and AIDS recently published a *Guide to Resources on Women and AIDS.* The guide is a collection and assessment of information on existing state and local, public and private efforts dealing with women and AIDS. The guide also includes case studies of successful interventions and instructions for establishing programs for women. Other publications planned include: *Issue Brief #1,* a review of research literature on women and AIDS; *Issue Brief #2,* an assessment of media coverage of AIDS as it affects women; Women/AIDS Kits; and *Women/AIDS Alert,* a monthly news bulletin.

Office of Minority Health Resource Center (OMH-RC).
Information Specialist, 1-800-444-6472;
301-587-1938
P.O. Box 37337, Washington, DC 20013-7337

The Department of Health and Human Services Office of Minority Health established the OMH-RC in 1987 to maintain information on resources available at the federal, state, and local levels related to minority health. OMH-RC staff are available to answer mail and telephone requests from consumers and professionals. Callers from all 50 U.S. States and Puerto Rico can reach the center through a toll-free number. Information specialists will refer callers to appropriate organizations, locate relevant materials, and identify sources of technical assistance. Staff members fluent in both Spanish and English are available to respond to telephone and written requests. The center concentrates on the six minority health priority areas, associated risk factors, and crosscutting issues identified by the Task Force on Black and Minority Health established by the secretary, DHHS. The priority areas are: cancer; cardiovascular/cerebrovascular diseases; chemical dependency; diabetes; homicide, suicide, and unintentional injuries; and infant mortality. Crosscutting issues include: health professions development; statistics/data; health education; and health care access and financing.

PUBLICATIONS: The OMH-RC produced *Closing the Gap,* a series of publications that includes fact sheets on the health status of minority groups in each of the priority areas outlined earlier. A fact sheet on the OMH-RC is also available.

DATABASE: The OMH-RC has developed a computerized database on minority health-related organizations, programs, publications, and audiovisuals. In addition, the center has established a network of knowledgeable professionals active in a variety of disciplines to offer technical assistance to OMH and OMH-RC staff and others interested in minority health issues who require assistance.

Office of Minority Health Resource Center (U.S. Department of Health and Human Services)
PO Box 37337
Washington, DC 20013-7337
Toll-Free number 1-800-444-6472

Maintains information on health-related resources available at the federal, state, and local levels that target Asians and Pacific Islanders, Blacks, Hispanics/Latinos, and Native Americans. Project activities include: information services, a computerized database of health-related publications and programs on minorities, a resource persons network, and publications to increase public awareness.

Patient Education Resource Center (PERC)
415-821-5404
PO Box 40519, 995 Potrero Ave.
San Francisco, CA 94140

The PERC was founded in 1984 to meet the great demand for easy-to-understand patient education materials appropriate for the consumers of public health services in San Francisco. PERC staff offer consultations on how to develop health education programs and how to use computers in health education settings. PERC staff can also assist with development of materials for populations with low levels of literacy and in finding translators for print materials. PERC staff pay special attention to the cultural appropriateness of each piece.

PUBLICATIONS: PERC distributes publications on a wide variety of health topics, including AIDS, cancer, nutrition, smoking, and substance abuse. Many of the materials available through the PERC are also available in non-English languages, including Spanish, Chinese, Cambodian, Laotian, Vietnamese, Korean, and Tagalog. A catalog of materials is available.

SERVICE LIMITATIONS: PERC provides services and health education materials for free to all programs of the San Francisco Department of Public Health; however, the center charges a small service fee to other health care and public service agencies. PERC activities are geared specifically to San Francisco consumers.

Public Inquiries Section, Office of Cancer Communications (OCC), National Cancer Institute (NCI), National Institute of Health, U.S. Department of Health and Human Services.
Public Information Specialist, 301-496-5583; 1-800-422-6237 (Publications)
Bldg. 31, Room 10A-18, 9000 Rockville Pike
Bethesda, MD 20892

The NCI conducts and coordinates federally sponsored research on the diagnosis, treatment, and prevention of cancer. NCI's efforts to control cancer in the U.S. include encouraging the prevention or cessation of cigarette smoking and modifications to diet to prevent cancer, early detection of cancer through effective screening, and widespread application of the latest findings of treatment research. The NCI maintains statistics on the incidence of cancer in the U.S. through its Surveillance, Epidemiology and End Results (SEER) Program. In addition, the institute has established a national Cancer Prevention Awareness Program. Minority-specific activities include the Black Cancer Control Program and the Hispanic Cancer Control Program. The NCI's Comprehensive Minority Biomedical Program provides support to minority scientists and encourages them to choose careers as cancer investigators. The OCC responds to requests from cancer patients, consumers, and health professionals. Staff fluent in both Spanish and English are available.

PUBLICATIONS: The OCC provides consumer materials on the causes of cancer, cancer prevention, breast self-examination, asbestos exposure, quitting smoking, x-ray exposure, DES exposure, testicular self-examination, the immune system, and the progress various types of cancer research. In addition, the OCC distributes *Good News for Blacks About Cancer*. Patient education materials are available on the many different types of cancer, cancer treatment, and cancer diagnosis. The OCC has also prepared special publications on coping with cancer, recurrent cancer, cancer in children and teenagers, clinical trials, and resources for individuals with cancer. Spanish language materials are available on the causes and prevention of the disease, smoking cessation, breast self-examination, the Pap test, chemotherapy, control of cancer pain, radiation therapy, facts on various cancer sites, anticancer pharmaceuticals, and health promotion for women. For health care practitioners, booklets are available on diet and cancer, radiation-related thyroid cancer, vinyl chloride, and prenatal DES exposure. The OCC distributes kits designed to assist physicians and pharmacists in encouraging patients to quit smoking. Special resources are available for program planners and communicators, including: a speaker's kit on cancer prevention; information on developing effective public service announcements; a report on smoking programs for youth; and audiovisual materials on breast cancer and breast self-examination. The OCC can also provide statistical information on cancer incidence, mortality, and survival in the general population and in minority populations. Other materials for professionals include several resource directories and detailed information on the NCI's functions and services. Annotated publications lists are also available.

SERVICE LIMITATIONS: Telephone orders for publications and consumer requests should be made through the Cancer Information Service, (1-800) 4-CANCER.

Report of the Secretary's Task Force on Black and Minority Health
U.S. Department of Health and Human Services
Washington, DC: U.S. Government Printing Office, 1985, 8 Volumes

This report presents the findings and recommendations of the Task Force on Black and Minority Health convened by the secretary of the Department of Health and Human Services (DHHS) in 1984. The task force analyzed and synthesized the information on major factors affecting the health status of Asians/Pacific Islanders, Blacks, Hispanics, and Native Americans, factors that account for the health disparities between minority and non-minority populations in the United States. The report also identifies minority health problems that require priority attention, including cancer. In addition to the priority health problems, the report identifies several crosscutting issues that affect the health status of minorities including access to health care, the development of and training for health professions, data development, and health education. The task force's report is arranged in eight volumes; the third volume deals with cancer, and the eighth outlines Hispanic health issues, and provides an inventory of DHHS programs and a survey of nonfederal community programs. In Volume I the task force recommends activities that the DHHS should initiate to improve minority health status; this volume also contains summaries of the information and data compiled by the task force. The other volumes contain the complete text of the reports prepared by the task force subcommittees and working groups, as well as extensive background information and data analysis to support the findings and proposed interventions. Many of the papers commissioned by the task force subcommittees accompany the reports. The reports contain a wealth of statistics gathered from sources such as the Bureau of the Census, the National Center for Health Statistics, and the task force's subcommittee on data.

Copies of volumes I-VIII are available through the Office of Minority Health Resource Center, P.O. Box 37337, Washington, DC 20013-7337, (1-800) 444-6472. Copies of volume I are available for $9 from the Superintendent of Documents, U.S. Government Printing Office, Washington, DC 20402; (202) 783-3238. GPO S/N 017-090-00078-0.

SRx Regional Program
1182 Market Street
Suite 204
San Francisco, CA 94102

This organization offers a wide selection of medication-education materials in several languages for senior citizens. There are fact sheets that explain the prescription drugs most commonly taken by seniors, handbooks that discuss medications and health, and compliance aids to help seniors to correctly maintain their medication regimen. Materials available include: "For Seniors Only: A Guide to Using Drugs in the Later Years" (English, Spanish), $1.25 to $1.00 depending on quantity ordered. "Over-the-Counter Medications and Chinese Remedies" (English, Chinese), $1.95 to $1.50 depending on quantity ordered.

Medication Fact Sheets (English, Chinese, Spanish, Vietnamese), $.20 to $.10 depending on quantity ordered.

Technical Information Center, Office on Smoking and Health (OSH), Public Health Service, U.S. Department of Health and Human Services.
301-443-1690 (Technical Information Center);
301-443-5287 (Public Information Center)
Park Bldg., Room 1-10
Rockville, MD 20857

The OSH offers bibliographic and reference services to researchers through its Technical Information Center. The OSH publishes and distributes a number of publications on the topic of smoking and health and, through its Automated Search and Retrieval System, can generate comprehensive computer printouts on topics of interest in smoking and health. The OSH also collects, analyzes, and maintains statistical data on smoking prevalence and behaviors in minority populations in the U.S., including Asian/Pacific Islanders, Blacks, Hispanics, and Native Americans. Also available are statistics on the incidence, morbidity, and mortality for cancer and other tobacco-related diseases among U.S. minorities. The OSH designs and conducts national surveys on smoking behavior, attitudes, knowledge, and beliefs among adults and teenagers on a periodic basis; it also works with other individuals and organizations interested in incorporating questions on smoking behavior into their survey research activities. The Technical Information Center is open to the public during business hours by appointment.

PUBLICATIONS: The OSH offers consumer publications on smoking and teenagers, smoking and pregnancy, and smoking cessation. Materials for professionals cover cancer, heart diseases, and lung diseases associated with smoking. Spanish-language materials are also available on smoking cessation and smoking during pregnancy. The office also produces the *Smoking and Health Bulletin,* a bimonthly abstract journal of the current literature, and the annual *Surgeon General's Report on the Health Consequences of Smoking.*

Transcultural Nursing Society of Illinois
Contact Person: Maggie Spielman, RN, Community Health Specialist at Health Care for the Homeless in Chicago
(312) 281-6689

This is a nursing support group for delivering culturally appropriate care.

Index